Real Life Diaries

LIVING WITH GASTROPARESIS

True stories, questions and answers by 15 women about managing and living with gastroparesis and other motility disorders.

LYNDA CHELDELIN FELL

with

MELISSA ADAMS VANHOUTEN

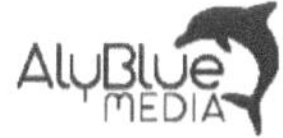

Real Life Diaries
Living with Gastroparesis – 1st ed.
Lynda Cheldelin Fell/Melissa Adams VanHouten
Real Life Diaries www.RealLifeDiaries.com

Cover Design by AlyBlue Media, LLC
Interior Design by AlyBlue Media LLC
Published by AlyBlue Media, LLC

ISBN: 978-1-944328-80-1
Library of Congress Control Number: 2017911400
AlyBlue Media, LLC
Ferndale, WA 98248
www.AlyBlueMedia.com

PRINTED IN THE UNITED STATES OF AMERICA

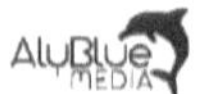

Living with Gastroparesis

DEDICATION

This book is dedicated in loving memory
of all who died from motility disorders

CONTENTS

BY LYNDA CHELDELIN FELL

PREFACE

One night in 2007 I had a vivid dream. I was the front seat passenger in a car and my daughter Aly was sitting behind the driver. Suddenly the car missed a curve in the road and sailed into a lake. The driver and I escaped the sinking car, but Aly did not. My beloved daughter was gone. The only evidence left behind was a book floating in the water where she disappeared.

Two years later, on August 5, 2009, that horrible nightmare became reality when Aly died as a back seat passenger in a car accident. Returning home from a swim meet, the car carrying Aly and two of her teammates was T-boned by a father coming home from work. My beautiful daughter took the brunt of the impact and died instantly. She was fifteen years old.

Just when I thought life couldn't get any worse, it did. My dear sweet hubby, Jamie, buried his grief in the sand. He escaped into eighty-hour work weeks, more wine, more food, and less talking. His blood pressure shot up, his cholesterol went off the chart, and the perfect storm arrived on June 4, 2012. Suddenly and without warning he began drooling and couldn't speak. My 46-year-old soulmate was having a major stroke.

Jamie survived the stroke but couldn't speak, read, or write, and his right side was paralyzed. Still reeling from the loss of our daughter, I found myself again thrust into a fog of grief so thick, I couldn't see through the storm. Adrenaline and autopilot resumed their familiar place at the helm.

In the aftermath of losing Aly and my husband's subsequent stroke, I eventually discovered that swapping stories helps us feel less alone. Our written words become a portable support group; it's comforting to know others understand the shoes we walk in and the challenges we face along the way. And thus, Grief Diaries and Real Life Diaries was born.

Helen Keller once said, "Walking with a friend in the dark is better than walking alone in the light." This is especially true when one lives with chronic, severe health issues. If you have gastroparesis or another motility disorder, or love someone who lives with one, the following true stories are written by courageous people who share your path and know exactly how you feel. Although no two journeys are identical, we hope you'll find comfort in our stories and the understanding that you aren't truly alone, for we walk ahead, behind, and right beside you.

Warm regards,

Lynda Cheldelin Fell

CREATOR, REAL LIFE DIARIES
www.LyndaFell.com

CHAPTER ONE

The Beginning

> It's hard to explain to someone who has no idea. Feeling pain and sickness on the inside while looking fine on the outside. -ANONYMOUS

Motility disorders are indiscriminate and affect millions of people yet no two journeys are the same. To fully appreciate the unique perspectives throughout this book, it is helpful to understand the different journeys from the very beginning.

*

MELISSA ADAMS VANHOUTEN
Melissa was diagnosed with
gastroparesis in 2014 at age 47

One cold February morning in 2014, my life was forever altered by a chronic illness. For me, the change quite literally occurred overnight. In the blink of an eye, my life transformed in ways I could not have imagined. One day, I could eat an entire buffet of food if I so desired, and the next day, I found myself unable to tolerate all foods and liquids.

I was rushed to the emergency room, hospitalized with severe stomach and abdominal pain, and nonstop vomiting, and put through a battery of tests (including one particularly terrible one where they forced a tube down my nose and pumped my stomach). After about a week's stay, I was diagnosed with an incurable illness of which I had never heard but which would become a central part of my new life: gastroparesis. I consider myself fortunate to have been diagnosed so quickly, since many people spend weeks, months, or sometimes even years searching for an accurate diagnosis. What is unfortunate is that, upon my release, I was sent home with very little information regarding my condition and was told simply to follow up with a gastroenterologist in about six weeks. I had no detailed diet plan, no medications to try, no real treatment plan, and no idea what to expect.

I went home believing my condition would improve, but instead it deteriorated. I was initially placed on a liquids-only diet, and was told I would gradually work my way up to soft foods and then eventually solids. Unfortunately, nothing like that occurred. Within a couple days I started vomiting again. The pain worsened, and I became so weak that I honestly could not lift my head up. I told my family goodbye, and I truly believed I would die. I had no idea what to do.

I finally mustered up the courage to call my doctor and told him that despite the risks, I thought I should try one of the few available medications that I had researched online. He agreed, but due to FDA requirements associated with this particular medication, it was two horrendous weeks before I could begin taking it. Without a doubt, it was the longest two weeks of my life.

Since starting the medication, I have stopped vomiting for the most part, but I still cannot eat without pain. It is clear to me now that this is a life-altering disease and that I will likely never again be able to eat normal foods in normal amounts. I have experienced levels of fatigue I previously thought impossible, endured unfathomable pain, and have come to realize the horrors of hunger and malnutrition. I had no idea I would face this, yet every day since my diagnosis, this is exactly what I have had to do.

It's amazing how a serious illness can change your perspective. After initially being diagnosed, I told myself I would not let this disease define or control me—it simply would not be the center of my life. But as time passed, I began to see how foolish that was. Every single second of every day, I think about food. I see it, smell it, cook it, and feed it to my family but cannot have it. I look in the mirror and see a skeleton. I try to eat even small amounts of food, and I am in agony. I am weak and fatigued to levels I did not think were possible. Some mornings, I do not think I have enough energy to get out of bed. I can barely concentrate and function enough to do everyday tasks. Almost every night my husband must help me up stairs to bed because he's afraid I might fall down the stairs. My thirteen-year-old daughter has seen me vomiting, screaming in pain, lying on the floor crying, and on the verge of passing out. At times, it has frightened her so much that she has asked me to get Life Alert. I grieve over the fact that I can no longer travel or get out of the house much. I grieve over missing family events, my daughter's activities, picnics, concerts, and other functions. I worry that I will not get to see all the significant milestones to come.

I am not on the verge of death today (at least I do not think so), but when I look in the mirror I realize that people who live with this do not have long life spans, and it bothers me. I worry about what will happen to my family when I am gone. I fear my daughter's reaction to my death and the consequences that might result from her growing up without a mother. I want to be there for her when she is sick, scared, or needs advice. I want to see her turn Sweet Sixteen. I want to hear about her first kiss. I want to see her grow up, graduate, get married, and have children. I want to know that she has a good career and a loving family. I cannot bear thinking about the pain my death will cause my husband, and I am concerned that he might not be able to function when this occurs. I want to grow old with him. Facing the strong possibility that none of these things will occur is anguishing.

I get frustrated because people do not understand how my life is affected by gastroparesis. If you saw me on the street, you would likely not realize I am sick. I do not look sick. People frequently ask me if I am better now. I cannot seem to convince them that I am never going to be better, not in the sense they mean. I am told I just need to eat, or that if I would try yogurt, I would heal. My own doctor labeled me as anorexic and advised my husband to watch me. And though I know people mean well, it still bothers me.

I am angry because I am a control freak, and I do not like being a slave to this disease. I am fiercely independent, and I do not enjoy being helped with everyday tasks and always having to rely on others for aid. I have screamed at, smacked, and pushed my husband away for simply trying to assist me more times than I care to count. I have thrown things (including food) across the room in fits of anger. I have intentionally gone without eating, even though I know I should not, just to show this disease who is in control. Mostly, I am angry because I do everything I am supposed to do: eat the right foods, exercise, and ingest the known medications, and I am still sick.

There are times when I am in such agony that I can do nothing but cry, lie on the floor, and beg God to just let me die. He does not, and I am thankful for that. I think about others who have this disease who are much worse than I am. I know many people who have sought treatment for dehydration, pain, and malnutrition, who have undergone major surgeries, and who have had to resort to feeding tubes for nutrition. I sometimes look at them and think that this will surely be my future too, and it scares me.

I don't understand why I have this disease, but what I do understand is that it's important for me to share my experiences and let others know that despite my challenges, I mostly have a good attitude about my circumstances. In fact, I believe I have been blessed because of my illness. Since my initial diagnosis, I have become heavily involved with online gastroparesis support groups. I have also created and now co-administer several support and advocacy groups that seek to foster awareness and change for my community. I feel connected and bonded to others in ways I had never dreamed possible a year ago.

I have discovered a whole new purpose and meaning to my life. Over the course of my journey, I have seen unimaginable suffering and need. I am overcome with compassion and concern for the people I have met, and I am likewise overwhelmed by the kindness and support they have shown me. I tell you, honestly, every person I know has aided me in some way. They have visited, called, assisted with chores and tasks, and simply cheered me up with their stories. Please do not ever be convinced that you can do nothing to help or that you do not matter. To those who are struggling, your efforts to understand, your cheerful words, your helpful attitude, and simply your willingness to contribute and be present, make a difference. I tell people all the time that I hate this disease, but I dearly love the people I have met because of it. This is a new life—one which I did not invite and which I do not welcome, but one with which I have come to terms, nonetheless.

*

SAMANTHA ANDERSON
Samantha was diagnosed with idiopathic gastroparesis in 2012 at age 26

One morning at the end of April in 2011, I woke up with what I thought was the beginning of a stomach bug. I had bad cramp-like pains, and felt sick. I had been out the night before and had been very tired leading up to my night out, so thought nothing of it and continued on with the day and subsequent days. I continued feeling unwell over the next few days with bloating, stomach cramps, a few vomiting episodes, and lethargy, yet I still went to work. About a week later, my mum persuaded me to go to the doctor as I continued to feel unwell, and was getting worse. I managed to get an appointment for Monday morning.

I hated the doctors at that point. Although I loved going to the gym and exercising, I was about size eighteen—a big girl—and the doctor would always go on about my size. The doctor did mention my weight, said I probably had indigestion, and prescribed lansoprazole, and made me feel like it wasn't that bad.

Over the next few weeks the nausea, cramps, bloated feeling and stomach pains worsened to the point where I was vomiting most of my intake. I took only a few days off, but being my active self and not wanting to let anything keep me down, I somehow went back to work.

I ended up at the emergency room a few times over the next month, once in an ambulance and once to the walk-in center. One doctor said I had just a urinary tract infection, gave me antibiotics and sent me home. The other doctor said it was constipation, gave me an enema and sent me home. They didn't seem to understand or wouldn't believe me that the sickness came before either of these. Again, I went back to work feeling very rough. I tried to drink more water, and to not get sick in front of my class.

I went back to my general practitioner's office and saw a different doctor after I finished the antibiotics. She was the first doctor who examined me, investigated the symptoms I was experiencing, and seemed concerned. She didn't go on about my weight, did all the necessary tests for blockages, listened, and referred me to a gastro-intestinal specialist at a London hospital with an appointment a few weeks later. Once again, I persisted to work although I had booked off my appointment and had a day or so off after having to go to the emergency room for some IV fluids and pain relief.

The day with the specialist finally arrived and I was hoping for so much: just help with what was going on, just to know. I had to be weighed and was eighty-one kilograms (178 pounds), although I wasn't sure of my original weight. I went in with the registrar and he questioned me about what was going on. Because of my measurements, he didn't believe I had lost any weight, and it felt like he didn't really want to help me. He sent me away saying he would see me in a month's time and to see if anything got better. He also ordered a CT scan and endoscopy. Obviously I was feeling a little deflated but hoped things would get better before then.

They didn't! I had managed to get cancelations on the CT scan and endoscopy before the next appointment, so was hopeful for some news about what was going on, and that I could get some help: a cure. The CT scan wasn't too bad. I didn't mind injections, so that was okay, and I didn't have to go all the way into the machine like you do for an MRI. It moved me around a bit like a fairground ride. The endoscopy wasn't nice at all. I didn't know it at the time, but this wouldn't be the only one I would have. They explained the procedure, saying I could have throat spray or partial sedation, but after seeing the size of the tube they were putting down my throat into my stomach, I went for the partial sedation—not that it seemed to work; it was a very uncomfortable experience, but nothing I couldn't deal with.

A month later I went back and was ten kilograms (twenty-two pounds) lighter. This time, seeing how much weight I had lost, the consultant listened. He gave me a combination of domperidone and cyclizine, as he was told I was going away with my family for two weeks to Turkey. The results from the tests hadn't yet come back so the doctor still had no idea what I had. He told me he would order more tests including a twenty-four-hour nasogastric tube test and a head MRI, as I was getting headaches, and that he'd see me in six to eight weeks, in September or October.

I loved my holiday, but not like I did on holidays before. I was sick whenever I ate and drank; people noticed, and it was embarrassing. I got dehydrated often. I also had some trouble with bowel movements after a week of not going (before this I was very regular, more than twice a day), but as I wasn't keeping much down I didn't think much of it. The anti-sickness tablets weren't helping. In fact, they made the vomiting episodes even more violent.

I returned home and got a cancelation for the nasogastric tube test for the beginning of September and my first day back at work. I managed to get in touch with my boss and told her I would be in but late. I had the tube inserted up and down my nose and throat. It was uncomfortable but I was more worried about being sick and bringing it up with the water before it was in place. Luckily it was okay, although a bit uncomfortable. Then I had to eat some food to test it and my swallowing. I had to eat cornflakes, but being lactose intolerant, had to eat it with water—yes, disgusting—but months of being constantly sick was nothing unusual really. I was a bit sick while in there, but they sent me home with it in and the machine to record it. I went off to work, with everyone noticing me as being ill. Normally I would hide it, but it was obvious. My day was a usual day of being sick and in pain but getting on. The next day I went and had it taken out and carried on as normal—well normal, as in with sickness, so far from normal really. I also had an MRI over the next couple of weeks.

When I returned to the consultant in October, I had lost more weight and was struggling. However, the endoscopy and CT scan came back normal. The MRI wasn't back yet but would be within the next week, and the nasogastric test I had a longer wait for. He then asked about my job, and insinuated that my illness was due to stress as many teachers get stress-related illnesses. He made me feel it was in my head and this started me doubting myself. I questioned myself every time I ate, every time I was sick, what led me to it, how long had it been from eating, what had I ate or drank, how was I feeling at the time and after, what was it that I was doing! It made me feel very low and if it wasn't real, how could I stop myself?

I was given different antisickness medications at my appointment as well as medication for constipation relief, as getting less food and drink apparently doesn't mean you should go to the toilet less. However, keeping the medication down was an issue in itself as I was getting more nauseous, more bloated and had more stomach pains, which were hard to explain. As a young adult, I had experienced bad periods, and had also at one point suffered from constipation, but this was nothing like that.

At my November appointment, the consultant said the MRI and nasogastric tests came back normal. But again, I had lost more weight and he was worried (medics worry when you lose weight and seem to worry much more when you aren't overweight). I understood losing weight could be worrying, but just because you were big didn't mean being ill wasn't horrible. I felt for others who were bigger than me and got ill. Once again, he gave me a different anti-sickness medication.

Again, he reiterated that it could be just stress. I again tried to explain that yes, being unwell was making me feel stressed, but before I got sick, it was the happiest I had been.

Luckily my mum questioned the nasogastric test result, and this time he actually looked at the screen. He then questioned me about belching, "You belch a lot?" His body language changed and it seemed liked he had an idea about what was going on. He said he was going to order another test which was essentially eating radioactive mashed potatoes and then being scanned for at least seventy-five minutes to see how it moves in the stomach. I got this test about a month later, and it was awful because I had to swallow my sick to make sure the test was accurate. They could see the sickness on the screen going in and out of my stomach. After an hour they stopped the test, I was unsure why. I had to stay in the room for about an hour longer as I was sick when I stood up, and it was radioactive. Even though I was still sick, they seemed to be okay with me going after about one hour.

I didn't have another appointment until the end of January, so I had about a six-week wait over Christmas. It wasn't fun like Christmas was before being ill, but it was always good being around family. I managed to get double ear infections over this period. My face was neck were swollen, and I couldn't keep the medication down long enough for it to help. They gave me some eardrops, but my ears were swelling shut and the drops weren't really getting in, and I ended up in the emergency room again. They got me in to see the ear specialist quickly, who cleared the ears slightly which was painful—extra pain on top of the stomach pain and headache. They also put wicks in my ears to attract moisture from the drops. I went back about a week later and although I still had a slight infection, my ears were open enough to have the wicks removed. I wasn't one to complain and wriggle about too much with pain, especially in procedures as it only prolonged them, but the ear specialist still commented on it. My parents told the specialist about my pain threshold and just wanting to get things done.

At the end of January 2012, I saw the consultant again. This time he smiled and told me he knew what I had. In the radioactive mashed potato test, radiation should digest and leave the stomach within seventy-five minutes even if the mashed potatoes don't. However, no mashed potato or radiation left my stomach at all. He diagnosed me with severely delayed gastric emptying or gastroparesis. He wanted to do another test to see how bad it was, but already knew it anyway. He said there was no cure, that it just had to be managed, and medications don't always work. He prescribed erythromycin for at least a month to see how that worked first. However, he didn't really explain to me what it was and the proper implications for it. I looked it up myself and joined various Facebook groups for support, (usually American, as UK groups were very hard to find).

It was nice to have a diagnosis and know it wasn't me. It took a long while for me to properly get out of questioning and blaming myself. It was idiopathic, which meant that the cause is unknown. My gastroparesis had caused such mental and definitely physical distress. Little did I understand that it was to continue, and a diagnosis wasn't the end—only the beginning.

*

JOLI ATKINS
Joli was diagnosed with
gastroparesis in 2015 at age 36

It was July 4, 2015, and I had gone to my dad's for a cookout. It was a normal day with no indication that there was to be any trouble. Two days later my entire world changed. I began having nausea and vomited everything I ate. For days I tried to eat, but even chicken soup wouldn't stay down. I knew it was not food poisoning because no one else who had been at the cookout was sick. I went for a week like this.

I made an appointment with my family doctor and when I went to see her, she took blood and gave me another acid reflux medicine thinking that it would fix the problem. It didn't and the blood results showed that my lipase levels were elevated. I messaged her a few days later because I was starting to have pain in my side. I had pancreatitis before and the symptoms were starting to resemble that, and I was starting to get worried. I was still unable to eat and still throwing up. She suggested that I go to the emergency room. I put it off for days and finally on a Friday I gave in. When I went in, I was of course dehydrated. My lipase levels were still elevated so they admitted me with a pancreatitis diagnosis. No food for a few more days, pain medication, and fluids. I went home a few days later.

I was able to eat a little before I left the hospital but after I went home I was not able to add foods I had been eating before, and it concerned me. I contacted my family doctor and she referred me to a gastroenterologist. The GI doctor did an endoscopy and colonoscopy, sent me to a pancreas specialist, and ordered an MRI. He could not find anything wrong, however I was still not able to eat anything of any real substance and was continuing to lose weight. His first answer for me was irritable bowel syndrome. I did not believe that, and demanded more tests.

At this point, he ordered a gastric emptying study to look at how fast food empties from the stomach. This was where the diagnosis for gastroparesis came from. When the diagnosis came back, I spoke with the GI doctor and he had no answers for me, and didn't know how to treat me. After this, I spoke with my family doctor and asked to be referred to the University of Virginia in Charlottesville to speak with a specialist. After a few months of waiting and still losing weight, I finally got to see another GI doctor. He ran a few more tests and confirmed the diagnosis.

No one at this point knows how to treat me. My family doctor tried some medications that are supposed to be good for this type of disease, however they haven't helped. I have come to understand that I just have to learn what my body will take and what it won't. If I can eat it, then I do. If I can't, then I just don't.

*

MEGAN BOGGS
Megan was diagnosed with
gastroparesis in 2017 at age 38

I woke up with sharp pains in my stomach. I started to feel nauseated and I thought, "Oh, God, not again." For the next six weeks, I threw up everything I ate and drank. This was the beginning of the end of my life. I clung to the toilet like a mother holding her baby, begging God for it to just end. Doctor after doctor, hospital after hospital, no one really had any answers for me. I had what seemed to be every test known to man to figure out that I had gastroparesis.

*

TRISHA BUNDY
Trisha was diagnosed with
gastroparesis in 2013 at age 35

I have been having gastrointestinal (GI) related issues for many years. None of the episodes have been anywhere close to being as severe or long-lasting as the issues I've had for the past four years. Prior to 2013, my GI problems seemed to disappear as quickly and unexpectedly as they began. During high school in 1992-1993 I had a really bad episode of nausea, abdominal pain, and being unable to eat or drink. I had numerous tests run and was even referred to a university hospital to rule out Crohn's disease. (One of my family members had a horrible time with Crohn's for many years before dying from pancreatic cancer). Nothing was ever really diagnosed except a few peptic ulcers. Eventually things improved and I was able to function normally.

Since then I have had numerous sporadic episodes of being unable to eat due to pain, nausea and vomiting, many resulting in diagnostic testing such as colonoscopies, endoscopies, and CT scans with no results. The symptoms would last a few weeks and then improve with no true answers as to why I was feeling so horrible. I have had problems waking up with nausea for the majority of my life. It has not been uncommon for me to begin the day with vomiting, dry heaving, or both, but then feel normal the remainder of the day. I am unsure if these episodes are related to what has been going on with me recently, but it's definitely a possibility. Unfortunately, during these years I was doctor-hopping as I could not find a doctor who I fully trusted or a doctor who was able to provide any assistance or explanation during these awful spells.

In early February 2013, just after my thirty-fifth birthday, life as I knew it completely changed. This time I did not improve after a couple of weeks. I became extremely sick with what we thought was the norovirus stomach bug being passed around the school and our family. I was unable to eat or receive an adequate amount of fluids orally, due to the severe abdominal pain, extreme nausea, and vomiting. A couple days later, I visited my local family doctor as I progressively continued to get weaker and the symptoms kept increasing in intensity, with no signs of relief. Initially my doctor diagnosed me as having possible diverticulitis (I had an elevated white blood count), and instructed me to go to the local emergency room if my symptoms continued to worsen. He cautioned me that the pain and tenderness in my abdomen could also be caused my appendix. That night, I was in severe abdominal pain so my family and I decided that it was time to visit the emergency room. In the emergency room, they ran a CT scan and said that I had gastroenteritis and sent me back home.

Days passed by and I continued to become weaker while also suffering with being dehydrated, as I was still unable to eat or drink anything without vomiting and pain. Once again I returned to the emergency room to receive no answers, but was able to receive some much needed IV fluids for my dehydration. A week later, I was forced to return to the emergency room once again because nothing had improved symptom-wise. Instead, I had additional abdominal pain. All of the pain medications and evident dehydration had led to stool impaction. I was scolded by the nurses and doctor for allowing myself to become so impacted. Talk about adding misery to my already depleted body! I hadn't planned on getting sick, hadn't planned on being unable to drink fluids, I was trying my absolute best to feel better. But when everything that you try to eat or drink does not stay down or creates intolerable pain and distress, how can you keep motivating yourself to keep pushing? Regardless, here I was in the hospital emergency room having enemas placed in my already painful and irritated rectum. If I only knew then that this was just the beginning of an exhausting and frustrating health journey.

Weeks kept passing and I continued to go through each day without eating and minimal amounts of fluids. My family and I knew that this was no longer a stomach bug and that my health was deteriorating quickly. Therefore, it was decided that the time had come to visit a gastroenterologist for my issues. I was sent for a number of imaging tests: MRI, barium swallows, CT, colonoscopy, endoscopy, etc. They could not find anything that would be causing my inability to intake nutrition without pain or nausea, or a reason for my lack of appetite and vomiting.

A couple months went by and I continued to get weaker and lose weight while the awful symptoms persisted. My gastroenterologist didn't know what else to try, and referred me to a urologist for a ureteroscopy, and to a gynecologist for a pap smear and vaginal ultrasound. Both came back fine and neither could come up with a reasonable diagnosis to explain my symptoms. I was then referred to a surgeon for a diagnostic laparoscopy. They were going to surgically look within my body to see if they could visually see anything wrong. However, I never made it to that appointment because my husband had had enough of me going from doctor to doctor with no results. I was not improving, was still unable to eat months after initially getting sick, vomiting or heaving over anything that went in my mouth, and struggling with lots of abdominal pain. All the while I was trying to maintain my responsibilities of parenting and teaching.

Fed up, one morning in late April 2013, my husband drove me to a nearby university hospital to be seen by their emergency room team. At first they did not seem concerned and were actually going to send me home. Apparently, being unable to eat while being overweight or obese is not taken seriously. However, after seeing that I could not even handle one cracker without vomiting or heaving, I was admitted. I went through various tests including CTs, and MRIs. We attempted a variety of medicines to try to find a mixture that would help ease the nausea and pain. We even tried Reglan, which is known for horrible side effects and carries a black box warning. Initially, one of the doctors tried to say my condition was stress related.

Thankfully, the hospitalist that took over my care while inpatient was compassionate, concerned, and willing to search for answers. He listened to my family and me, truly listened. It was during this hospital visit that I met my first consistent gastroenterologist, whom I was very pleased with. A week later, after becoming more stable, I was sent home to see if I could maintain improvements. I was placed on a liquids-only diet and told that I had to gradually work my way up to soft foods, and then eventually solids could slowly be reintroduced. They figured that my body was trying to heal from damage or sensitivities created as a result of the virus, postviral gastroparesis. They were pretty sure that with time my body would recover.

Unfortunately, nothing like that occurred. I was able to drink diluted Gatorade in tiny amounts, but it became clear that it would be a long time before I would be able to eat normal foods or drink normal amounts of fluid. As the week went on I was unable to drink an adequate amount of fluids, became dehydrated again, and was facing awful side effects from the Reglan that I was once again attempting. Therefore, I had to return to the hospital as an inpatient once again. More tests were run: a HIDA scan to check my gallbladder function, and a gastric emptying study. Since my nausea, pain, vomiting and heaving were so severe and it was evident that I'd be unable to eat a solid meal (it was May and I still had not and still have not eaten a meal since early February 2013), I was asked to drink about six ounces of Boost laced with a radioactive dye. I was only successful at drinking about three to four ounces, which was extremely uncomfortable, followed by four hours of x-rays and intense nausea with heaving. In addition, I had a brain MRI. In order for me to regain strength, I had to receive nutrition and it was clear that I wouldn't be getting it orally.

In May 2013, I had to have a GJ feeding tube placed in my small intestine, which I still have today. I have a machine that pumps formula into my body throughout the day. I wear a backpack to carry it or push it around on my IV pole with my other fluids.

I was diagnosed as having gastroparesis, a GI motility disorder with no cure. There was only one FDA approved medication (Reglan) which could lead to lifelong neurological side effects. Knowing it was the only medication for gastroparesis, I took the risks and attempted it numerous times until I began having side effects. Everything else was trial and error symptom management medications, many being used for off-label purposes.

I am guessing most people have never heard of this. I know I hadn't prior to my diagnosis. I was also labeled as having a functional GI motility disorder since I had been unable to perform the gastric emptying test with solids due to my inability to eat. It's not uncommon for some patients with gastroparesis or functional GI disorders to flip-flop between the two, since test results can change day-to-day, and some days are more symptomatic than others.

Since then, I have continued to work with my medical team to try to determine the most effective treatment plan. This has not been easy as there are very few options, side effects or efficacy of medicine changes. Other issues have arisen such as pelvic floor dysfunction and colonic inertia, and my body continues to physically change. I've become tolerant to some medicines that were previously helping, etc. It's an uncertain journey in that we continue to make adjustments as we try to find which treatments mays be most beneficial for me.

When I began this health journey, I was caught off guard. I had never heard of digestive motility disorders. I was not familiar with the demands that living with chronic illness can have on one's body and loved ones. I was not a regular in doctor offices, I did not know how to advocate for my health needs, and I thought I was alone. I didn't know anything about feeding tubes nor anyone who had one. All I knew was that they can be used when someone is on their deathbed. I didn't know anyone who had an ileostomy. All I knew about central line ports were that they were used by cancer patients. However, becoming ill has opened my eyes to a much wider degree. I've learned how these tools can help sustain life, and even improve the quality of life for many. With this knowledge, I choose to blog about my health experiences online at GastroparesisCrusader.weebly.com. I have found writing to be very therapeutic for me as well as an outlet to hopefully help others.

*

LISA COLANDREA
Lisa was diagnosed with
gastroparesis in 2016 at age 42

In 1999, I was twenty-six years old and married, with two toddlers. Life was good and I felt proud to be a mom. But like many women, I struggled to take the pregnancy weight off. Diet failure after diet failure, I gave up. I needed help. Over two hundred pounds sat on my five-feet-one-inch frame and I was miserable. I began researching gastric bypass surgery after I had heard about Carnie Wilson having it done. I needed this and I found the best bariatric surgeon in Boston and scheduled my first appointment. I spent the next several months attending informational seminars, appointments with their psychologist and dietician. It was an intense process but I was desperate and determined. The day of surgery came and for a minute I questioned my decision. I was waiting in the preop area, my surgeon came in all ready to go and so off I went!

Immediately after surgery, I questioned what I did to myself. I don't think any amount of preparation could have prepared me for what I was about to face. During the first several months following surgery I had to basically learn how to eat all over again. I followed a strict diet, took all prescribed medications and necessary supplements and the weight fell off. I did everything I was supposed to do. About six to eight months after surgery, my labs began to show low levels of vital nutrients. I became anemic and needed iron infusions three times a week. I began having gastro-esophageal reflux disease and bleeding ulcers. Over the next five years I had more bleeding ulcers, blood transfusions, and suddenly blacking out. My doctors prescribed more medication for GERD and ulcers following many endoscopies. I was tired all the time, and everything I ate made me sick.

My health became worse in 2014 after my family and I moved to California. I was so fortunate to find a doctor who finally listened to me and found a problem. All these years of being sick, and finally it was found that I had a large hernia pushing my stomach up into my chest. I questioned how this was missed. My surgeon scheduled me for a gastric bypass revision and felt it would resolve my issues. It didn't. I wasn't able to keep anything down. I even had a hard time with liquids. My weight dropped to ninety-three pounds.

At that point, we discussed a gastric bypass reversal in hopes I would be able to eat again and put weight back on. But in order to have the reversal, it was crucial to get nutrition in and put some weight on. I was placed on TPN (total parenteral nutrition) for a few months and monitored closely by my doctor and home care nurse.

My reversal was scheduled for December 2015, exactly sixteen years after my original surgery. I was petrified. I was warned of all the complications, and because it had been so long, there was a good chance my original stomach wouldn't work correctly. The first two weeks after surgery were very difficult. I was in a lot of pain and it was difficult to eat even soft foods or protein drinks.

Things became worse. The nausea, pain and vomiting were constant. A trip to the emergency room resulted in an admission. My doctor scheduled tests to check for any obstruction. The final test was a gastric emptying study which showed severe gastroparesis, a rare and chronic disease with no cure that I will have as long as I'm alive.

*

TAMMY DOWNS

Tammy was diagnosed with Crohn's disease, irritable bowel syndrome, spastic colon, gastroesophageal reflux disease, and gastritis in 2006 at age 46, gastroparesis in 2015 at age 56, and motility dysfunction disorder of the rectum and pelvic floor in 2016 at age 58

Back in 2006, I was diagnosed with Crohn's, another disease that caused me to quit work. I had worked for several places and ended up in the hospital five times, and it caused a situation with my jobs that I could not continue. Over the years I continued to have other medical problems. Seven years ago when I had my gallbladder removed, I thought everything was going to feel better. For the last three years, I started running into major stomach problems. When I ate it felt like my gallbladder had grown back. I had pain and nausea, and because of the Crohn's disease, I had severe diarrhea.

I did not understand what was going on until I ended up in the hospital again in October 2015 after being put on Remicade. I went for my second IV for my osteoarthritis and Crohn's and I had a severe reaction that placed me in the hospital, so I can no longer have this medication again. I had a very bad upper respiratory infection, pains in my stomach and chest, and a hard time breathing. I went to the hospital and they thought I was having a heart attack. The bloodwork was bad. After getting out of the hospital, I went to a cardiologist who ran all kinds of tests. My heart was fine but breathing tests revealed early COPD, narrowing of the bronchial tubes. My doctor was also concerned because my bloodwork wasn't looking good; my red and white blood counts were very low.

I was sent for a gastric emptying test which showed gastroparesis. I was having nausea and vomited up everything I ate. It felt like I had a rock sitting in my stomach. My weight started dropping rapidly so I was sent to a cancer doctor. I underwent a bone marrow transplant because of leukopenia and hypogammaglobulinemia, and they thought I had the start of leukemia. It turned out that mercaptopurine, a medication I had been on for twelve years for Crohn's disease, had damaged my bone marrow. An anti-cancer chemotherapy drug, I had to discontinue it immediately.

I was sent to University of Florida Health Shands in Gainesville to start medication for gastroparesis. I was seeing someone who was a motility gastroparesis specialist, and hoped that this was my answer. Instead, my insurance wouldn't cover a lot of the medication the doctor tried to get me on. I had a lot of severe side effects from some medications until I finally found two that worked. Some of the medication was very costly and I didn't have insurance.

Thanks to the gastroparesis support group, I found smoothies, soups, protein drinks, and a lot of ideas that I am trying. I'll see if these ideas will help with my stomach and put some weight on so I can feel better, so that I do not get dehydrated and malnourished. Dealing with my Crohn's, irritable bowel syndrome, gastritis and acid relax was difficult, plus having the fusion and six screws in my neck that cause migraines and interstitial cystitis. I also have sleep apnea and wear that darn CPAP mask every night. Plus I have mild COPD, osteoarthritis and neuropathy, along with recurring shingles.

I've had good support from my doctors, and I've also experienced no support from doctors who leave you out in the cold to fend for yourself. I learned really quick that gastroparesis does not have a lot to offer, and it makes me wonder whether doctors know what to do with their patients. I'm sure for some, it is just as frustrating for the doctors as it is for the patients who go through this.

*

SKYE FALCON

Skye was diagnosed with gastroparesis and other autoimmune diseases in 2006 at age 25

I've been sick my entire life. Adopted at birth in a closed adoption, any records were sealed about my bloodline's medical history.

Whether it was a respiratory illness, constant bouts of strep, or some violent stomach bug, I was always sick. Always on medications. Antibiotics. Cold medications. Always trying to feel normal. Every holiday it seemed I was stricken with some new issue, and everyone always made a fuss over it. In my late teens, the stress from school, trying to fit in with all of my weird issues, bad relationships, and life had caught up to me, and many believed I had an eating disorder. That just was not ever true, and getting people to understand was impossible. My issues were not with not wanting to eat—I always wanted to eat. Everything, in fact!

My appetite was always voracious until my teens. I was still hungry then, so I'd eat. And then I'd bloat, and more often than not I'd end up throwing up part of whatever I'd eaten. Trying to explain that to family members who only heard what they wanted, saw what they wanted through tunnel vision, and believed it to be true because I was thin, was impossible. I ended up attending support groups for bulimia, because that's what everyone assumed was happening. But I did not fit in with those groups, either. I did not have the same mental aversion to food that they did. My aversion was only to the physical reaction of vomiting and pain after I ate. I realized I would have to make people listen to get anywhere, and I was not in the right headspace for that. I was just a teenager. That was my first taste of people not really listening, both in my personal life and in the medical world, when I reached out for help.

Over the years, I did normal teenage things. I swam a bit and was in the marching band, and then grew into doing normal adult things.

Or at least trying to. There were always jokes and side comments about my health, but these were mostly brushed off on my part. Even back then, all of the signs were there. If I swam at practice or meets too long, I would end up vomiting for hours afterward. People would say, "Oh, just relax. You're making yourself sick." If I practiced too long with band, same effect. "You're fine. Just take a break." If I tried to match my friends by staying out late at a party, I was down for a week after. "Oh, you must've drank too much last night!" even though I'd only had water and iced tea.

It was not until I was entering my twenties that the autoimmune discussions really began, and once I was in the middle of my first solid pregnancy and diagnosed with hyperemesis gravidarum and hooked up to tube nutrition unable to keep even the smallest cracker down, we knew something was wrong. I was put on every known nausea medication, questioning every pill and its safety with my growing fetus still inside. No one had answers, not real ones anyway. I made it to the thirty-seventh week, where all hell broke loose with a stuck baby head, emergency C-section, and my NICU baby boy. After that birth, I was still on all the same stomach medications because keeping food in was still proving to be an unexplainable problem.

Life wasn't going to stop for me, and I wasn't going to slow down to figure it out right then. With my second pregnancy came two months of preterm labor and a whole host of other hospital-stay issues. She arrived four and a half weeks early. After this, there seemed to be a break in the symptoms, and nothing was worsening. As long as I remained gluten-free and ate smaller portions, I was able to function and thrive. My weight plateaued, energy came back in spurts but my immune system struggled more than ever. I was hospitalized often for severe lung issues, pneumonia, and respiratory distress. There were not a lot of answers, but the growing concern was felt with each specialist visit, and the wrinkled-brow look that fell across my primary doctor's face every time I saw her.

And then I was pregnant again. My husband and I had discussed it as a possibility, especially if my body was already starting to decline even more. As an only child, I had always dreamed of having a handful of kids. Why wait? There was a moment early on in this pregnancy when I knew my body was again shifting. Things that calmed my pregnancy-related issues prior to this point were no longer working, and desperation was setting in. In my sixth week of pregnancy, a PICC line was installed. There was no nutrition getting to either of us, and we were in bad shape.

I remember listening to the doctor argue procedures, insurance problems, and even whispering about my sanity just outside the hospital room door. They made it sound like I wanted to be there rather than home playing with my kids. Like I would rather be trapped in a bed, being fed via tube instead of eating tacos and watching Twister. Sure. They could not wrap their heads around why I could not even keep liquids inside. "There is no reason…," and "Makes zero sense to me," still roll through my dreams to this day. Some things just stick with you, and those two doctors are forever in my head, always making me second guess a symptom, or feel the need to verify that my symptoms were real.

The PICC line saved the day and allowed the pregnancy and myself to continue thriving until the fourth month, specifically the eighteenth week, when trouble again rose. My first pregnancies were extremely rough, but this time around was incredibly different. I could feel my insides ripping apart, literally, and thankfully my doctor knew to listen. I had intense moments of spotting throughout the thirty-three weeks I was pregnant, and internal physical therapy for weeks until the end. The ripping and tearing happened frequently, first with an under-the-skin burn, that changed into external bruising, redness, and intense heat on my skin. I would then go see my physical therapist, where they would try to weaken the scar tissue in my abdomen via external and internal therapies, some of which the details are just too risqué for this book. Even with all of the intervention, things were still turning south. I knew then that 2007 would be the turning point in my physical health. I could feel it in my bones.

I woke on the morning of February 28, 2007, to an intense burning across my lower belly I had never felt before. One eerily calm call to my doctor, and I was in her office. Within the hour, I had ruptured; my uterus tore away from my body, also tearing apart in multiple places, and my premature baby girl and I were in the fight of our lives. It was this point when my doctor saw the progression of heavy scar tissue, fibrous tissue, and the adhesions connecting everything in my abdomen together, and the real beginning of my autoimmune journey was upon us.

The copious amounts of scar tissue in my abdomen had flipped and frozen my uterus and reproductive organs and attached to everything it could, causing the violent rupture. I had an emergency total hysterectomy at age twenty-five, which led to more scar and fibrous tissues building and attaching everything left in my abdomen together. The issues I had before worsened quickly after the hysterectomy, first with complete dietary changes and lifestyle changes. Then again with the sudden hormone fluctuations, and everything was suddenly a hot, sweaty challenge. With three small children, the youngest of which had serious heart problems requiring multiple surgeries, GI issues, and was then diagnosed with celiac disease just before her first birthday, my focus turned from myself, to them. All while I ignored the constant vomiting, pain, diarrhea, bloody stools, gagging, and inability to swallow, inability to breathe, chronic bouts of pleurisy, and extreme pinpoint pains. All the adhesions were growing, thickening, and worsening inside my own body with little sign of slowing down.

Years passed, and I did what most moms do: forgot about myself. I put myself on the back burner to ensure my children had the best lives they could. Looking back over the past ten years from where I sit now, I wish I had taken more of a stand for my own health. I wish I had made the doctors listen, and pushed back at them as hard as they pushed me away. In all of the appointments, tests and re-tests, one doctor took the time to listen, although I was nowhere near his specialty. He studied, researched, and found a medication regimen I could try, and lucky for us both, it seemed to keep me steady for a while. Although, no matter what we tried, my immune system just could not handle the stress and germs that public teaching introduced daily. The number of mutated child-germs I was exposed to was even giving the hospitals a run for their money.

After a long nine-day stint of life-threatening pneumonia, I had to make the hard decision to back out of public school teaching. Thereafter I opened my own in-home private home school and tutoring business. This allowed me to continue with my passion, kept me healthier, and away from the mega-germ load. My kids loved it too. As super-smart introverts, they could now learn in their own comfort, PJs, and excel at their own rate. Plus, we had a few friends join us over the years at random times throughout the school year.

It was during this time when I also picked up an old hobby once again: writing. Leaving the career field I had studied hard and set my life up for was hugely defeating, and I knew I needed to pick up the extra slack with another thing, or I would die inside a little every day. Head first I dove back into writing, pouring emotions and life out onto the pages of books, poetry collections, novels, anthologies, cookbooks, and more. Seeing the continued interest in my work and publications made me want to work even more, and it was around this time I began "OH, Forks!" which is my health food business. Ten years ago, living a gluten-free lifestyle because one had to was pretty unheard of. There were not yet loads of premade foods on the market to suffice, so my recipes, cooking skills, and food knowledge were widened immensely. All the classes, the hospital education books, and all my stellar cooking skills were being put to the test, and it turned out that everyone loved them. Writing and helping people learn to cook in a healthier way gave me purpose, and reignited my fight for health.

A few years ago, things took another turn. My body began rejecting everything that was put in it, and the weight began to fall off once again. I've never been a big person size-wise, and never one to focus on my weight, or anyone else's, for that matter. But for whatever reason, everyone else became obsessed with my weight and my body, which made dealing with my issues a must. So, I did. Right then. I was referred instantly to a major hospital's gastroenterology department where they began a myriad of tests. They were quick to pinpoint the scar tissue buildup and lung function that had been altered from the scleroderma, and Raynaud's phenomenon and Sjogren's syndrome were present too, each causing special issues of their own. Next was the paraesophageal hernia, and scar tissues attaching my stomach to my chest cavity through the hole, causing my breathing troubles and constant lung sickness. Then another test showed probable early Barrett's esophagus from the loads of heavy proton pump inhibitors I had been on for a decade to ensure I could attempt to eat.

That began the steady stream of bad news, diagnoses, and learning what was to come, like learning how to avoid aspirating stomach acid into my lungs, or planning ahead for violent bloody blowouts in public. And finally, the gastroparesis diagnosis, which they say was most likely caused by damage to my vagus nerve from multiple abdominal surgeries, and the scar tissue and fibrous tissue buildup that was brought to life after every baby was born via C-section, surgery, injury, internal infection, and the like, hardening my intestinal tract just like everything else from the other autoimmune diseases. I was labeled as having multiple autoimmune syndrome.

In this timeframe, I played sleuth detective, and located some of the blood-biological relatives. And while it was not a reunion like the Lifetime movies make adoption stories seem, I learned that most every female in the bloodline had some form of autoimmune issue, or serious medical issue. Although they really wanted nothing to do with me, it was comforting in a twisted way to know that these issues did come from somewhere, and it was starting to make sense.

For the past two years, I've been in limbo. The gastroenterologists do not agree with my other specialists, and everyone wants to try the latest test, or medication. No one can make a decision to save my life, and I am so incredibly tired. In dramatic trial and error fashion, we find out I can't tolerate or have severe allergic reactions to most medications. After the allergic reactions, I am left worse than before whatever attempted and failed treatment it was. Side effects seem to stick with me for years.

I am what my doctors label "anti-tubes and pills," and we go around and around about treatment. Sometimes I am pretty sure they hate my semi-holistic approach, and their own big pharma plan, too. I live on liquids and softs, handfuls of medications I do not want to take just to ease the issues, and struggle constantly with chronic pain and burning throughout my abdomen. The doctors tell me it's the scar tissue tearing, growing, and changing form. All I know is it feels like my abdomen is a constant ball of fire, and pain medications are all on my "caution: allergic reaction" list. My weight steadily decreases; sometimes I can regain control to put back on a pound. Which would be great except that the next week I lose three. Ingesting anything by mouth is a hellish risk, as any pressure inside of my immobile intestines causes more tearing, ripping, bruising and burning. There is no rhyme or reason, or any immediate fix as I, and so many others, wish there was.

In all that, I'm still a mom. Now they're preteens and teenagers, no longer nonvocal infants, and I read and see the worry scroll across their faces when I freeze in place, and declare I have to go sit down for a bit. That I need to rest and am three-shades of white, with my head suddenly in the nearest trash can, all because I emptied the dishwasher. Or when I pass out unexpectedly, and they wait patiently next to me, ready to assess the situation and see that I'm safe, or saved.

I'm still a wife. I love my husband, and I need him in ways I should not have to. I'm still a woman. I have needs, wants, dreams, hopes, desires, and everything that healthy humans do. I'm a business owner who wants to grow, expand, and meet more people. And I'm a chronically sick human who pushes through every day the best I can.

In all these years and constantly morphing illnesses, I have chosen the path of utmost honesty with my children. My youngest, now ten, faces her own medical woes like the true champion I always knew she was. I think, in some ways, she might be better at all this than I am because she never knew any other way. Sometimes I wonder if things would be different for me now if when I was little I would've known more about why I was always sick. If my medical records would not have been sealed. If there were tests that could have diagnosed me sooner. If I would not have been exposed to the chemicals, fumes, and toxic things we know today are carcinogens. If I would not have taken quadruple doses of cancer-causing proton pump inhibitors for over a decade with no hope of losing my dependency on them. With gastroparesis and other autoimmune diseases, those what ifs are hard.

But what is there to wonder about really? This is the life I've been given, and this is my every day to drive through. I can't step away from my illness, as it's joined my life, my marriage, and my remaining friendships as the invisible yet excruciatingly loud, third wheel. So, I take every day for what it is. I make my lists, stick to my goals, push on in my work, and see to crossing things off those lists as I am able. I'm embracing my slower life, and hoping I can continue to work on my own inner peace for as long as I can. It is all I can do to hope for less judgment from those who should support me, and to not lose those I love because my life is such a heavy, uncontrollable medical disaster. I did not choose this, and if there were some magical fix, you can bet I would be on it. But things just do not work that way with these types of illnesses. I have learned to accept the bad, and let the pain push me on, drive me to do better, be better, and help others. This is just another day in my #ChronicallyAwesome life with gastroparesis.

*

ROBIN MCNAMARA
Robin was diagnosed with
gastroparesis in 2013 at age 55

My problems all began with a bad tooth infection that needed a root canal. After the first treatment from the dentist, I was given a prescription for an antibiotic, amoxicillin, which little did I know would change my life forever. I'm a foodie (or was) and loved anything that involved food. I'm also a food buyer which means that part of my job involves eating. My round of antibiotics was in the early spring, and as the summer rolled in, I was having bouts of nausea that would just come and go. I didn't really give it much thought because on any given day, I ate many different foods. Other times, I'd lay down flat and sit up fast as I could feel acid rushing up my throat. The other thing that was happening frequently was that I would get dead tired and need to take a nap; some naps lasted three to four hours.

These odd symptoms continued for five months when I found myself on vacation. Every day I had a "drink of the day," which was usually a pina colada. After three days of pina coladas, I saw someone with a strawberry daiquiri and thought that would be good for a change. About halfway through the drink, my stomach soured and I grew extremely tired. I went to grab food for lunch thinking it would help, but I didn't eat much and then discarded it.

I went back to my room and fell asleep hoping. It was getting later and my sister was hungry so we went to dinner. We shared small tapas plates. I ordered a glass of wine. After eating I felt as though I was perking up a bit. I ate some food, finished my wine, and on the way to the casino I started to get really tired again, and could feel acid rolling around in my stomach. I skipped the casino and went back to my room. When I tried to lay down I could feel acid rushing up my throat. I grabbed a San Pellegrino sparkling water from the mini bar hoping it would help to get a burp up. I sat upright on the bed, leaning against the headboard and fell asleep.

I'm not sure how much time passed but I woke up feeling as though I was going to vomit—I hadn't barfed since I was six years old. I ran to the bathroom and kept saying, "No, no, no," but vomited twice. No food came up, just red wine with dark speckles in it. I went back to bed, got up the next morning, didn't feel great but did take it easy on what I ate and drank, as being sick like that was pretty traumatic.

I had a checkup with my gastro doctor and all seemed fine. But as time went on, I dropped a fast ten pounds without trying. I went back to my gastro guy who said I was having issues with reflux and thought maybe it was time for a change in medication. I told him I thought Nexium would work better than the Protonix, and he just wrote the script and off I went.

I started that day in November feeling fine. On the way home, I stopped at Whole Foods and got a cream puff and a nice hot latte. By the time I finished both, I grew dead tired and all I wanted to do was go home and go to bed. I fell asleep in a chair and woke up a few hours later with my chest and throat on fire from acid, and feeling as though I was going to vomit. I was cold, shaking, and felt like I was going to die on my bathroom floor. And did I mention scared?

I texted my sister, who is a registered nurse, thinking she was home, telling her what was happening. She texted me saying, "You know you are not having a heart attack right?" I explained what was happening, and she told me to call my doctor for some anti-nausea medication. When I called my doctor around 8:45 p.m., he was more than agitated with me. What did I want? What was wrong? I told him what was happening. He was getting pissed at me as I was on my cellphone and it was breaking up on him. He agreed to the anti-nausea medication and asked me to call him back with a twenty-four-hour pharmacy number. I thought I found one, and called back to give him the number. Then this arrogant little man called me, angry as hell that it wasn't a twenty-four-hour pharmacy, and he didn't want me calling him later in the evening. I asked him to call my regular pharmacy and that was that. In the meantime, my sister texted me and told me to take another Nexium, which I did. After a couple of hours sitting upright against a wall, I went to bed.

The next day when I got up, I seemed to be okay. I brewed a cup of coffee, lit a cigarette, and after three gulps of coffee the nausea rolled right back in. I made another appointment with my gastro guy and told him something was very wrong. He wasn't saying much, and said my stomach seemed fine when he touched it. I told him I was down over ten pounds since my last visit, which wasn't long before this appointment, and he didn't say anything. His young nurse said, "Wow, you are right," and he still didn't say anything—he handed me a script for Carafate and sent me on my way.

Things remained horrible. The burning acid, more weight loss, and I couldn't really eat anything. I made another appointment and he looked pissed to see me again. I told him I needed an endoscopy to see what was going on. It was November, and he told me, "You are due for that and a colonoscopy next month." I told him I couldn't wait, so he agreed to do it.

When they wheeled me into the room, this horrible man was pacing, mad that the anesthesia guys were behind and he should have had four more people done (and how professional is this?!). My sister was the one who had said to get the scope done so I could get into a new GI doc. He prescribed Reglan as well, and seemed as though he had an idea of what was going on. But when I asked him what I had, all he would say was, "You need to heal." So I asked him, "Heal from what?" He just looked at me with a blank face like a deer in headlights.

Before I got into my new gastroenterologist, I had visited the hospital emergency room where my sister worked. They ran a bunch of tests to check my gallbladder and whatever else could be causing the issue. I went for a few visits there. My stomach hurt, which I couldn't tolerate, it was the round-the-clock nausea that I just couldn't live with. It took a bit of time to get into the new gastroenterologist, but he saved my life, and I believe he kept me from becoming a tubie.

The new doctor had me going to outpatient for an IV stomach medication along with an anti-nausea cocktail. He was kind, patient, and just beyond wonderful. He kept telling me he needed to get the acid pumps to settle down. He also told me that he didn't think I was crazy or depressed, but he wanted me to take a low dose alprazolam, and Remeron, which he called a sleeping pill, but it's one of those magical antidepressants (without all the horrible side effects). After a bit of time, things started to settle down and here I was, twenty-five pounds lighter. When I couldn't eat, I told my sister I was going to die without food. She reminded me that as long as I kept hydrated, I could live quite a while without food.

My new doctor ordered a gastric emptying test though I never asked about the results. Eventually he brought me in for another scope and diagnosed me as having gastric atony. I had to look up what that meant. I didn't realize at that point that my life would be changing forever. It turned out that my doctor is more than familiar with gastroparesis. I have been blessed to find this man. He still says to me, "Kid, you scared me for a while. I thought I was going to have to lock you up for a bit."

With the Remeron giving me seven to eight solid hours of sleep, I know that was part of my getting out of the woods. My old doctor? I don't think it's a coincidence that his office is right next door to a funeral home.

*

TAMMY PITTMAN

Tammy was diagnosed with gastroparesis and irritable bowel syndrome in 2014 at age 34

I had a terrible problem with irritable bowel syndrome and reflux that started when I was pregnant with my daughter in 2000. I had exhausted every option for medication when I saw a gastrologist in 2013. Multiple tests were done, including an esophageal motility study that determined my lower esophageal sphincter had atrophied. I was sent to a surgeon who did a Nissen fundoplication on March 7, 2007. There were multiple errors made during the surgery that caused me to develop a subphrenic abscess the size of a football in my abdomen and a 1600 milliliter pleural effusion.

*

TAYLOR SCHMITZ
Taylor was diagnosed with idiopathic gastroparesis in 2014 at age 22

In 2012, during my deployment to Afghanistan, I started noticing digestive problems. I was nauseous a lot after eating, and I seemed to get full quickly. It didn't really faze me, because I barely slept four hours every other night, and ate on the go. I was a truck driver, and we were always busy. Unfortunately, the symptoms worsened when I came home, and with my pregnancy. After I gave birth, things stayed pretty much the same. Nausea, heartburn, diarrhea, and early satiety were all just a part of life. After the pregnancy, the army pressured me to lose weight as fast as possible. They measured my hips and weighed me every month. They let me know I was too fat to be in the military, so I needed to lose the weight as fast as possible. I was dieting, eating as healthy as I could, and exercising, but the weight wouldn't come off.

In October 2013, after my wedding, we got food poisoning from our dinner! Myself, my husband, and my father all had it at the same time, in our brand new house. It took me weeks to get better, but I honestly never recovered after that.

Finally, in late 2013, my symptoms hit their peak. I was on a trip to New York with my mother-in-law, her mom and mother-in-law, and my sister-in-law. I had recently turned twenty-one that year, and never consumed alcohol, so they wanted to show me a good time. I had a few drinks but was still very alert. I was hit with extreme stomach pain late in the night. Running to the bathroom, I had severe diarrhea, and thought I was going to vomit, even though I never did.

Weeks later, I was still unable to eat anything without being in pain and sick all night. On New Year's Eve, I drove myself to the emergency room, because my husband believed I was overreacting. Ten hours later, I returned home with the diagnosis of gallstones. I went to a gallbladder specialist, and he ran several tests. We decided on surgery, but I couldn't get in until Valentine's Day! I had to miss several drill weekends, and my leadership was so fed up with me. I was so very sick.

After I got my gallbladder removed, things only got worse from there. The doctor referred me to a gastrointestinal specialist, and he ran many more tests. Late in March 2014, he discovered idiopathic gastroparesis after a very long gastric emptying scan. I was devastated. He told me there was no cure, and quite frankly, there was little I could do. He told me to eat Jello, applesauce, bread and yogurt, but that he couldn't see me anymore. He didn't know enough about the disease to treat me, so he referred me over to the Cleveland Clinic.

*

DEB SHRADER-TROTTER
Deb was diagnosed with
gastroparesis in 1999 at age 37

We were at the very initial stages of many tests. There had already been one psych exam because of the confusion caused by this disease. The top gastrointestinal specialists in Memphis back in 1998 and 1999 ran a battery of tests but couldn't solve the puzzle. They then leaned toward spousal abuse because they were confused. By the time I arrived at the tail end of testing, I was severely dehydrated. A gastroenterologist who was on duty at the hospital said I should see this motility specialist he knew. Now, mind you, by this time I was questioning my own sanity! I asked him, "Please, can you just tell me if you think I am crazy?"

He said, "No, ma'am! I believe you have motility issues. Your stomach and gut don't move right. Will you let me refer you to this doctor?" I agreed. He recommended Dr. Abell who proceeded to save my life with three days of testing, which determined the diagnoses in 1999, including gastroparesis, colonic inertia, and chronic intestinal pseudo-obstruction syndrome because my large intestine wasn't moving my bowels at all. Dr. Abell recommended the colectomy after consulting with Dr. Lahr in South Carolina. I had that done in 2000.

*

JESSICA SPENCE
Jessica was diagnosed with
gastroparesis in 2016 at age 25

I first became sick in the spring of 2005 when I was fourteen. We had just moved to a new town and I was in a new school. I would wake up in the morning and race for the bathroom to vomit the contents of last night's supper. My mother took me to the local doctor who treated me for the next eleven years. Every test said I was fine—constipated, but fine. The doctor said it was anxiety from my new school and sent me on my way. I was not satisfied because this was the umpteenth new school I had been to; I was a pro at this.

My symptoms seemed to come and go every few months over the next three years. At seventeen I enlisted in the Guard and was sent to

Relaxing Jackson for basic training the following summer. My body couldn't handle the heat and humidity. I started passing out every week and throwing up after every meal. I tried to stay strong and tough it out until my drill sergeant accused me of bulimia. It broke me.

Couldn't they see how hard I was trying? Why didn't they believe me when I said I wasn't doing this on purpose? Why were they accusing me of trying to get out? I wanted this. Couldn't they see how badly I wanted this? I was assigned a battle buddy to ensure I ate everything on my plate, no matter how much it hurt. Sergeant would smoke the platoon if I didn't finish my meals. I cried through my meals trying to finish. I was put on a deadman's profile. They discharged me during the last few weeks of basic.

When I got home I was diagnosed with vasovagal syncope. My doctor dismissed my stomach issues as anxiety and body image issues. He didn't believe me when I said I wanted to gain weight. A few more years went by with flares coming and going. I went through several gastrointestinal doctors who all came to the same conclusion: I was a young woman with body image issues. No one believed me.

I started to think they were right, that somehow I was making it all up in my head without even knowing I was doing it. I prayed for a doctor like Dr. House to come and figure out what was wrong. I didn't care what it took. I just wanted a name for this monster. I wanted to know if it was all in my head. I didn't know what to believe anymore.

When I was twenty-four, a colonoscopy was finally ordered. I drank that whole bottle of disgusting stuff with my wonderful fiancé at my side. He camped out in the bathroom with me and watched

Netflix. I knew then that I had found the one. He believed me. He gave me hope. Then the test came back inconclusive because I still had stuff in my small intestine. In front of my fiancé and mother, the doctor accused me of not drinking all the prep juice. He told my mother I needed a head transplant because I was a hormonal young woman, and nothing was wrong with me but being crazy. My mom thought my small intestine must be necrotic because it just wasn't working. He assured her I was crazy.

I begged my doctor to send me to another specialist, the fourth gastroenterologist I would see, to test my mom's theory. That doctor took one look at my history and the colonoscopy results, and told me he thought I had gastroparesis. He wanted to do a gastric emptying study to see if he was right. I cried the whole way home. I had found my Dr. House.

The first GES I did was incomplete because I couldn't keep the meal down. He wouldn't give up and had me repeat the test. Sure enough, my stomach was lazy. Over half my food was still in my stomach three hours into the test.

After eleven years I finally had a name for the monster I had been battling for almost half my life. I had no idea that my battle had just begun. I had fantasized about this day, and imagined that once we knew what it was, it would be easy to fix.

I had never been more wrong about anything in my entire life.

*

NICOLE STARZYNSKI
Nicole was diagnosed with gastroparesis in 2016 at age 33

I was diagnosed with gastroparesis in 2016, but my journey started long before. I realized while writing my story that I had blocked so many things out of my mind. When you are battling a disease, sometimes the only way to keep fighting is to forget, or take every day as a new day. The bad memories through your journey become a foggy nightmare. I've cried my eyes out so many times because I felt like I was completely alone, and that I was never going to find answers or get the help I needed. No doctor would ever be able to make me feel better.

Gastroparesis is different for everyone, but the one thing most of us have in common is being misdiagnosed, ignored, disrespected, left to feel helpless and alone. Most doctors make us feel like we are crazy. They say gastroparesis isn't painful, a diet will fix all of your issues, eat smaller meals. Most of us have questioned ourselves: I don't really have this, I'm not as sick as other people, maybe the doctors are right that there isn't anything wrong, I'm just making a big deal out of nothing. It's sad but as different as many of us are, most of our journeys start the same. The biggest issue is finding a doctor who actually understands gastroparesis or even has close to a clue. That's why sometimes the diagnosis can take years.

I guess when I think back, I have always had problems with my stomach. My mother said when I was a baby, I used to puke up breast milk and they said I was lactose intolerant. Once I was on formula, they said I had iron issues and that was causing me to have severe constipation issues. My mother remembered being scared that she had to take me to the emergency room because I used to scream in pain from not being able to go the bathroom. As a baby and as a kid, I used to have severe issues with constipation and would vomit up food. Back then they said I had a lactose allergy and put me on soy. Growing up, I used to vomit up stomach acid frequently. However, I ignored it since I felt okay afterwards.

I was always a little overweight growing up. When I was a teenager I always had diarrhea and had accidents. In high school, I carried Imodium on me because it was the only way I could make it through the day. Kids used to call me Poop Break as a joke. That nickname stayed with me into my twenties. I remember throwing up stomach bile in the mornings. Since I was overweight and puking up meals, I was accused of being bulimic. For a while I believed that I was but I didn't understand that I wasn't forcing myself to vomit. I was just vomiting up my food after I ate. Back then nobody really seemed to think there was anything else going on with me. There was no internet back then, so there wasn't a way for me to research anything. How would I or my family know any different from what the doctors told us? My mom just recently learned I was never bulimic.

In my early twenties after graduating from college, I took a job in Daytona Beach, Florida. I continued to have problems with diarrhea and vomiting. Sometimes I would eat and have to go the bathroom immediately. I was young and my new career was keeping me pretty busy. I worked out every day and went on the Atkins diet. I finally lost some weight and while I was not skinny, I was wearing a size ten and felt good about myself.

In 2004, when I was twenty-three years old, I became pregnant with my daughter. I had an awful pregnancy with severe nausea and vomiting that lasted the entire nine months. I used to get dizzy and pass out. I had gestational diabetes and preeclampsia, and when I was twenty-eight weeks pregnant I was put on bed rest for eight hours a day. I watched my sugars and was able to keep them low enough that I did not need insulin. I had ankles so swollen I couldn't even walk.

A week before I gave birth, I had a large painful mass in my right breast. I went to the doctor and they tried to aspirate it, but decided that it was too deep and it would need to be surgically removed. So, ready to pop, I had to have surgery awake. It was a clogged milk gland. Only I would have a clogged milk gland while pregnant! The surgery was something I would sooner forget, but after that it definitely led to other obstacles. My daughter was born by vaginal birth with no complications on March 4, 2005, a healthy eight-pound four-ounce baby.

Over the next few years I still had the same symptoms I always had but started throwing up stomach bile more often. I also started to experience stomach pains that were completely debilitating. I gained a lot of weight after the birth of my daughter and in 2008, I weighed 220 pounds. Between 2005 and 2008, I had a number of ankle surgeries and pushed my stomach issues to the side. There were just too many other things going on. I was working full-time and trying to keep up with a busy toddler. My family had a history of irritable bowel syndrome, ulcerative colitis, and digestive issues, so I did not think that it was imperative for me to see a gastroenterologist.

It wasn't until after my divorce in 2008 that I really started to experience increasing symptoms. My daughter and I moved in with my parents, I had just taken a new job and I was going through a nasty divorce. The perfect storm of stress! That sent me down a path I never seemed to recover from.

In 2009, I was so sick that I was missing work and it constantly felt like I had the stomach flu. I was experiencing severe stomach pains, vomiting up food and stomach bile, had body aches, was constantly tired, had severe bloating, and I was never hungry. I would only eat every few days. One day, I vomited up blood and had blood in my stool; that was finally enough—at twenty-seven years old this was not normal. I scheduled an appointment with a gastroenterologist.

The next few years were somewhat of a blur. I had over twenty tests between 2009 and 2011. I had bloodwork, two endoscopies and colonoscopies, barium x-rays, ultrasounds—an endless list of tests that lead to no helpful solution. At every doctor appointment I felt worse than the appointment before. I started to feel like I was crazy, and that going to the doctor was pointless. A complete waste of time.

During this time I went to the emergency room about fifteen times in two years for severe stomach pain, vomiting up blood, or both. Sometimes I was treated like a drug addict looking for pain medication. They would do an x-ray or ultrasound of my stomach, tell me they did not see anything wrong and send me on my way. They also could never find where the blood was coming from, whether in my stool or my vomit. It was very frustrating. My poor mom took me to the emergency room every time. After enough visits with no relief I decided that unless I felt like I was ready to die, there would be no more emergency room visits.

I decided to go see my gynecologist and they did ultrasounds and sonograms to rule out any cysts. I had my regular doctor order a complete workup of any blood work he could think of. Still no answers. Due to my frequent trips to the emergency room, my gastroenterologist was trying to get a SmartPill test approved, but the insurance company denied it six times between 2009 and 2011. We even appealed it, but they refused. In 2010, I was diagnosed with celiac disease, irritable bowel syndrome, and ulcerative colitis. My doctor at the time told me I needed to cut gluten out of my diet, lose some weight and prescribed me Asacol for the ulcerative colitis. At that point, I was tired of all the doctor visits and tests. I had a treatment plan that wasn't helping. I felt defeated and completely hopeless, so I stopped going to the gastroenterologist.

In 2012, my symptoms picked back up but I decided there was no point in calling a doctor, since I had previously spent almost four years and it went nowhere. I just stuck to the few things I could eat and for a while I was okay. Not a normal person okay, but I was less stressed than I was when I was having pointless tests done. Since no doctor was of any help, I created my own treatment plan. I basically found a few foods I could live on that didn't make me sick. I ate those and I only ate a few times a week. I wasn't really hungry. I pretty much had lost my appetite, didn't want to eat, and started to lose weight.

In 2013, I briefly went into remission for a few months and my symptoms were manageable. I was coaching my daughter's softball team and felt the best I had in a long time. This was a constant up and down cycle that went on for a few years. I would feel somewhat okay and functional and then something would trigger a flare up. Since I had been diagnosed with ulcerative colitis, the flare ups seemed normal. Almost daily I had severe diarrhea; sometimes I would wake up and throw up my food, or stomach bile. I was constantly picking up colds, bronchitis, and the stomach flu. One thing I found over the years is that every blood test since 2007 showed an elevated white blood cell count. Like I was always sick.

The one thing that was my biggest issue was bathroom attacks. I had so many explosive diarrhea attacks at work and I did not always make it to the bathroom. Talk about the most embarrassing conversation to have with your boss. "I just pooped my pants and need to go home to change." It was awful, and something I still wish did not happen, but it does.

When my symptoms would get worse I would start to think about calling a doctor, but then I would either feel a little better or decide it was not worth the time or energy. I spent every holiday in the bathroom or on the couch in pain for as long as I can remember. Nothing like camping out on your aunt's toilet while everyone was eating their Thanksgiving dinner. Your mom yelling up the steps, "Are you okay in there, do you need anything?" Thanks, Mom. Everyone was eating their dinner, I was sick as a dog and you called attention to that. That used to bother me but not anymore.

The next few years I basically accepted that I could not eat most foods and just dealt with feeling sick all the time. I had a daughter and a job. It did not really matter if I was sick. Life had to continue.

In 2013, I bought a house and my daughter and I moved in. For the first time we were on our own, out of my parents' house. The next two years we were pretty busy fixing up our new house and getting settled. Over the next few years my symptoms slowly progressed. They really picked up in 2015. Even my safe foods started to make me sick. Some days I was okay, others I would wake up and feel like death. Body aches, tired all the time, but overall food was just not even possible most days.

In October 2015, leading up to my diagnosis there were some stressful things going on at work. I was working about eighty hours a week. I was only eating a few times a week, sometimes two meals in an entire week. That was the only way I found I could function. At the time I could eat hummus, pizza and burritos. I know, right? Out of all foods why could I eat those? There's no explanation. Eventually I couldn't eat the pizza or the burritos. I was waking up every morning and vomiting up food that I had for lunch the day before. I was exhausted all the time and felt like I had the stomach flu. My body ached. I started working from home more and more because every morning for a few hours I would puke my guts out. Every day, it didn't matter if I ate the day before or not.

In December 2015, I started having a problem with holding urination. A cough or sneeze, and I peed my pants. At my regular gynecologist visit, she ruled out any issues with cysts or anything else that would cause abdominal pain with a sonogram and ultrasound. My gynecologist suggested I see someone to schedule a colonoscopy. I found a gastroenterologist in my area and scheduled an appointment.

At my first appointment I really liked the doctor. She seemed really nice and listened to all of my concerns. She immediately scheduled blood work, a colonoscopy and endoscopy. She mentioned a radioactive egg test that she might have me do because I mentioned the undigested food I was vomiting up. The week leading up to my colonoscopy and endoscopy I was really sick and didn't eat anything. I also didn't want to make the day before the procedure any worse. That awful jug of liquid they make you drink: Yuck! In this day and age, nobody should have to drink that stuff. Some I was able to get down, some of it I puked up. Either way I don't think I will ever like anything flavored with lemon as long as I live.

My mom took me to my procedure. Everything went well and when I woke up the doctor came over with a smile on her face and told me they didn't find anything wrong. I immediately broke down in tears. Anesthesia had made me emotional in the past but she looked at me like I was crazy. Let me be clear. I did not want something to be wrong but because I had been so sick I wanted answers, so I wouldn't be sick any longer. The nurse seemed to understand, but the way the doctor acted made me feel different about her.

I left the hospital that day with a prescription for Protonix and was told to start taking MiraLax twice a day for the constipation I was having. I was frustrated, here we go again, and now this doctor thinks I am a basketcase because I had a meltdown. My mom calmed me down and I decided to try to be open minded, so I started taking the Protonix. A nightmare.

I wrote this message to my doctor's office: "I started the pantoprazole 40 mg tablet and MiraLax on Saturday. On Tuesday I was nauseous in small waves throughout the day. On Wednesday I was so nauseous, extreme diarrhea. I had to take the day off of work because the nausea wouldn't go away. I woke up at 5 a.m. sick with diarrhea. The nausea was pretty consistent until about 6 p.m. I did not puke but I couldn't do anything. Today I did not take either medicine. I puked twice and have diarrhea but I would rather feel like today than how I felt on Tuesday or Wednesday. Should I continue not taking either one?"

The nurse replied back and asked if I had the flu or a fever, and if my symptoms had improved. I called their office and explained that the medicine was making me sick, so they prescribed Pepcid. I told the doctor's office that I drank Coca Cola with my food because if I didn't, I would puke it up. I told them that I don't have a lot of stomach acids or produce enough digestive enzymes and this type of medicine was not going to help me. They ignored me and I took it anyway. I will never forget taking that medicine in combination with the fiber filled MiraLax.

I wrote this message to my doctor's office after the nightmare I had taking Pepcid: "The Pepcid makes me nauseous. Is there something I can be prescribed to take for nausea with the Pepcid? Also both nights I took it I could not fall asleep. I don't know if Pepcid can keep you awake when you take it at night or not, but nothing else changed and I never have a problem sleeping. Right now my options are take no medicine and vomit, but be somewhat functional for the day. If I take the medicine, I don't puke but I am so nauseous that I can't function. So the medicine by itself doesn't help me. I would rather vomit everyday then feel like that. Again, that isn't a solution. The doctor talked about doing a gastric emptying study with an egg. Is that not an option? I don't feel that I have a solution to my issues. I am still in severe pain, still have diarrhea, and bad enough that sometimes I don't make it to the bathroom. When I had my colonoscopy and endoscopy last week, I cried when I heard the results. Not that I was upset I didn't have anything, but that I would be stuck again with no help. Pepcid doesn't help someone not poop their pants. I am eating very small meals, staying away from fiber and foods high in fat. None of these things are even making a difference in any way."

They were brushing me off and I wouldn't stand for it. For the first time in my life, I stood up for myself and my right not to suffer. Shortly after the nurse called me, the doctor ordered some new tests. They told me I needed to schedule a gastric emptying study, small bowel follow through, ultrasound, and more blood tests. The nurse even asked me on the phone if I was still taking the Pepcid, Protonix and MiraLax, which made me angry because they obviously didn't update my chart that those medications were like poison to my body.

I was able to get the tests scheduled rather quickly. I had the gastric emptying study and abdominal ultrasound scheduled the same day. The ultrasound went well and then I went over to nuclear medicine. Radioactive egg time. I was nervous. I had no idea what to expect. The thought of eating anything in the middle of a nasty hospital room with machines everywhere was very odd to me. The fact that I had to wear latex gloves and an apron made me nervous. What was I eating? No worries, there is less radiation in the egg than any x-ray. I ate the eggs and jelly bread, and drank a glass of water. For four hours I had to have pictures taken. What a long test! I had no idea what any of the tests meant.

A few days later I had the small bowel follow through. This is where you drink the barium and they take photos. You have to roll around, and they take pictures while you are drinking it. There are different drinks you drink at different times but the main thing is barium. This test took six hours. I was ready to lose my mind. When I got home that night my stomach blew up. I was in so much pain. It felt like I was filled with concrete that had hardened. I couldn't sit, I could barely walk. I remember awkwardly sitting on the couch with my head back, breathing in and out to get through the pain. It took eight long days for my stomach to deflate and thirteen days to go to the bathroom. I was miserable, felt completely alone, and was angry with the care I was receiving from my current gastroenterologist.

Then the day happened when I received a call from my doctor's office with test results. My gastric emptying study showed a severe delay and I was diagnosed with severe gastroparesis. The nurse explained that while the disease wasn't that common, it was usually easily controlled with diet; in rare cases medication would be needed. She said I would receive a call from a nutritionist to figure out a meal plan. I had no idea my life would never be the same.

*

JENNIFER ZUBIK
Jennifer was diagnosed with idiopathic gastroparesis in 2010 at age 27

I first became sick on Christmas Eve 2009, fourteen days after becoming engaged to my best friend, who is now my husband. I was on my way home from my aunt's house and started feeling severely nauseous. After eating Tums, thinking it was just indigestion from overeating, I struggled but eventually went to bed. I then woke up Christmas Day to begin preparing everything for the holiday. I was entertaining my family at our house that day. It was challenging to prepare the ham and turkey because I couldn't even stand the smell of the meat. I felt so nauseous, I had the hardest time preparing for our feast. Thinking I may just be getting the flu, I continued with the day, eager for it to be over so I could just go to bed.

My symptoms continued, and I was so sick I was unable to eat and could barely drink fluids. I took a pregnancy test, but the result was negative. After two weeks of being sick, I had lost twelve pounds. Within two months, I drastically transformed and had lost forty-five pounds and weighed only eighty-seven pounds. I was beyond scared, and feared I was going to die. This was supposed to be a joyous time of my life with the excitement of planning a wedding and enjoying everything about life with my daughter and soon-to-be husband. Not only did my life come to a drastic halt, but theirs did as well.

I was evaluated by several doctors and gastroenterologists, and was first diagnosed with irritable bowel syndrome and given medications. My symptoms were not subsiding at all, so I then had tests done that determined my gallbladder was not functioning properly. I underwent gallbladder surgery thinking it would end my agonizing pain and sickness, but after weeks of recovery, nothing improved and seemed to be getting worse. At that point, I was no longer able to work, was afraid to leave my house because of the fear of getting sick in public, lived and slept on my bathroom floor day and night, my anxiety had sky-rocketed, and I was eating nausea pills like candy. Before long, I lost all hope, fell into a deep depression, and felt it was necessary to create a living will, medical and general powers of attorney, and my last will and testament with an attorney I had previously worked for.

*

CHAPTER TWO

Learning the Diagnosis

Warning: I'm having one of those "I don't know which part of my body to cry about first" days.
-ANONYMOUS

For many, diagnosis and treatment of motility disorders can be delayed by years from the beginning of symptoms. For some, the diagnosis comes far later. What brought about your diagnosis?

*

MELISSA ADAMS VANHOUTEN
Melissa was diagnosed with
gastroparesis in 2014 at age 47

My gastroparesis actually came on quite suddenly, though that is not necessarily typical. Many struggle with symptoms that gradually worsen over time, and then spend months or even years seeking a proper diagnosis. Prior to 2014, I never had any serious stomach. My gallbladder and appendix were removed in late 2002, after a brief series of attacks, but I suffered no ill effects from that surgery, and my life improved drastically upon removal of the offending organs.

My life from 2002 to 2014 was relatively uneventful in terms of health issues. I was eating healthy, exercising, had no major health concerns, and believed myself to be in perhaps the best state of health I had ever been. I had no food-related issues, no nausea, and no pain.

February 11, 2014, was a typical day for me, and I ended the evening feeling normal with no discomfort of any sort. But that changed suddenly and drastically on the morning of February 12, 2014. I awoke to a minor tummy ache, which very quickly turned to excruciating stomach and abdominal pain. This was followed by intense and sudden nausea, and then nonstop vomiting. The pain and vomiting continued for several hours, and I finally became so weak and frightened that I called my husband and asked to be taken to the emergency room. My daughter, then ten years old, witnessed this and, though worried and afraid, did her best to comfort me, offering pats on the back, bottles of water, and a warm blanket.

I vomited all the way to the hospital, which thankfully was only fifteen minutes from home. I was taken back to a room immediately but told that I could not have any anti-nausea or pain medications until I had been seen, so that my symptoms would not be masked. By the time I saw a doctor, my symptoms had subsided, and though I was still experiencing pain and off-and-on vomiting, my situation had improved slightly. I refused the pain medications but was helped immensely by what I have come to view as a wonder drug, an antiemetic known as Zofran. My labs indicated a high lipase level and a high white blood cell count. This, according to the assigned doctor, was cause for hospital admission. So, off I went.

For the next week, I was forced to undergo every test known to man, including one particularly awful test in which a tube was forced through my nose and into my stomach. I refused this at first, but the nurse enlisted the help of the on-call gastroenterologist who convinced me that he needed to empty my stomach of all liquids if we wanted to get closer to diagnosis. I hope to never endure this procedure ever again. Placing the tube was not simply a matter of slight discomfort. Instead, it was excruciatingly painful and frightening. Throughout the long week, I endured an ever-present IV, daily bloodwork and labs, CT scan, upper endoscopy, and finally a gastric emptying study. On February 14, a not-so-pleasant Valentine's Day, I was given the diagnosis of gastroparesis.

At the end of the week, I was released from the hospital and directed to follow up in six weeks with the gastroenterologist who had treated me. Despite following a liquid diet and all the other guidelines, my symptoms worsened after returning home. The vomiting, which had all but ceased in the hospital, returned and the pain rose to intolerable levels. But I was a stubborn one, and I did not wish to return to the hospital, so I persisted. Eventually, I became so weak that I honestly could not lift my head off the sofa, and I truly believed I would die. I called my gastroenterologist, who agreed to see me as an emergency appointment, and he ordered domperidone, a prokinetic which helps with motility but due to FDA restrictions, it was two weeks before I could begin the medication. Those were, without a doubt, the longest weeks of my life. However, once the medication took effect (a week or so for me, but it can take up to six weeks for many people), my pain decreased to tolerable levels and my vomiting and nausea nearly disappeared.

Today, I am on a mostly liquid diet with a few soft foods thrown in when I can tolerate them, and my nausea has largely been kept at bay. The stomach and abdominal pain is still ever-present, but I address it the best I can, and it has not risen to the send-you-to-the-emergency-room levels I experienced immediately after diagnosis. I frequently experience extreme bloating and early satiety. Those symptoms have not lessened. In fact, they have grown worse.

No one is certain what caused my gastroparesis. I have been labeled idiopathic, a term I have grown to detest. The doctor theorizes that perhaps I had a virus that brought about my gastroparesis, but he tells me we will likely never know for certain. He once told me that if this were due to a virus, I had a chance of recovering within the first year or so after diagnosis. I held out hope for that for a very long time, and I still think about that possibility from time to time now, but I recognize that this is likely not to be. I continue to undergo tests which could lead to the discovery of the underlying cause, but I have had to come to terms with the fact that I will likely never know. That is tough. I want to know the reason my life was upended overnight. I want a reason for this madness. But, for now, knowing gastroparesis is my diagnosis must be enough for me.

The last three years have been harrowing, but in the midst of my nightmare, it has been comforting and reassuring to know there are people who care and who seek to help me through my most difficult days. For that, I am grateful.

*

SAMANTHA ANDERSON
Samantha was diagnosed with idiopathic gastroparesis in 2012 at age 26

I always describe my symptoms to people as the sickness or stomach bug that never went away. I started off feeling like I had a stomach bug with really bad nausea and cramps. At that point, I didn't have actual vomiting or problems going to the toilet. I felt awful; I was bloated, and couldn't eat or drink much. Then I started to vomit. The vomiting got worse—I couldn't eat or drink without being sick. I would vomit up food hours after eating, even the next day. I was nauseous and in constant pain. I felt bloated and full after the smallest bit of food or drink, and it hurt. I felt weak, exhausted, fatigued, and my sleep pattern had become disrupted. I woke up from pain and vomiting, and a few times from choking too. It was disgusting.

Feeling faint became a regular occurrence, but I tried to do as much as I could to not end up in the emergency room for hydration and pain relief. Not wanting to eat because of the nausea, hours of vomiting, and bloating, I suppose in many ways was a blessing and almost became the norm. The diagnosis took over a year, and I had to have many tests that were horrible, especially ones that involved having to swallow my own vomit in the hope that it would help the test. Doctors diagnosed indigestion, a mystery along with stress, and me doing it to myself, before they diagnosed gastroparesis. Even then, I still had to prove it to different doctors. The diagnosis wasn't the end, and treatments to help had started before the diagnosis was given.

*

JOLI ATKINS
Joli was diagnosed with
gastroparesis in 2015 at age 36

I got my diagnosis in December 2015. It was just weeks before my thirty-seventh birthday. The doctors have not been able to find a reason for my diagnosis. At this point they are listing the cause as idiopathic. I had problems with my stomach for many years, however the symptoms for this attack came on very suddenly. My main problem was nausea and vomiting. I was able to eat some solid food at first but it was very limited, and over time that changed to a mainly liquid diet. I have been on this type of diet for almost a year now.

*

MEGAN BOGGS
Megan was diagnosed with
gastroparesis in 2017 at age 38

Bloating, gas, vomiting and pain. I was thirty-eight years old and my life was over. I was an independent, strong woman who was crumbling slowly, and losing her mind to top it all off. The diagnosis was like a death sentence, or so I thought.

*

TRISHA BUNDY
Trisha was diagnosed with
gastroparesis in 2013 at age 35

I was diagnosed with gastroparesis in April 2013, after being unable to eat anything or drink an adequate amount since February 2013. I had just turned thirty-five years old. Constant severe abdominal pain, vomiting or heaving every time I attempted to eat or drink anything, recurring dehydration, and fatigue kept my doctors (when I found a team that listened and didn't dismiss my condition), family, and I perplexed and searching for answers. In May 2013, I became dependent on a gastrojejunostomy feeding tube for nutrition. It helped for a while, but then I began struggling with my tube feeds. My constant nausea was being managed with dissolvable Zofran and Remeron, while my pain was being helped with Bentyl and later dissolvable Levsin. Neither the nausea nor my abdominal pain were completely eliminated but were toned down enough that I was able to return to teaching the following fall.

I honestly believe that I would have been taken seriously earlier if I was not so overweight. Being overweight, some medical providers were not concerned about me being unable to eat or my weight loss because I had plenty to lose. My amazing hospitalist was aware that I could still be extremely sick, malnourished, and dehydrated even when overweight. He saw me as a person, not just a chart, and listened empathetically to my husband and I as we discussed and explained the past few months, my symptoms, and our concerns. I will remember and appreciate him always! When he was my hospitalist again in later hospitalizations, he was shocked at the amount of weight that had been lost as a result of illness.

We are unsure of what actually caused my illness and digestive issues. It may have been a result of a viral stomach infection or simply idiopathic (meaning they don't know why). However, other digestive and gastrointestinal motility issues began appearing soon afterwards.

In October 2014, I was hospitalized and diagnosed with pelvic floor dyssynergia after once again becoming severely impacted with stool. After completing an anorectal manometry study, they determined that some of my constipation issues were a result of my rectal sphincter not relaxing or functioning correctly.

In December 2014, I underwent gallbladder surgery for gallstones and inflammation which were causing extreme upper right abdominal pain. Next, I began having trouble with choking when trying to drink liquids. During the summer of 2015, an esophageal manometry test revealed that my lower esophagus sphincter was not relaxing. This test required me to have a tube placed down my nose and throat. Then I had to drink water while the technician assessed muscle movements. The results found that I was having sporadic esophageal spasms and that my lower sphincter was not relaxing correctly. Therefore, I had my esophagus dilated during an endoscopy. This did help decrease the choking feeling, and I had the dilation repeated once more with the knowledge that it may need to be repeated again in the future.

I also suffered from chronic constipation, lightheadedness, dizziness, continued abdominal pain, continuous nausea, and dehydration issues. After completing the Sitzmarks study in 2015, we discovered that I also had colonic inertia, which led to having my colon removed and the creation of an ileostomy, a bag on my abdomen. In addition, small intestinal bacterial overgrowth (SIBO) still occurs at times and has to be treated with antibiotics. SIBO can cause increased bloating, pain, and gas. So basically, my digestive system sucks.

At first I felt relief. I finally had some answers and hope. However, when the symptoms continued month after month and then year after year with little to no improvement, I began to feel disbelief because there was no cure or immediate treatment that could make all of my symptoms or illness go away. As newer issues began and the severity of my symptoms and the negative impact on my quality of health increased, so did my fears.

*

LISA COLANDREA
Lisa was diagnosed with
gastroparesis in 2016 at age 42

The symptoms I had leading up to my gastroparesis diagnosis included debilitating nausea, vomiting, pain in my abdomen, diarrhea or constipation, and not being able to empty my stomach at all for days or weeks. I was diagnosed at the age of forty-two in January 2016. Since then it has gotten much worse.

*

TAMMY DOWNS
Tammy was diagnosed with Crohn's disease, irritable bowel syndrome, spastic colon, gastroesophageal reflux disease, and gastritis in 2006 at age 46, gastroparesis in 2015 at age 56, and motility dysfunction disorder of the rectum and pelvic floor in 2016 at age 58

I had my gallbladder removed around seven years ago. Well, if I did not know any better, it felt like it had grown back. When I ate, it felt like my food had turned into a big rock sitting in the pit of my stomach. I got very nauseous after eating, and the pain would be so bad that I would throw up. This horrible feeling occurred day and night. It was to the point where I found myself not eating and I started to lose weight.

*

SKYE FALCON

Skye was diagnosed with gastroparesis and other autoimmune diseases in 2006 at age 25

I often describe my years of symptoms as a giant snowball. Once the ball started going down the hill, it just kept getting bigger, and bigger, and bigger. Knocking down trees (plans) and wiping out entire cities in its path (life-changers). I was sick my whole life. My immune system was never up to par, and I spent the majority of my time on antibiotics. I'd always been prone to vomiting, and illnesses that seemed to revolve around my gastrointestinal tract and how well it was functioning. But it was not until after my first successful pregnancy when other issues were finally brought to light, that any of this started making sense.

After being diagnosed with scleroderma in 2002 and beginning to deal with the internal scar tissue, adhesions, and fibrous tissues hardening my insides, something began to change with my gastrointestinal tract. I call these times "the shifts." At first, the shift was chalked up to the autoimmune issues and just having a flare. My flares seemed to happen more frequently, and were not touched or hindered by the prednisone and other drugs they used to treat my other ailments. I was on three different proton pump inhibitors, blood pressure medications to calm my Raynaud's phenomenon, Plaquenil, a gamete of medications to keep my scar tissue at bay, immuno-suppressors, and other stomach medicines to ease the issues, but it was not working. This was all happening so much more severely months after my emergency hysterectomy in 2007. And then the weight just started to fall off. At first, the doctors and specialists just went along with it. I was still close to 155 pounds. After a C-section and hysterectomy, experimental scar tissue prevention surgeries, and another major surgery on my small five-foot four-inch frame, getting back down to around 130 pounds was the goal. "Just continue to let your body adjust," they told me over and over again.

That's what I did and was doing, until the constant vomiting began and the constant pain again increased. With now confirmed gluten issues, I just kept thinking I had glutened myself, tripping an autoimmune reaction, throwing my body into internal fits of rage. Over and over it happened with the frequency speeding to what seemed like everyday issues. This seemed too regular and too frequent to be a gluten-induced flare. The weakness, physical and mental, was more than I had bargained for. I was not ready to be held down like this in life. I was not done living and growing. The pain was, and continues to be, relentless, life-altering, and world-changing. The localized, specific intense pain that crept up after ingesting any sort of food item was breathtaking and heart-stopping. With each meal, and the progression of the food bomb stagnating through my intestines, came more of the abdominal scar tissue ripping, tearing, and burning.

One day, after I had eaten a delicious cobb salad, I went to the bathroom thinking that I had to simply urinate, and I was greeted with some intense rectal bleeding and a pain I had never felt before. A few hours after, the blame was placed on a lodged bezoar with a small intestinal bacterial overgrowth infection.

Now my weight teeters between 100 and 105 pounds, and I am lucky if I edge above that. That began the long process of testing, biopsies, motility tests, and more, which brought me to gastroparesis. They believe my gastroparesis is caused by vagal nerve damage from multiple abdominal surgeries compiled with the complications of scleroderma, and the buildup of scar and fibrous tissues in my entire abdomen. Hearing the official diagnosis of gastroparesis brought relief, but the fear of learning how to live with yet another setback and illness is something that keeps me close to the edge.

*

ROBIN MCNAMARA
Robin was diagnosed with
gastroparesis in 2013 at age 55

Extreme nausea that was leaving me hanging over the toilet, but not getting sick, feeling the burn of acid in my chest and having it creep up my throat, a bloated abdomen and pain all over my stomach and intestines. Anything I tried to eat resulted in horrible acid, nausea, sweats and chills. And with the acid, I slept on my couch so I could keep myself propped up and the acid down.

My gastroparesis is idiopathic. However, the more I've thought about it, it was a slow seven-month slide down to the pit of hell, stemming from a round of antibiotics for an infected tooth and root canal.

I was fifty-five years old when officially diagnosed by my new gastroenterologist. My first doctor had no explanation. He said, "You need to heal." When I asked from what, he stared blankly into my eyes and said nothing, gave me a script for Reglan and Carafate, and sent me on my way.

My new gastroenterologist tried giving me injections of Protonix and nausea medication, which made no difference. Then he did an endoscopy and called it gastric atony. I looked up what this meant and became more and more frightened. I wondered if I would survive, because in the beginning I was so sick I thought I would die. There was no relief knowing I would never be eating all the great foods I once enjoyed as a foodie. I was miserable and sad. I tried not to be angry, but it was hard not to be at times.

*

TAMMY PITTMAN

Tammy was diagnosed with gastroparesis and irritable bowel syndrome in 2014 at age 34

I had a terrible history of reflux since being pregnant with my daughter in 2000. It was so bad at night that I had to force myself to throw up just to sleep. I had exhausted every option I had for medication when my gastrologist started more intensive testing, which included an esophageal motility study in late 2006. This showed that my lower esophageal sphincter had atrophied. My doctor sent me to see a surgeon for a Nissen fundoplication. This was done on March 7, 2006, and was a nightmare. There were multiple errors made during surgery that caused me to develop a football-sized subphrenic abscess.

I developed a 1600 milliliter pleural effusion that went unnoticed for two weeks. Adhesions collapsed my lower left lung. I continued to have problems with my bowels and reflux.

Within a year, I started vomiting more and more. Back on medications I went. I was in the worst pain. My second surgeon (I transferred myself to another hospital out of state) sent me to multiple pain clinics. I would describe the pain, and I heard over and over that my pain was medical and the surgeon needed to fix something wrong. Finally, I was forced to deal with it. I finally got my gastrologist to see me in 2013 for further testing because I was in terrible shape. He finally ordered the gastric emptying study.

*

TAYLOR SCHMITZ

Taylor was diagnosed with idiopathic gastroparesis in 2014 at age 22

When I was twenty-two years old, I was diagnosed with idiopathic gastroparesis. The doctors had no idea what caused it, and quite frankly, they didn't try to find out. When I was diagnosed, it devastated me. My doctor was very vague, and didn't really have time to explain anything to me. Nausea, heartburn, indigestion, pain after anything I consumed, and panic of thinking I was going to die was at every turn.

*

DEB SHRADER-TROTTER
Deb was diagnosed with
gastroparesis in 1999 at age 37

I began to have migraines, which evolved into a stomach flu off and on, with endometriosis. After a hysterectomy, appendectomy, sinus surgery, walking pneumonia, and numerous tests to find out why I had constant diarrhea and constipation with pain, I was diagnosed with motility disorders. I was diagnosed with gastroparesis, colonic inertia, and chronic intestinal pseudo-obstruction syndrome. Later I would be given additional diagnoses of postural orthostatic tachycardia syndrome (POTS) and mitochondrial malabsorption.

*

JESSICA SPENCE
Jessica was diagnosed with
gastroparesis in 2016 at age 25

My symptoms started when I was fourteen years old. We had moved to a new area, and I started to throw up every morning before school. I would feel sick for most of the day and start to feel better when the sun was setting. I would be absolutely starving at dinner and after a single bite would be totally full. Sometimes I would crave something, take a bite, and throw it right up. After a few months the nausea subsided, and I pushed it from my mind. A few months later it would start all over again. This cycle continued for a decade.

After a decade my symptoms stopped being cyclic and started to get more severe. There were more and more foods that triggered me that had never been a problem before. The pain and nausea became constant. So at the age of twenty-four I was given a colonoscopy. The test was inconclusive because I still had stool in my colon. I was accused of sabotaging my prep and told I was a crazy little girl who needed a head transplant.

When I was twenty-five my mother pushed me to see a fourth gastroenterologist. He took one look at my colonoscopy and said he thought it was gastroparesis and wanted to do a gastric emptying study. I threw up after thirty minutes of the test, so we rescheduled and that test came back conclusive. I had gastroparesis. When I was first diagnosed I was so happy. I had been fighting to prove I wasn't crazy for eleven years, and I had won.

*

NICOLE STARZYNSKI
Nicole was diagnosed with
gastroparesis in 2016 at age 33

I have always had stomach issues for as far back as I can remember. However, it was not until after I gave birth to my daughter that I really started to experience issues. Although I do not have diabetes now, when I was pregnant I had gestational diabetes which I was able to control with a strict diet. I had previously been diagnosed with celiac disease, ulcerative colitis and irritable bowel syndrome. For a few years, I just dealt with feeling worse because nobody had helped me before.

Over the years I became more and more sensitive to different foods. I would experience severe bloating, diarrhea, vomiting of food in the morning, vomiting of stomach bile, and stomach pains. Over time this progressed and I became more limited with what I could eat. I had cut out everything from gluten, dairy, preservatives, and sodium but eventually I couldn't eat any food without becoming deathly ill.

After numerous tests that ruled out such illnesses as diabetes and autoimmune disorders, I was diagnosed with idiopathic gastroparesis at age thirty-three. They had no idea if I was born with gastroparesis, if something caused it, or if having gestational diabetes while I was pregnant caused it. This caused a trickle down effect.

Gastroparesis is hard enough to treat when you know what's causing it. With idiopathic gastroparesis, it's harder to group everyone together because without the underlying cause, the same treatments may not work. I worry if gastroparesis can be shown as hereditary. If it is hereditary, what are the chances of my daughter having it?

Prior to my diagnosis, I'd never heard of gastroparesis. When I received the call from my doctor's office, it was bittersweet. I was excited and relieved that they finally had a name for what I had. This was followed by a rush of feeling overwhelmed and scared. I cried just because I had waited so long to actually know what was wrong with me. As soon as I searched for gastroparesis on the internet, a thousand different thoughts and fears started rushing through my head at once. Maybe I was better believing I had something else. For once, while reading about a disease everything fit; that was exactly how I felt. I saw a picture that said, "My stomach feels like there are shards of glass inside." It brought tears to my eyes because of all the years when the doctors didn't do tests, told me nothing could be causing my pain, and that I needed to lose weight.

Then I was filled with a lot of anger. I was angry at the insurance companies that years earlier had denied me a test that could've given me the correct diagnosis. What if I had known then? Would I be in a better place now if I knew six-plus years ago? I was really scared. I read so many horrifying stories about what this disease had done to others. I joined a few online support groups, which both helped and scared me even more. I immediately felt a connection to so many people I had never met—people who were experiencing the same issues as me.

You hope that once you learn more about a disease, it will ease some of your fears. With gastroparesis, information is scarce and most doctors don't know enough about the disease. The ones who do can't even tell you if the nerves will continue to die, and how you'll respond to treatments. It's a luck of the draw. Even after multiple treatments fail, you have to convince yourself to fight for your right to live, be your own advocate and never give up.

I decided to do my own research. I read through procedures and clinical studies all over the world. I talked to fellow warriors in online support groups. In less than four months I had appointments at Cleveland Clinic and Johns Hopkins. I had to cyberstalk some doctors, writing countless emails to them. I was persistent and stayed strong. I wasn't backing down until I was heard.

My quality of life is awful and I feel like a prisoner in my own home. Most days I wake up vomiting and dry heaving. Sometimes the nausea lasts for hours or all day. Sometimes it will go away, sometimes it feels like it's never going to end. There has been no significant difference in the severity of my symptoms on a liquid diet versus solid food. I barely go to the bathroom. Sometimes I feel like my stomach is so bloated it is ready to burst. The sad thing is that I still feel this way after consuming only liquids for weeks. It doesn't matter. The pain is unbearable, like I am being stabbed from the inside out.

*

JENNIFER ZUBIK

Jennifer was diagnosed with idiopathic gastroparesis in 2010 at age 27

My symptoms started suddenly one day without any warning, rhyme or reason. I had severe nausea, extreme pain and rapid weight loss. The first night I experienced anything, Christmas Eve 2009, I thought I just had a belly ache from eating too much. The next day I did not feel any better and assumed maybe I had the stomach flu. Yet it just continued and would not stop. I was extremely nauseated and had stomach cramps. The pain was not nearly as bad as the nausea. I felt horrible and could not eat, drink or even stand the smell of food. The nausea was so overwhelming that I spent almost all night and day in the bathroom. This was difficult for my household considering we only had one working bathroom while the other was slowly being renovated by Lou, my boyfriend at the time.

New Year's Eve was difficult. We had plans with our friends and other couples to go out to dinner and then drinks for the evening. I always told Lou that New Year's Eve was important, and we had to always have a great night together, to start the new year right and make the year a great one. A bad night would jinx us with a bad year; a great night would give us luck and hope for all to come that year. At first, I was alright at the restaurant, even with the smells of all the food. It felt good to be out of the house, the first time since Christmas Eve.

However, when they brought out my soup and the aroma of it was directly under my nose, I had to run to the restroom. I then spent the rest of the dinner outside, in the cold, smoking one cigarette after another, trying not to vomit in front of everyone there to dine. Needless to say, Lou had my meal packed to go and we went home after the others were all done with their dinner. We were unable to celebrate the new year happily. That was the beginning of what I thought at one time was the end.

Within two weeks of the first day of symptoms, I had lost twelve pounds. I didn't even realize until I was trying to get ready for a family member's birthday party and my pants were falling off. I was so nauseous that I could not eat anything and could barely even drink for days. If I could eat, I felt full almost immediately, after very few bites of food. Not eating anything resulted in malnutrition, which made me tired and weak and unable to function. Fatigue, hair loss, achiness, nonstop cold flashes, anxiety, and depression manifested as well.

The pain I experienced at first wasn't too unbearable, but I think it was overshadowed by the overwhelming nausea. The feeling of having to vomit, or doing so, was the worst thing in the world. When I was little, I rarely got sick with the flu, but when I did it was the worst thing. I would just cry and cry for my mom, and do anything possible to not throw up. My mom would always be with me to hold my hair back and tell me I would be okay. Of course, being on my own and not living at home anymore, my mom wasn't there to do that.

I then began my adventure of seeing numerous doctors and having several tests done. The first gastroenterologist I saw tried to tell me I just had irritable bowel syndrome, even though I wasn't eating or going to the bathroom and was losing weight. I didn't have medical insurance at the time, so he did not want to run any tests due to the high costs. He gave me a handful of prescriptions to try, and basically said good luck. I then saw a different doctor who did run tests, and said my gallbladder wasn't functioning properly. In February, I had my gallbladder removed, and hoped that I would feel better soon. At that point, I had lost even more weight. Within two months after Christmas Eve, I had lost forty-five pounds, and only weighed eighty-seven pounds. I didn't have any improvement at all after the surgery. Instead, my symptoms intensified.

After many more tests during the next few months, I finally had a gastric emptying study in May 2010, one month before my twenty-eighth birthday, which showed a severe delay of emptying. I was finally diagnosed with severe idiopathic gastroparesis. The doctors didn't know why it happened. I had always been healthy without any major medical problems. I very rarely even got a cold or flu. I didn't even experience morning sickness when I was pregnant with my daughter. I was not diabetic, and I did not have any major abdominal surgeries prior, or anything that would have caused this damage. When they finally gave me a name for what was wrong with me, I was happy, and almost relieved. Since the start, nobody listened to me that something was actually wrong, and they would all look at me and act like I was crazy. I started feeling and thinking that I was crazy, but I knew something was wrong. When the doctor told me he figured it out, I finally had hope that I would soon be well again and the nightmare would end.

*

CHAPTER THREE

Describing the Pain

"Yes, hello, I'd like a refund on my body. It's kinda defective and really expensive." -ANONYMOUS

Living with motility disorders means pain. Some days it's better, some days worse. Some days it requires medical attention to manage. Because pain is an invisible symptom, it can be difficult to describe. Is it stabbing? Dull and aching? Is it constant or intermittent?

*

MELISSA ADAMS VANHOUTEN
Melissa was diagnosed with gastroparesis in 2014 at age 47

How to describe my pain? It is difficult to find anything which compares. It is the most excruciating, debilitating pain I have ever experienced. It would be difficult to overemphasize the severity. It stops me in my tracks and keeps me at a standstill, unable to perform the most basic daily tasks. Every time I eat even a few bites, even foods considered safe for most gastroparesis patients according to the recognized diet plans, I experience severe, sharp upper stomach pain that gradually works its way down to my abdomen. It begins almost immediately after I eat and can continue for a few hours on bad days. There is nothing that can prevent it, nothing that completely takes it away, and little I can do but bear it until it passes.

The good news is that I can lessen the pain a bit with my medication and by using a heating pad—lessen it to the point that I can survive it, that is. I can also avoid it by not eating. That is the dilemma, of course. I must constantly balance my hunger and nutritional needs with the pain. It is a never-ending choice between eating and enduring the pain or skipping food and living relatively comfortably. These are not lovely options. I find that, most often, I refuse food until I am weak and drained and must resort to eating; then, I struggle to survive the pain that I knew would ensue, and the vicious cycle begins again. I am weary of this pattern, but it is what I must do to survive.

The pain that results from eating is difficult to bear, but the larger burden, by far, is the mental and emotional pain that accompanies gastroparesis. I feel guilty when I eat because I know it will lead to pain, and guilty when I do not because this leads to fatigue and long-term malnutrition. Food is a poison, but it is also life-giving. How does one make these decisions? Moreover, the fatigue and weakness from not consuming enough calories, from the malnourishment, prevents me from engaging in activities I once relished. I can no longer attend most family gatherings, frequently miss my daughter's school events, and am largely confined to my home. When I choose and am able to enjoy a day or evening out, I must go without food entirely. To eat, even a tiny amount, means my time out will come to an abrupt end.

And when I do indulge in an outing, I pay dearly. The price is pain, fatigue, and misery for sometimes days afterward. Again, I must choose: home in relative comfort, or out with physical suffering as the consequence.

The pain resulting from my choices is the most agonizing pain of all. It harms not only me but my family and loved ones as well. It hurts to let people down. It stings to constantly fail them. This... the disappointment in my daughter's eyes when I miss her latest play, her tae kwon do promotion test, or her choir performance... the discontent my husband tries so hard to mask when I cannot accompany him to corporate events, family gatherings, or even an evening at the movies... this is the most excruciating pain of all.

*

SAMANTHA ANDERSON
Samantha was diagnosed with idiopathic gastroparesis in 2012 at age 26

I could honestly write many essays about my gastroparesis journey but I think it would include a lot of repetition.

My gastroparesis stomach pain is constant and dull. It is more on the left side of my stomach but radiates around my whole abdominal area. It almost feels like my stomach is exploding at times. Sometimes it feels like a big rock is in my stomach pushing at all sides, and there is a cramping feeling that it is being squeezed and stretched. Before I had the gastric stimulator fitted in March 2016, I had pain patches which took the edge off the pain. However, the surgeon and doctors wanted me to get off them as they are opiate based and they didn't want me addicted. As well, they don't help the stomach because they slow it down and cause constipation. So I came off them after having the pacemaker fitted. It's not that I'm in less pain—the pain is still very much there and at times worse at the site of the pacer, but I can keep more down. It's still not great, but much better than before.

Now I'm on Pregablin and the dose is increased when the consultant feels like it should be. Like all tablets, I try not to be reliant on them, though. However, while the pain dampens slightly, it doesn't disappear. As I say though, every little bit helps. I will get on and do as much as I can and more, maybe too much at times, in ridiculous amounts, in pain or not. I think I often work my body a little too hard, but know it quite well. I know when I need to sit down and kind of relax for a while.

There are times when the pain goes right through my stomach to my back, which makes it hard for me to do my normal activities, and to be on autopilot and just getting on with it all. Standing up is more difficult, as is sitting. I find in general the pain is hard to properly get comfortable with, but I've learned to ignore it as much as I can. I want to have a normal life somehow, and at some point I will hopefully get there. Nothing really helps, but hot water bottles can at times slightly soothe it. The pain often wakes me up in the night and getting comfortable enough to sleep is very difficult. Having a full night's sleep has become almost impossible but, to be fair, it's not just the pain.

*

JOLI ATKINS
Joli was diagnosed with
gastroparesis in 2015 at age 36

I am very lucky that I do not have a lot of pain. I do get pain in my right side sometimes and the doctors have not been able to determine what causes that pain. The pain can double me over. There is no rhyme or reason for the pain and I have no warning when it is coming. I just have to deal with it because nothing that I have tried makes it better.

*

MEGAN BOGGS
Megan was diagnosed with
gastroparesis in 2017 at age 38

The pain of this is debilitating. There are sharp pains shooting from my stomach and I want to curl into a ball and cry. I can't work, and I can't do what I want to do. I have tried every homeopathic solution to calm the nerves. I have tried yoga, meditation, acupuncture, chiropractic care, the list is endless. My symptoms would, and still do, get worse when I am stressed out.

*

TRISHA BUNDY
Trisha was diagnosed with
gastroparesis in 2013 at age 35

Gastroparesis is an individualized destructive disease. Everyone is different, yet the pain is still there. My journey with gastroparesis began in mid-February 2013, and will continue until someone is able to come up with a cure or at least better treatment options. Everyone's pain is different, some better managed than others. Some similar to mine. And yes, some much more severe. Hopefully, I can give you an idea of how disabling gastroparesis pain can be.

Upper abdominal pain. For me, this pain is an unbearable, hard to breathe, nuisance. It occurs whenever I try to be brave and eat or drink real food. Something as simple as a couple crackers, a cup of delicious hot chocolate, a slice of grilled toast, yogurt, or a bite of scrumptious cheesecake can send me into almost immediate pain. This isn't a normal little stomachache that lasts a few minutes, or even an hour, and then goes away. The pain lasts for numerous hours. A full flare can last continuously for days, sometimes even weeks, without a break. The pain is horrendous, and I'm unable to function. I try to hold back tears while attempting coping strategies. And as if the pain isn't horrible enough, bloating and nausea usually accompanies it hand in hand. Eating something as simple as one banana can make me spend hours feeling like I have overeaten at a buffet and contracted food poisoning. Only the pain and nausea doesn't pass quickly, and stemmed from only a small amount of food or liquid. Some of my friends also have distention, luckily I don't. They can eat a few bites of food and their stomach will literally expand. One minute they are thin, the next they look and feel like they are nine months pregnant.

Lower abdominal pain. The pain in this region used to be continuous and accompanied by bloating and intense nausea. I had no control over pain in this region. It didn't matter if I chose to eat or drink a little something or not. I seemed to constantly have consistent pain in the lower abdomen. It could range from a nagging dull pain at times to intense fetal position pain at others. If I had to rate it on a number scale, I would say that I was always at least a level four on the pain scale with varying degrees higher, often seven or higher as the day went on.

I am unable to receive adequate nutrition orally due to my upper abdominal pain issues. As a result, I am dependent on a GJ feeding tube. Throughout the day, I am required to run formula which used to create more lower abdominal pain and discomfort. Usually, I could handle the pain of this region first thing in the morning. However, as the day progressed so did my pain. Unfortunately, my doctors and I couldn't figure out a successful remedy for this pain. The nausea medication and intestinal cramping medication that I used throughout the day (Zofran and Levsin) were at their highest dosage available. They could be taken every six hours but only lasted for about three to four hours. While they did offer some short-term help, they created new issues and later more pain in the form of severe constipation.

My doctors and I worked together to figure out the best medicine regimen, weeding out those whose benefits did not outweigh the risks. Sometimes, I was lucky to suffer the pain in the lower abdominal region solely on its own, but other times I had to suffer the pain of both the upper and lower region together, with relentless nausea regardless. I struggled entire days with pain that was over the top.

Eventually, we decided to do a Sitzmarks study and defecography. As a result, we learned that I was experiencing colonic inertia and chronic constipation. Basically, my digestive system came to a complete halt when reaching the colon (large intestines) and my rectum was not functioning correctly when expelling waste. Relief from the colonic inertia and constant aggravations of severe and chronic constipation was finally achieved when we had the colon completely removed (colectomy) and an ileostomy created.

Feeding tube pain. I have a GJ feeding tube. The G portion enters my stomach. If my nausea or bloating is really bad, sometimes I can get lucky and vent my stomach. This means I can allow the contents of my stomach to run out of the tube into a container or the sink. I have been instructed to be very careful with this, as it can cause electrolyte problems. I resort to venting only when my nausea has me at the point of vomiting or heaving. The J portion of the tube enters my small intestine. This is where the formula that is pumped in my body goes. Currently, I am running formula at forty to forty-five milliliters per hour for about eight to ten hours a day. This is my sole nutrition. I am unable to run it any faster or longer, as the pain, nausea, or both become too awful; at times it's unbearable.

Besides the intestinal pain and cramping, I also have sporadic pain around the tube. The stoma, the hole under my breastbone for the feeding tube, sometimes becomes extremely sensitive and irritated. I have to be careful to ensure that it doesn't become infected. I have heard horror stories about the pain and life-threatening nature of infections around the site or in the tube. The stoma pain can be rough, but thankfully I can usually find measures to improve the cause and shorten the duration of pain. Tubie pads, cloth pads to place as a bumper between the tube and my skin, have helped a lot.

Every three months, unless sooner due to unexpected issues, the feeding tube is replaced by an interventional radiology. The procedure itself isn't too bad. I am under conscious sedation, yet can still feel the tugging and, at times, short-lived pain. I am usually sore for the rest of that day and possibly the following day as well.

All over physical pain. As a result of receiving inadequate nutrition and fluids, even with a feeding tube, I stay dehydrated and occasionally have vitamin deficiencies. Therefore, I must deal with all over muscle pain, cramps, and fatigue. Even though I have a regular sleep pattern, I do not always wake up refreshed. I toss and turn during the night on most nights, due to the unwanted nausea and difficulty getting comfortable. The dehydration also puts wear on my body. It makes me feel very weak, tired, and creates restless arms and legs. Dehydration causes additional intestinal issues as well, such as constipation and colonic inertia prior to my colectomy with ileostomy. Both the colectomy and ileostomy procedures added even more cramping and razor blade pain with defecation. Additionally, the dehydration causes concentration issues, lightheadedness, dizzy spells, orthostatic hypotension, and at times heart palpitations. Often my body remains in some sort of allover fatigue with general achiness. It is more problematic when I overextend my energy or when my electrolytes or minerals are deficient.

Power port pain. To help with dehydration, a port was surgically placed in my chest for IV fluids. A port is a central line that runs in a vein that enters the top of the heart. In order to receive the hydration that my body requires, I depend on IV fluids at home five days a week.

During 2016, I had a port surgically placed in my upper right chest. Unfortunately, as a result of an infection, I had to have it removed. After a couple of months with a PICC line in my arm, I was able to have a new port placed in my upper left chest. The first week after the port was placed, I experienced some pain and soreness. Now it only hurts for a moment when my home nurse accesses my port. A nurse comes by every Monday to take the needle out and then replace it with a new needle. Having IV hydration at home has been extremely helpful in keeping me hydrated.

Emotional pain. I can't even begin to make you understand the emotional pain that I endure as a mother, patient, and friend thanks to gastroparesis. It's truly too difficult to explain, but I will try my best. As a mother, I always felt as if I had to be strong for my children. I still do, though my vision of what strong means has been altered. I used to believe that being strong meant showing my kids that everything was under control. However, having gastroparesis has proven to me that being a strong mother means showing your kids that things are not always under our control. Sometimes we have to be strong enough to ask for help. We have to be strong enough to accept help from others. I have realized, and hope my kids have as well, that strong mothers have unconditional love for their children and will always fight the battles worth fighting, by never ever giving up.

Being a mother isn't easy. I worry about my children; it's only natural. It pains me to see them hurt. Unfortunately, when I see them hurt, I hurt too. I hurt when I see their disappointment and the tears in their eyes, because they feel helpless from being unable to help me with my physical pain and struggles with illness. It is so painful to see them create a special magic hug or piece of art to try to help me feel better, only to see no change. It's heart-wrenching to hear them tell me they understand if I can't make it to a ball game or special event, when I know how important it is to them and how badly I want to be there. I feel emotional pain, sadness, and guilt knowing that they are missing out on exciting vacations because I can't physically handle them. Painful tears slide down my face as I hurt for the energy and strength to actually play outside with them and create fun lifelong memories before their childhood years disappear. It's painful as a mother to realize that before long my kids will be on their own, and will be left with memories of me as a patient in pain instead of a mom who actively enjoyed life with them.

Not only do some of my friends and I suffer from physical and emotional pain brought on as a result of gastroparesis, but we also have to deal with numerous medical providers. I will not deny that my initial gastroenterologist and primary doctors were awesome. My current gastroenterologist is phenomenal. He has been everything I expect and need from a doctor. I am afraid about who my next gastroenterologist will be as he is moving out of the state at the end of this month, June 2017.

I have been very blessed with having some open, respectful, and knowledgeable physicians. Unfortunately, that is not the case for everyone, and hasn't always been the case for me. It still isn't the case at times when facing emergency rooms and hospital stays. I hear complaints every day about the experiences that others have with their doctors. So many physicians, including some of the emergency room doctors and my immediate care doctors, just don't get it. Either they are unfamiliar with what gastroparesis is, unfamiliar with how to treat it, or unfamiliar with its debilitating nature. It is not uncommon for someone living with gastroparesis to be told from their doctor that it's all in their head, that there's nothing wrong, that the pain is not real, that they don't know what else to do, that they have run out of options, or that they simply can't help them. I've experienced this myself and I read about it every day in the support groups online.

In the groups, I have witnessed the confusion, loneliness, and heartache of not having supportive doctors. I have witnessed and experienced the darkest hours of this disease, the feeling of being alone, being a burden, or being helpless. My heart also aches each and every time I hear of someone who lost their life to gastroparesis complications. Many have died from such things as malnutrition, infections leading to sepsis, organ failure, and even suicide.

Luckily, I was rescued from those deep waters. God, family, and close online friends rescued me. I know that there is hope. I am in this fight and I will not give up! Unfortunately, others are still struggling, still drowning. I do my best to help and I share their pain. I can't describe how difficult it is to hear others talk about struggling to survive yet unable to find a helpful and compassionate doctor. The pain and anguish is an even higher magnitude when kids and babies are the ones struggling with gastroparesis yet unable to receive appropriate treatments. This is why I participate in online support and advocacy groups, write openly about my health experiences in a personal blog that is shared publicly, and agreed to be a part of this book. If my story and experiences can help one person survive this journey, decrease the emotional pain they face, or help give them ideas of what to discuss with their own personal physician, then my struggles have at least achieved a purpose.

*

LISA COLANDREA
Lisa was diagnosed with
gastroparesis in 2016 at age 42

Every day I face some level of pain on and off, but the nausea is a constant. Individuals with gastroparesis often compare the illness to having the flu every day, but most days it's much worse. Some days I can cope and other days I feel like giving up altogether. The pain is very debilitating. It is also emotionally and physically draining suffering with gastroparesis every day. The only thing that helps me cope with the pain is knowing that I have a family who I want to wake up to every day. I also go to pain management and take medication to manage some of my symptoms. The pain clouds my mind so bad that most days I can't even gather my thoughts or focus.

*

TAMMY DOWNS
Tammy was diagnosed with Crohn's disease, irritable bowel syndrome, spastic colon, gastroesophageal reflux disease, and gastritis in 2006 at age 46, gastroparesis in 2015 at age 56, and motility dysfunction disorder of the rectum and pelvic floor in 2016 at age 58

Because I have Crohn's disease and irritable bowel syndrome, I'm on dicyclomine for pain and cramping, and promethazine for nausea.

I also have acid reflux and gastritis. Whenever I eat, pain soon follows. My stomach feels like it is on fire and bloated, like I had eaten something that did not agree with me and I'm coming down with a bad flu. Then the nausea comes, and then the pain gets worse. I took dicyclomine because I thought it was helping, but it got to the point when nothing helped and it was the most uncomfortable pain. I didn't eat because I did not want to be nauseous and in pain all day and night. I did not want to throw up after eating to get rid of feeling like I had a rock in my stomach. I ended up in the hospital once because I thought I was having a heart attack. It can really mess up your day. On days when I felt good, I would use all my strength to do what I could.

*

SKYE FALCON

Skye was diagnosed with gastroparesis and other autoimmune diseases in 2006 at age 25

When my pain is the worst, my entire body burns, I lose focus for and on everything except the pain, and everything I see is tinted red. Literally. Maybe I've taken the correlation of being in hell a bit too far, but when my brow is furrowed and my face stern and angry, I am most likely facing one of my worst pains. Those are usually split pretty evenly between the gastroparesis pain and the pain that comes from internal ripping and tearing of scar tissues and adhesions. One pain always seems to trigger another, and any amount of stress makes everything one million times worse. Some days all I can do is sit, stare at the wall in a quiet room, and try to control the number of tears pouring from my eyes because let's face it, sobbing and lung issues do not usually work well together.

Some days I truly wonder if I will see the next morning, because I am sure I cannot live through another night of the intense, never-ending pain. Knowing that one bite of the wrong food could knock me down for an entire week, and cause blinding pain makes wanting to eat a challenge in itself. It is hard to face each day when, before I have even moved to get out of bed, my entire midsection is screaming at me and in fiery pain. Knowing that I have people depending on me, commitments to keep, and jobs to complete, I have learned how to hide most of my pains, push through the worst, and still be productive regardless of how hard it truly is, or the toll it is taking.

The changes that have occurred due to the lack of nutrition, body changes, and morphing illnesses are not only a burden physically, but also mentally. On my worst pain days, my patience level is almost nonexistent. I remind myself every minute to force that fake smile, really focus on and listen to what others are saying, and play it off the best I can so no one notices my struggle. The pain causes cluster headaches which then prevent me from working on the computer or tablet either to write or on social media to entertain myself. There are times it is so intense I have to go silent because I cannot handle looking at the screens of anything, even my cellphone. Other times, I have been known to combat my chronic pain with more pain, in the form of tattoos, or even purposely eating something I should not. I spend my days rotating from heating pad to heating pad, and using natural oils and meditation methods for relief. I am taken down by this pain multiple times per week. My pain robs me daily of things I want to do. Things I need to do. Things I could do. Things I am determined to do.

On the flip side, my pain is a large driving force in my life now. The past few years of dealing with the worsening illnesses, I have accepted that every day will include this red, searing pain, and that in order to be a proper functioning human, I need to learn coping mechanisms to push through not only for myself, but for my family.

Being able to have businesses that revolve around my passions truly helps keep me going, and allows me to focus on growth and the future. I try to not focus on the negative daily aspects, but also keep them in the forefront, as well. I acknowledge my issues, good and bad, but keep moving because there is no time to stop. I grab on to the intense pain, and I squeeze it harder, pumping out whatever energy I can muster.

While the physical symptoms and ailments of gastroparesis are not ignorable by any means, the mental side of illness can be controlled. It can be adjusted, corrected, and changed to fit where life is taking you, and where you need to go. It was not, and is not, always easy to stay positive and focused. You really, really have to want to and work at it. Thankfully I get to face my reasons every day, which helps keep me moving forward.

*

ROBIN MCNAMARA
Robin was diagnosed with
gastroparesis in 2013 at age 55

In the beginning, I had sharp pains that traveled down my left side, along with a constant ache in my chest. I texted my sister, a registered nurse, a lot and ended up in the emergency room a few times where they gave me anti-nausea medication and painkillers via IV. Today, I have occasional pain, nothing debilitating, and have never taken any narcotics (except in the emergency room) for pain. Now it's mostly nausea. To cope with minor pain and nausea, I pace back and forth, sometimes out on my deck in the dead of winter, and try to stay occupied to keep my mind off the nausea.

Allergies mess my stomach up so flares occur more often now than they were. It's not predictable with me. I can be feeling good and then all of a sudden I get that certain feeling and know I need to get near a bathroom. I pop a Zofran and hope it works.

*

TAMMY PITTMAN

Tammy was diagnosed with gastroparesis and irritable bowel syndrome in 2014 at age 34

The pain was very intense stabbing and cramping in my abdomen. If I started cooking, sometimes it was just the smell alone that caused me to double over. At times, it was the first bite. So I stopped eating because I felt it was better than the pain.

*

TAYLOR SCHMITZ

Taylor was diagnosed with idiopathic gastroparesis in 2014 at age 22

I experience daily pain every time I eat, even if it isn't something that is harmful. Even if it's liquid! I use a heating pad a lot, Epsom salt baths, and relaxation techniques to deal with the pain. Sometimes I fall to the floor in pain, but I try not to let it stop me from doing things.

*

DEB SHRADER-TROTTER
Deb was diagnosed with
gastroparesis in 1999 at age 37

My pain is intense at times, and feels almost like I'm having a heart attack with the esophageal spasms. The migraines stop my life. The pain in the epigastric and lower intestine can double me over.

*

JESSICA SPENCE
Jessica was diagnosed with
gastroparesis in 2016 at age 25

It's hard to talk about the pain. I don't know where to start because everything hurts. My stomach is either so empty it hurts, so full it hurts, or feels like it is full of acid that's trying to climb to freedom. There is severe pain in my intestines every time something tries to move, making bowel movements the bane of my existence. Since I'm not eating properly, my arms and legs constantly ache like I just did the Iron Man Triathlon.

I was taught from a young age to push through the pain and work. Pain wasn't an excuse. So as an adult it was easy to ignore the pain and just push through. Everyone hurt and I wasn't special. Focus on a goal and push, push, push. Just like everyone else. It wasn't until recently that I learned how flawed this logic is.

It's the emotional pain that eats away like necrotizing fasciitis, knowing there isn't a cure to fix it or make it better. Knowing that I will never eat like friends and family. The pain of feeling defeated by my own body. Of realizing that everyone doesn't hurt like me. Feeling like I was tricked into distrusting myself because I was emotionally unstable and really not sick. Realizing that at the age of twenty-six I have no idea how to take care of myself, and will still question whether it is real or all in my head. This pain that infects your mind and tears you apart is something that I am still figuring out how to deal with. What I have learned is that I need to respect my body as well as myself.

*

NICOLE STARZYNSKI
Nicole was diagnosed with
gastroparesis in 2016 at age 33

Sometimes the pain in my stomach feels like I am being stabbed from the inside out. The excruciating pains take my breath away. I make jokes to people when my stomach is making noises, that the war at Hiroshima is going on inside, because my stomach makes the loudest, most awful noises. It's embarrassing. It sounds like I could explode at any time, and most of the time it has nothing to do with going to the bathroom. I experience stomach spasms after I eat; my stomach becomes angry because the food won't move and it starts freaking out. You can actually see it move when this happens. Usually shortly after the stomach spasms comes the excruciating stabbing pains from the inside of my stomach. Sometimes they are so awful that it is worse than labor pains. The only way to get through them is to shut my eyes and breathe in and out. I have to completely relax and focus on nothing but the breathing.

I have spent many hours in the emergency room only to end up frustrated and upset. I find ways to deal with my pain. Sometimes even while I am breathing through the pain, tears will fall from my eyes because no matter how hard I try, the pain is so bad it's impossible to ignore. I had been told for eight years that nothing was causing my stomach pain. I was sent to my gynecologist more times than I can count for abdominal scans and to rule out any ovarian issues. For years I had no idea why I experienced pain that took me off my feet if I ate too much food.

Oh, and the bloating! How can I forget about the bloating? As I am writing this I am ready to explode. I can watch my stomach grow from being able to see my ribs, to looking like I am ready to give birth. I have been keeping a picture diary for my doctor to show him how bad it blows up. My daughter thinks it's crazy when after we eat and bam! I look like I am going to explode. Have you ever watched Charlie and the Chocolate Factory when she blows up like a giant plum? It's awful. Sometimes I can barely walk so I shuffle around my house like a little old lady. Sitting, and especially lying down, is so uncomfortable. Besides being uncomfortable, it is extremely painful and sometimes feels like my skin is just going to rip apart. If you push on my stomach it's hard as a rock. Sometimes I am just bloated but normally I have stabbing pains. I can't forget about being nauseous, which seems to come and go whenever it feels like it.

I have tried hot baths, heating pads, and lidocaine. Sometimes they help a little bit. I have also tried laxatives when I am extremely bloated because sometimes I haven't had a bowel movement in days. The most ever was thirteen days—what a nightmare that was! Sometimes even if I have had a recent bowel movement, it still feels like I have to go. The laxatives have helped to deflate me on some occasions. I have tried monitoring my diet by keeping a food journal to see if there were any particular foods that triggered symptoms. At one point I thought I had a good grasp on what was safe and what wasn't. Then everything pretty much became unsafe. No matter what I eat, I end up nauseous, in pain and bloated.

I have lived on clear liquids for months at a time. When I still feel awful every day and yet so sick of chicken broth, sometimes I say, "Screw it. I'm going to be sick anyways. I'll go for the gold." I get to the point when if I'm going to be sick anyway, I might as well eat a meal that is delicious and deal with being sick later. Every time I've done this, I've regretted it and promised myself I wouldn't do it again. Only to continue the same cycle over and over. It's hard to live on mashed sweet potatoes, applesauce and chicken broth.

Sometimes the thought of leaving and getting sick somewhere besides my house makes me panic. I have had total meltdowns because I feel awful and I have a meeting or something I cannot miss, when my daughter needs me. I'm her only parent and I can't let her down. This triggers a panic attack. When is this ever going to end? I have probably asked myself that question a million times. At the same time, I feel like a prisoner in my own home. During the wintertime while it snowed, I felt like I was in a snow globe. The entire world moved around me while I stayed still in the center of it all.

Sometimes I feel I have to hide the pain because I am finally around other humans outside the compound of my homebound prison—I mean, house. Sometimes it's because people's sympathy makes me feel awkward. Sometimes it's because I want to pretend that nothing is wrong with me, especially on the rare occasion I am having a good day. Sometimes in groups of people there is always that one butthead that thinks the disease you have is made up and you're just over dramatic. The list is endless. Sometimes it's easier to pretend to be doing okay than to be honest with people. I find myself constantly saying my pain is better than it is, maybe even to convince myself that the pain isn't that bad. Then the pain hits and I am immediately reminded that, for who know how long, I will feel the awful pain.

I have had dizzy spells and completely blacked out from being malnourished. In 2016 as my symptoms progressed, blackouts happened a few times. One day I was in a store and felt dizzy. Next thing I knew, I had blood all over my hand and face. I had blacked out and bashed my face on the floor. A few days later, after my daughter got on the bus, I started puking, and next thing I knew I woke up on my bathroom floor. When I looked at the time, three hours had passed. After running tests, my doctor believed that the blackouts could be from malnutrition, but there was at least not anything serious that was causing them.

Tired of being tired, I can honestly say that this disease does feel like you wake up with the stomach flu every day of your life. You can feel great and then for no reason this sudden wave comes upon you and you're sick. I get ulcers inside my mouth from vomiting. At times it will be fine, other times it will be severe to the point when the entire inside of my mouth is raw with ulcers. I have had eight root canals on teeth that never even had cavities—all from vomiting.

*

JENNIFER ZUBIK
Jennifer was diagnosed with idiopathic gastroparesis in 2010 at age 27

The pain I had was an extreme cramping feeling. My stomach burned too. I guess it was because there wasn't anything left in there except for stomach acid. The burning pain was so much worse and uncomfortable to me than the cramping. I also sometimes felt so bloated and full of air that it hurt to breathe any more in. I was always immensely uncomfortable. Anything I ingested, liquid or solid, increased the pain and discomfort. My stomach was not happy.

I couldn't find much that would help give me relief, other than sleeping and not having to experience it for that period of time. I mostly spent my days and nights sleeping in my bathroom and I had to sleep sitting up the majority of the time. I would wrap myself up in my electric blanket and just sit or lie down until I fell asleep. Then I would wake up and feel alright for a little while, until I would feel too bad and try to sleep again. Heating pads and electric blankets became my buddies during this time. They were the only source of comfort I could find. The symptoms of this disease overtook my life. I could no longer work, I could barely take care of the household chores, I couldn't cook for my family, and I could barely leave the house due to the anxiety and fear of getting sick while out in public.

*

People who need help sometimes look
a lot like people who don't need help.
GLENNON MELTON

*

CHAPTER FOUR

Identifying Triggers

Your genetics load the gun. Your lifestyle pulls the trigger. -DR. MEHMET OZ

Although the exact cause of motility disorders remain unknown, there are a plethora of triggers unique to each person. For some, it's certain foods. For others it's stress. But before we can manage the triggers, we must first discover what they are. What triggers have you correlated to a flare of symptoms?

*

MELISSA ADAMS VANHOUTEN
Melissa was diagnosed with
gastroparesis in 2014 at age 47

The short answer to this is: food. For me, any food, even a few bites, causes pain. Liquids do not typically cause pain, but both food and liquids result in feelings of early satiety and extreme bloating. It is recommended that gastroparesis patients consume several small meals consisting of low fiber and low-fat foods each day, but following this diet has not helped my symptoms. I should note that I also live with a redundant and loopy colon, which exacerbates my issues. What is the treatment for redundant colon? A high fiber diet. And what is the recommended diet for gastroparesis? Yes, low fiber. This is a no-win for me. My best bet is to take tiny bites of food and sips of liquids, such as protein shakes, throughout the course of the day. This has kept me alive for the last three years. My family is quite understanding and tries to accommodate my needs whenever possible. Our lives no longer center around food, and we have learned to focus on being together and to enjoy one's company rather than living to indulge in food.

Second only to food as a trigger is stress. I believe a moderate amount of stress, when it is short-term and low-level, is actually desirable and beneficial. It can boost your energy and memory, act as a motivator, and even enhance your physical strength. But those of us with chronic illness often battle prolonged stress with few to no breaks, and this can be quite detrimental to our health. I find that my symptoms worsen during particularly stressful times. I've had to learn to recognize the signs of harmful stress: mental confusion, anxiety, worry, depression, fatigue, and altered sleep patterns. I do my best to prevent and lessen these by maintaining a routine, avoiding harmful stress when possible, managing it with relaxation techniques and distraction, and focusing on the good and being grateful for the small, joyful moments. My family assists me in maintaining low levels of stress by avoiding conflict, refusing to engage in harmful escalation of problems, and engaging me in enjoyable activities inside the home. Our lives have changed radically to better suit my needs, and I am blessed to have a family willing to accommodate me.

Finally, I have found that overdoing physical tasks and exerting myself to the point of exhaustion triggers symptoms. I find it best to engage in moderate exercise when I can, limit my household chores and outings, and get plenty of rest. If I am careful to reign myself in a bit, I can avoid the worst of the symptoms which result from overexertion. Fortunately, I have supportive, loving family and friends who assist me with chores, errands, and maintaining my household. My husband and daughter do their best to pick up the slack and complete chores. In addition, my husband frequently dons the role of mother, and acts as essentially both parents during activities outside the house, attending my daughter's every field trip, performance, and lesson. My friends and neighbors often assist as well. I am fortunate. Many in my gastroparesis community do not have this sort of support system and are forced to get by on their own the best they can. That is a difficult road, and I am thankful for the gift of companionship I have been granted.

*

SAMANTHA ANDERSON

Samantha was diagnosed with idiopathic gastroparesis in 2012 at age 26

The obvious symptoms get much worse if I eat. It can be from a bite of food to a quarter of a cup, and I pay for it. I experience nausea, fullness and bloating, extra pain, and hours of vomiting, but I eat just to get some nutrition to try to energize my body. Even now, with it being better with the pacemaker (I'm not vomiting as much), it's still hard work. I'm not complaining. Things were worse before.

I'm just working on my diet now. Before I was sick a lot more with solids and liquids, and working on a diet didn't work, but now I need to sort my diet out. I knew nine or ten years ago that I'm lactose intolerant, so I already knew to avoid dairy. I was then told by the consultant to cut out gluten as they are linked. That helped a little so I have continued that. However, so many foods trigger bad episodes. One day, I can tolerate a food, and the next day my stomach is literally saying, "No!" At the moment I can tolerate purees a lot more than proper solids, and if anything they are easier to bring up. I still tend to only eat at the end of the day though, just to try to get some life.

It's awful when my whole body seems to be gagging, when I'm trying to keep food down and breathe my way through it, but it is still happening. The acid in my stomach feels like it is burning its way out. My throat and mouth are sore from it. There are times when food gets stuck as it is coming up, and I feel like I am choking on it.

The mornings can be particularly hard (not saying the rest of the day is a breeze). Sometimes I'm sick from the previous night's food. I have to tell myself I can cope with the pain; I can and will get through the day and do some of the things I intend to. I tell myself the pain isn't as bad as it is. Although it's not every day now, I often still feel bloated and can be nauseous, have indigestion, heartburn and get bad acid.

It's not just food. Viruses and bugs can cause bad flares also. When symptoms are much worse, it is harder to cope with everyday life. Recently I had shingles and I felt like I wasn't in my own body because I felt so rough. I'm quite sure I am the type of person who continues until I drop. I'm lucky enough (although not always sure it's lucky) to have regular periods. However, life becomes harder during those cycles, as it is much more painful. My back and my whole abdominal area, especially my stomach, is always in pain, but during my period everywhere hurts. My head is much worse and it continues most of the way down my body. Having to deal with anything extra besides gastroparesis is so much more difficult. I cope with it and generally get on, but it feels like I'm on the edge of a tightrope, and it's literally step by step, breath by breath.

*

JOLI ATKINS
Joli was diagnosed with
gastroparesis in 2015 at age 36

My symptoms tend to get worse when I eat a lot of solid food. As long as I stay to a liquid diet such as Ensure, applesauce, and popsicles, then I tend to have less problems. When I do break down and eat solid food because I just can't take the liquids anymore, I will then spend days in bed because my stomach just can't handle it. I try to not make that mistake very often. My friends and family are very supportive and they understand why I have to limit my solid food intake. We limit eating out because not too many restaurants have liquid diet menus.

*

MEGAN BOGGS
Megan was diagnosed with
gastroparesis in 2017 at age 38

My triggers are increased sugar levels and not eating right. Sometimes I feel like no one understands. I always feel anxious. I pray every day for my life back. Stress triggers everything.

*

TRISHA BUNDY
Trisha was diagnosed with
gastroparesis in 2013 at age 35

I have learned to recognize some of my symptoms. Taking food or fluids orally is the main trigger for my symptoms. A few other triggers are exhaustion, lack of sleep, side effects of some medicines for normal sickness such as colds and antibiotics, running my formula too fast or too long, dehydration, or excessive stress.

To minimize my triggers I limit my formula intake, taking breaks when needed to allow my small intestine to rest. I am very cautious of what and when I try something orally. I usually try only one thing a day, aside from my safe liquids or foods, and at a very small volume. Even then, I do not attempt something by mouth every day. I often skip a day or more before trying anything by mouth again, especially if I'm having a symptomatic day. My feeding tube is my main nutrition source. I receive about 500 calories a day. On days when I am able to supplement with fluids, yogurt, or ice cream, I average a total of 700 to 800 calories a day.

It is not uncommon for me to overexert myself physically. I become severely fatigued very quickly, yet it's hard for me to stop when my exhaustion is beginning. My family has been extremely helpful and supportive, reminding and encouraging me to rest and consider the consequences. I am learning how to pace myself better and allow days of rest in between. Currently, my family drives me everywhere I need to go, which is usually medical appointments. I do go to the grocery store once a week with my daughters where I can drive the electric scooter. I also try to attend my youngest daughter's softball games when they're in town and the weather is nice (not too hot and not too cold), and I'm not already too exhausted. The majority of my days are spent at home on the couch attached to my IV bag and feeding tube. Even though that can be annoying, it has required me to take it easier and rest since it limits me from doing much physically.

Recognizing that very little activity fatigues my muscles, my family became concerned about my strength and endurance. I had a few falls and even more close calls due to balance and stamina, so my mom shared her concerns with my doctor. He, too, was concerned about muscle deterioration so referred me to a physical therapist. Together, my family and medical team work together with me to best minimize my key triggers while also better understanding, accepting, and managing the triggers and symptoms when they worsen.

*

LISA COLANDREA
Lisa was diagnosed with
gastroparesis in 2016 at age 42

What triggers my gastroparesis flares is usually stress related. Emotional and physical stress have really taken its toll on me. No days are ever the same. It's unpredictable and very hard to plan and organize your life around this illness. Some of the things that bring some comfort during triggers or flares are baths, a fan, heating pad, meditation and trying to focus on something else like watching a movie. It's not so simple most of the time to deter a trigger. It just happens.

I have found a lot of support through social media from others who suffer from gastroparesis as well. Some of my friends and family have been really supportive, and others haven't been as supportive as I thought they would be. Most people just don't understand, even if you try to explain it to them. I often think people don't really know what to say. I've been lucky to have the support of my wife and my children who get me through each day.

*

TAMMY DOWNS

Tammy was diagnosed with Crohn's disease, irritable bowel syndrome, spastic colon, gastroesophageal reflux disease, and gastritis in 2006 at age 46, gastroparesis in 2015 at age 56, and motility dysfunction disorder of the rectum and pelvic floor in 2016 at age 58

Eating food. Heavy food. Red meat. Eating ham, barbecue, anything with sauces, spices, raw veggies, ice cream, and fried foods. Green veggies, even if they are cooked because they do not digest. I could not even eat my favorite once in a while: M&M's. I would say to myself, "How can food become my worst enemy? How can food cause me so much pain and nausea, and turn into that big rock that makes me so uncomfortable all the time in the pit of my stomach?" Then it came to baked chicken, baby food, baked potatoes, sweet potatoes, and smoothies. I used almond milk, started making soups and went on gluten-free foods to help my foods not be so heavy. I had small meals and a boost for protein. Then I got dehydrated and my blood pressure started dropping. I had to drink Propel mixed in bottled water to help get my blood pressure up because it was dropping so low.

Thanks to my wonderful nurse, Amy, who I can call to ask what I should do for every situation, I was told what to try. I appreciated that because it was not that easy to get answers from my doctor. My doctor from Shands Hospital got me on bethanechol, a medication that has been helping so far. I still have issues being able to tolerate food a little bit though.

A circle started when if I ate food, it caused a problem called anorectal manometry dyssynergic defecation dynamics (type II) motility problems. I kept a lot of Calmoseptine ointment and panty liners around. That's right, in other words I got constipated when I ate food, and it caused more problems. So then I was back to baby food, liquid foods, and stuff that does not cause constipation. It was a vicious cycle. To stop going to the bathroom, I would not eat, flat and simple as that, which is no fun. Food was no longer my best friend; it became my worst enemy.

*

SKYE FALCON

Skye was diagnosed with gastroparesis and
other autoimmune diseases in 2006 at age 25

Air. Air and stress. Some days, I am almost positive all it takes is air to trigger another round of intense pain, throbbing, excruciating waves of cramps that travel through my abdomen, and for my gastrointestinal tract to just quit. Gastroparesis seems to create a vicious circle when stress controls and wins. The more stressed I am, whether it be from the debilitating, life-changing factors of the illness, or general life stressors, the worse my symptoms and pains are. This is true whether food is present or not. The more stress that is present, the easier it is to fall into a flare, and the harder it is to ignore the symptoms and ailments that arise. The trouble is, we cannot get away from the stress that gastroparesis and illness brings because it is so constant and ever-changing.

Extra medications. If I get a migraine, which happens more often these days with my influx of medication, and have to take something simple like acetaminophen, it causes an immediate flare. I have a very low tolerance for pain medication of any kind, and they all seem to react badly inside my body. In fact, any medication I take, I have to start on a low dose, and work up to the full recommended dosage. Many medications have never made it past a child-size dosage, due to reactions or horrible side effects. Pills, liquids, IV form... my body hates it all. Being pain-medication-free is a challenge.

I am often judged for being in a bad mood, or being a b**** when I'm really just trying to push through the day and the intense amounts of pain I try to hide from every person I run across. You truly never know the pain the person standing in front of you might be facing. The same can be said about the extra medications that I have when I feel an illness coming on, especially respiratory. "Captain Side Effect" was my nickname for the longest time at one of my specialist's office, and one I wished I could shake. Because of this, I have a very set regimen of medications that we very rarely veer from, until something shifts so much that it's truly warranted. I have become petrified of most new medications because these days the stronger the pill, the more side effects I am faced with.

Foods. These days, I do best on mostly liquids and softs, although I have days when I just cannot seem to adhere to what I know I should be doing. With celiac issues, avoiding gluten is a must, along with dairy and soy, which sadly cuts out most processed foods. Being that I have limited motility or ability to digest raw, healthy foods like fruits and vegetables, the days of running for a salad for nutrients and healthy, vibrant colors are over. Red meat is out. Boiled chicken and occasional fish, shredded, with some sort of sauce for extra moistness is all I can do. Funny thing is, the things I can eat change every day.

The rate of my digestion speed today seems to be determined by what I ate yesterday, and the week before. I never know what each day will bring, so every day I just start slowly and hope for the best. There are days, however, when no food or liquid helps, and the stomach issues rage on with emptiness. Other days, the pain in my abdomen is so great, that I risk a blockage and eat a cookie. I figure, what's a little more pain considering the amount I am already facing? So, why not have a cookie, even if it only stays in for an hour?

There are other things that heavily affect my days. Some are traveling, being active, smells and strong scents, and extreme weather temperatures. I learned two years ago, during a family getaway to the mountains, that I could not ever make the ten-hour drive again. The exhaustion, pain, and bodily repercussions from pushing myself too much lasted for weeks. The mental strain from carrying the stress of illness and travel was almost more than I could take. I felt that I ruined that vacation for my family and my kids, so that is something I consider when making any plans to this day. Even for work and author events, everything must be planned and include resting times. I only attend events that are within three hours away.

I have three kids, so being active is something that I do not get to step away from quite yet in their lives. They are amazing humans, and know my limitations sometimes better than I do. I adjusted my life to be able to make theirs grand by working from home, and having low-stress home-grown businesses to deal with. Staying in the home as much as I can allows me to stay calm, keep the body rested, and close to any medication or item I might suddenly need. And let's be honest, being in your own bathroom when any of the gastroparesis symptoms hit is usually best and helps calm the psyche.

In Indiana, more often than not, we have all four seasons in one day. With every trip of the Raynaud's phenomenon and the whitish discoloration of my fingers and toes, my gastrointestinal system freezes in place along with it—for days at a time. The Midwest cold has a way of creeping into my already shivering bones, and overstaying its welcome. Over the years I've learned to avoid winter, and the extreme heat. I am the lady who wears long sleeves and pants with a giant sunhat on a hundred-degree day, and fourteen layers of clothes with a heated vest when it's fifty degrees outside. I literally cannot function without the extra heat. Without the direct, focused heat, I can barely move past the pain.

If I'm being honest, support comes and goes, and sometimes it does affect my symptoms by adding stress to the mix. I can understand this aspect more because I cared for my ailing grandparents, and handled some of their life's wishes. It is incredibly hard for family and friends to face and deal with someone with a constant, chronic, or terminal illness. It is stressful, tiring, depressing, and really makes you face the real circle of life, that always ends in death.

All that said, we, the chronically awesome and ill, still need our people. Someone. Anyone. Having someone to lean on and share all the disgusting parts, the happy parts, and the triumphs and losses with is vital. But our people are busy, just like we are. Taking the time to learn about our illnesses takes time, and a certain required motivation that we cannot push for. They have to want to be our supporters, and want to continue to be our friends.

These illnesses, and the circumstances in my life have made me see life more openly, and know what I want out of it. I have lost friends I had hoped would always stay, and gained friends to whom I never dreamed I would give the time of day. Family has left, not ever looking back, when I could have used their hand the most. The same hand I extended to them in their own times of need. But then again, strangers have stepped in to their roles, proving to be better family than I could have imagined.

It is just life, and it is harsh in some way for everyone. I am always grateful for those who stick by me, even on the stressful days when I am completely unlovable. All that said, there are definitely aspects of my life that could be made easier by those around me changing simple, small things that would prevent flares, sudden sickness, and the like. But I realize that asking or pushing such things is not always right either.

*

ROBIN MCNAMARA
Robin was diagnosed with gastroparesis in 2013 at age 55

I try to get between seven to eight hours of sleep each night, as staying well rested helps keep symptoms at bay. Stress is also a trigger which I do my best to manage by staying busy with my pets, a movie, or a book.

Support from family is different. Although my immediate family members realize I'm sick, I don't believe that nieces and nephews fully understand, nor do they ask, and the same goes with most of my friends. It would be nice to hear, "Is there anything I can do for you?" from friends rather than hearing "ick" when I say I'm nauseous.

I'll be quite honest that at times I just spend time with myself to avoid all the bull. I'm tired of watching people eat all the foods I love when I cannot eat them. And to also hear, "Just eat it and see what happens." That doesn't cut it either, as there are so many foods I used to eat that my body will no longer tolerate. I remember being at a gathering once when someone put a plate of food under my nose and said, "You want this?" They took the food away, laughed, said, "Oh, ha ha, you can't eat this," and walked away. People putting desserts under my face do this as well. I now tend to retreat and not participate. These people think it's funny. My emotions waver between wanting to cry and punching someone.

Some of the stress is internal, thinking about all of these things that have gone down and even writing about them is hard. Do I feel supported? Some would say they support me, but in the big picture I don't really feel supported. My life has been confined to getting up, going to work, coming home, eating the same boring foods, taking medication and going to bed. Gastroparesis has stolen my life. Gastroparesis has also shown me who my real friends are and who really cares.

*

TAMMY PITTMAN

Tammy was diagnosed with gastroparesis and irritable bowel syndrome in 2014 at age 34

The smell of food, taste of food or eating a meal exacerbated the pain. My bowels started to act up worse than any irritable bowel syndrome symptoms I'd ever dealt with. I had to manually disimpact myself regularly.

*

TAYLOR SCHMITZ

Taylor was diagnosed with idiopathic gastroparesis in 2014 at age 22

I avoid anything fibrous, and anything heavy such as protein. I eat scrambled eggs, fish, and sometimes turkey for protein, but lately those have been too painful, so I've been backing off of them. My family and friends are such huge supporters of my condition. They all check on me, and do what they can to help and encourage me. Unfortunately, it gets to my husband, which is completely understandable, considering he is my caregiver round-the-clock. He hates to see me in pain, especially when he doesn't know what to do. Bradley is the best husband I could have ever asked for. He makes me laugh, he comforts me when I'm hurting, and supports me in everything I do. God has blessed me so tremendously with Brad, and my family. My grandma, my dad, and my few great friends support, encourage, and check on my well-being daily. I'm so surprised they aren't tired of me yet!

*

DEB SHRADER-TROTTER
Deb was diagnosed with
gastroparesis in 1999 at age 37

Eating is my trigger for the motility disorder. Sunshine, dehydration, and barometric pressure are my triggers for the migraines.

*

JESSICA SPENCE
Jessica was diagnosed with
gastroparesis in 2016 at age 25

I have a lot of food triggers, like pork, onions, tomatoes, or citrus. If I am unable to take my medicine I will not be able to eat at all, so I try to make sure I always have my medicine. I've learned to read full ingredient lists and avoid even the smallest amounts of foods that are bad for me. My fiancé will take me anywhere I want if it means I will be able to eat something, which is a huge relief. So I've started to enjoy going out for food.

As it turns out, restaurants care more about my dietary needs than some of my family. My father is of the opinion that if he can hide it, then it won't upset my "Timmy" (the Terrible Tummy). It doesn't matter how small you chop the onions, they still make me sick! My mother, on the other hand, is my crusader. She is constantly asking what she can make for family night that I can enjoy with everyone. She has been fighting for me since the beginning, doing everything she can to help me feel better. I am lucky and blessed to have the support system I have, even if not everyone is on board.

*

NICOLE STARZYNSKI
Nicole was diagnosed with
gastroparesis in 2016 at age 33

Every day is a science experiment: let me eat this and see what happens. Sometimes it takes days for a certain type of food to start war. It doesn't matter what I eat. If I am stressed, sometimes my stomach has a mind of its own. For no reason it will decide to kind of work, or it'll be out of order for the day, maybe the week.

Let's face it, there are some things in life we cannot miss. In these instances, I have learned to not eat for days leading up to events. I stay away from social media and separate myself from any added stress. I have found food coupled with stress sometimes is enough to create the perfect storm inside my stomach. It's taken a lot of self control but I have learned to not let myself get upset about little things either. I've learned there is a lot more in life and it's not worth the negative energy. Sometimes you have to think, "Is this going to bother me in a week, or in a month? Does it really matter?" Life, getting up every day and spending time with the people we love is what's important. So one thing is definitely learning to limit some of the stress in our lives.

Obviously it's not possible to avoid everything but it does help for everyday mental well-being.

Sometimes you wake up and you feel like today isn't so bad. You start doing some things around the house and then bam. You feel like death, you are nauseous and have stomach pains. These days are probably the hardest for me mentally. It makes me feel like there is no end, that I could feel almost normal for just that tiny bit, and then it's taken away again. But sometimes talking to my mom or my boyfriend helps. I have a friend I grew up with that has gastroparesis and we recently just started talking again. She has been a great person to talk to about how I feel, daily struggles, up and downs, and the nausea. She gets it and that has been an invaluable resource.

I feel pretty lucky that the people directly around me do everything they can to make sure I can eat or that they have options that I can eat. My mom makes every holiday meal around my needs and she always has. My daughter and my boyfriend adjust their diets to my diet, or not far off. My sister has made me special desserts so that I can actually eat them. I feel very supported at home and at family events. I read stories of others who have so many frustrations with their families, and I take for granted how lucky I am to have that support.

I tend to write to myself when I am upset. Lately I feel like my stomach has gotten worse. Until last week, my nausea and vomiting was usually in the morning. Recently, it has turned into waking up in the middle of the night to puke my guts out. I have had cold sweats, and chills. The last two nights I have barely slept. The pain is awful. I can't drink water without my stomach feeling like a fish bowl. I dread nighttime and I am so tired of being sick all the time. I want to feel good, but I live life every day revolving around this awful disease. I'm very frustrated.

Sometimes I eat things even though I know it's going to make me sick. Usually after I have felt sick despite not eating anything, I say, "Screw it. If I am going to be sick, I might as well make it worth it." Then afterwards I hate myself for making such a bad choice. Sadly I will do it again; I am just learning to not do it as frequently. I stick to the stuff that keeps me at a somewhat manageable level, which to most people would still feel like one of the worst stomach flus they ever had.

You learn to live with how you feel and take each and every day as a new day. If someone says, "How have you been feeling?" My reply is usually, "Today has been good so far," or "Today hasn't been such a good day." I try not to focus on the fact that maybe the past few days were awful. If the day is good, I focus on that. I push the bad out of my head. Even a good day isn't a good day, it's just a day when I feel well enough to actually function. Sometimes throughout the day there are bad times, and even on a good day I need a nap. It doesn't matter that I get enough sleep every night. I am tired all the time.

*

JENNIFER ZUBIK
Jennifer was diagnosed with idiopathic gastroparesis in 2010 at age 27

I didn't necessarily have specific triggers, as everything was a trigger. I learned that I could not attempt anything after 7 p.m. or I would definitely spend the rest of the evening in the bathroom. When I would actually find something I could tolerate for a moment, it wouldn't be long before I couldn't eat or drink that either. At first, I ate a lot of soup and broth, if having a good day. So much that I vowed I would never eat soup again once I was better. Then maybe a cracker or a bite of bread, just to get something in my stomach. Yogurt, Ensure drinks or any kind of protein shake—I tried all that stuff at some point.

As time passed and after many medications and procedures, throughout the years I could sometimes tolerate very bland foods like plain, boneless and skinless chicken, plain white rice, plain noodles, bread, unsalted and plain crackers. Nothing anyone else would want or choose to live on, but I didn't have a choice. That was all my stomach could handle at times, if any. There were many days I didn't even have an appetite and didn't want to try to eat. Then later it just got to the point that I was scared to even try to eat due to the fear of feeling worse.

The disease had really taken a toll on both my mind and body. My friends and family were supportive, yet very concerned. I felt horrible for what I was putting my family through and how I was making them feel. Everyone felt guilty for eating around me knowing that I couldn't enjoy the taste of what they were having. Yet everyone was as supportive as they could be and helped me in any way that they could, both physically and emotionally. They would always try to accommodate my needs. It was difficult for me, but difficult for everyone around me too. Gastroparesis has been a life-changing experience for all of us.

CHAPTER FIVE

Working with Practitioners

The good physician treats the disease; the great physician treats the patient who has the disease.
-WILLIAM OSLER

Knowledge, attitude, and practice with dysmotility pain can make or break relationships with our medical practitioners. Some are compassionate and understanding. Others have preconceived notions or stigmas about chronic pain. What emotions come up for you during doctor appointments? Do you feel supported or minimized?

*

MELISSA ADAMS VANHOUTEN
Melissa was diagnosed with gastroparesis in 2014 at age 47

Doctor appointments have never been something I relish. In fact, though they are necessary and often helpful, I despise them. I always have, but especially so since being diagnosed with gastroparesis. I will say, though, that I am a much wiser patient now than ever before. Gastroparesis is an excellent teacher, and I have learned to better explain myself and take control of my own care. This once shy patient has developed into one who accepts nothing less than collaboration from medical providers.

I actually abandoned my initial primary care physician after seeing her the day before my emergency room trip, which marked the beginning of my life with gastroparesis. I had not been having significant issues prior to that day, but my symptoms were worsening on this particular day, and so I opted to see my primary doctor rather than attempt an urgent care visit. I assumed she would be more helpful since she had been treating me for a few years and presumably possessed better knowledge of my medical history. It had been perhaps a year since I had seen her though, so I cannot say she was up-to-date on all that had been going on with my health.

I have never really been overweight or unhealthy, but for several years prior to my diagnosis, I had been eating healthy and had started exercising—running, mostly. I had lost weight but overall felt healthier than ever before. I thought my primary doctor would realize this, but instead she seemed to ignore my complaints about new stomach pain, nausea, and feelings of fullness. She further rejected my explanations about my weight loss. Without any sort of real examination or consideration of my statements, she determined that I was anorexic, and told me to go home and eat. She even warned my husband: "Watch her." She informed me I was simply a "skinny white girl." I was dumbfounded. This was possibly the worst doctor visit I had ever had. I knew I was not experiencing the effects of anorexia. This came on suddenly, and up to this point, I had been eating well. I felt completely ignored, dismissed, and patronized. I went home, complained to my husband rather loudly about the uselessness of the visit, and decided I would wait a bit to see if the pain went away. It did not, of course, and when I woke the next morning with excruciating pain and nonstop vomiting, I headed for the emergency room.

During my hospital stay, the doctors were far kinder and much more willing to listen and explore the possible causes of my misery. Based upon what I have seen in my support groups, I realize many of those with gastroparesis have not had such pleasant experiences. Diagnosis can be difficult, and hospital stays frequently end without answers. However, I was pleased with my treatment and felt as if the staff treated me with dignity and showed genuine concern and commitment to finding the source of my ailment. They did not belittle me nor behave as if I were faking my symptoms. They took my concerns and symptoms seriously and did their best to get me through the difficult days.

I've had the same experience with my regular gastroenterologist. He is my favorite doctor to date. Though not a motility specialist, he is fairly knowledgeable about gastroparesis, and when he does not have answers, he is willing to consult other sources. He's happy to consider suggestions I bring to him, and he's honest when he feels I need to see a different specialist or seek a second opinion. He's empathetic, demonstrates concern, and seems genuinely interested in my well-being. He talks openly about my care and quality of life goals and does not presume to know what matters most to me. He listens. Unfortunately, we recently came to the point where he informed me that he does not believe he has the expertise needed to help with some of my worsening symptoms, and he feels he has exhausted his options where treatment is concerned. He referred me to a specialist just a few months ago, and though I continue to see him for regular visits, the new specialist largely handles my gastroparesis care now.

I'm still deciding whether I am pleased with my new motility specialist. We got off to a rocky start at my first visit, but my second appointment went far better. The first appointment began with my new doctor's declaration that gastroparesis does not cause pain, and ended with him telling me to stay off the internet. Now, anyone who knows me is aware that those two phrases are the absolute worst expressions one can use around me. My pain is real. Pain from gastroparesis has been well documented by physicians and researchers. And the internet? Well, that is my life. I exist to serve my online gastroparesis community.

Nevertheless, I remained calm largely because he is considered the best specialist in my state (the "Holy of Holies" in the gastroparesis world, according to my regular gastroenterologist), and because I wanted to see where the tests would lead. He did, at least, seem interested in pursuing other treatment options and in finding alternative causes for my worsening symptoms and pain. He did not dismiss my pain but offered his opinion that my gastroparesis is not the ultimate cause. Based upon what I have seen and read, I do not agree with this opinion, but I am willing to entertain all possibilities. He also seems set upon finding the cause of my delayed stomach emptying and has not ruled out the possibility that something more than gastroparesis could be at play.

I left the first visit half-intending not to return. I felt as if I could barely get a word in, though I was not shy and did speak up, even arguing with his statements at times. My husband convinced me that perhaps I was being hasty, maybe the doctor was not having a stellar day, perchance he would be better during a second visit. This turned out to be accurate. I do believe doctors are human, and I do agree that it is sometimes a good idea to give them more than one chance. This seems to have been the case in this particular situation.

My Holy of Holies was much more open to conversation at my second appointment, and he seemed to listen to my concerns and try to evaluate them from my perspective. He helped me with referrals, ordered more tests, which he explained pretty thoroughly, and discussed with me the direction he thought we should head. I was far happier with his demeanor and am now willing to continue under his care, though I still see my previous gastroenterologist for regular appointments and some follow-ups.

My post-diagnosis health care attitude has changed much from what it was pre-diagnosis. Though I still dread the thought of doctor visits, I now handle them with greater care and skill. To begin with, I have learned how to communicate and prepare for visits. I keep better record of my medical history, track my symptoms, and record all pertinent treatments and procedures. I come to each appointment with questions and a list of the most important issues I wish to address. I also listen a little harder when the doctor is speaking, take notes of what transpires, ask questions when I do not understand, and make certain I know details regarding the follow-up measures I must take.

Further, I have learned it is acceptable, even advisable, to consider the doctor a collaborator, a partner of sorts, rather than a simple authority figure. His expertise is invaluable, but he does not necessarily know all, and he certainly does not get to set my life and health priorities. This is a matter for discussion and, ultimately, those are standards I must establish.

*

SAMANTHA ANDERSON
Samantha was diagnosed with idiopathic
gastroparesis in 2012 at age 26

I absolutely hated and still hate going to the doctor. I just wanted to know what was going on. A few doctors and people made me feel like it was all me, and had me questioning everything I was doing. I even blamed myself. Even now I often think about what I did that caused this, even though my gastroparesis is idiopathic. I'm so thankful that my mum or other family members were always with me, otherwise I really think I'd have been dismissed.

My tests kept returning normal, but after the twenty-four-hour nasogastric tube test, my mum asked him again to make sure it was okay. He read the results again and noticed I was belching a lot. A light bulb started to flicker in his head, and he sent me for other gastric emptying tests to confirm his suspicions.

As I was a big girl, just five feet tall but a UK size eighteen, the doctors didn't take much notice at first. They didn't believe I'd lost weight until I returned for a second time. They often made me think there wasn't an issue unless I was losing weight, even with all the other symptoms. I even had a doctor say when I was going through all this, "You do need to lose weight!" It was like she was saying that what I was going through was okay. To be fair, a letter of complaint was written to the doctor's surgery about her from my step-dad.

When I needed to go to the emergency room, whether it was for IV hydration and pain relief, a bug or collapsing, it could be hard. Especially when I first started going, as gastroparesis actually isn't an emergency; it is a long-term condition. However, hydration and infections can be emergencies. Many doctors didn't know what gastroparesis was, and there was nothing accident and emergency doctors could do for it. In the end, when I went to the emergency room, doctors realized that they generally needed to give me IV fluids and pain relief and then send me on my way. My mum made this so much easier.

Do you know how hard it is getting IV fluids and vitamins? Even when my consultant organized it, it was difficult for him to get done. I had to go to the hospital for a few days in a row. The extra traveling was tiring. I may be giving you too much information here, but this treatment often resulted in dumping syndrome, where I'd go from going to the toilet once a week to going to the toilet a couple of times after each treatment with IV fluids and vitamins.

Now that I have the gastric pacemaker, when going to the doctor or surgeon I feel like I should be saying everything is fine. This is far from the truth, though things are much better than before. I put on weight more easily, although at times it fluctuates. I just want more. I think I am different from many people; I would be so much happier if all I had to deal with was the pain. I'm slowly getting there. I obviously want, and striving to have, less symptoms. The doctors who generally know me are actually a little more understanding now. The new doctors are hard work. I feel like I have to prove feeling ill to them.

I seem to have this complex that I am not deserving of extra help, that there are people who need it more. This is partly due to how I feel about things. However, I believe it's also because of many doctors' initial attitudes toward me, and people's lack of understanding of gastroparesis. Unless you see it, I suppose you really can't understand it. I don't always look sick and people don't get that I can't keep anything or much down.

*

JOLI ATKINS
Joli was diagnosed with
gastroparesis in 2015 at age 36

I get very anxious when I go to the doctor. Most of my doctors don't know what to do with me or how to treat me. They know my diagnosis but that's all. They have no other answers for me. We have tried some medications to try to help with motility, but none of them have worked.

*

MEGAN BOGGS
Megan was diagnosed with
gastroparesis in 2017 at age 38

Doctors don't care. They do not know what to do. They do not know how to treat patients with empathy or common decency. They think they know it all, but they don't. I get angry, scared and confused.

*

TRISHA BUNDY
Trisha was diagnosed with gastroparesis in 2013 at age 35

The emotions that I feel surrounding my medical appointments depend greatly on the doctor and the circumstances. For the most part, I feel like I've had a supportive and compassionate medical team that understands and has been authentically concerned since my first hospitalization in 2013. I have full faith and trust with my current medical team, though I am still often nervous at appointments because I have a difficult time finding the accurate words to describe my plight. My current gastroenterologist (GI) and psychologist have been phenomenal, as well as one of the hospitalists that I've been fortunate enough to have a few times when inpatient. Unfortunately, my GI is moving, so I am very anxious and worried about how that transition and change will be. I like my primary physician and feel as if he has an empathetic ear and cares. However, he hasn't really been put to the test to see how he would handle situations, as all of my recent concerns have been related to gastrointestinal issues.

I'm aware that I have fears of dismissal, of losing medical support, and of being incorrectly labeled. Though for the most part I have no reason based on the medical team I have at the moment, I hear about these situations all the time. I don't want to be looked down upon. I don't want to be considered emotionally weak, even if I am at times, because I don't want to lose respect from my medical team or family.

I don't want to be referred to as a robot or artificial, even if I am currently dependent on a feeding tube, port, and ileostomy. I don't want to be given up on or have no more explanations or options available that can help me feel better, even if I feel like giving up myself at times. I'm scared of being hospitalized again, which leaves me walking on eggshells about when or even if I should reach out for help. If I do, I try to determine how much I should actually say to inform them of my reality without hindering my healthcare or landing me back in the hospital. I'm fearful of having no medical support, fearful they'll eventually no longer be willing to help me improve my health.

Many times, as result of past experiences and fears, I find myself downplaying symptoms or hesitating to reach out to medical providers. I don't want to be a nuisance or have to return to the hospital. I'm in fear of being mocked, misunderstood, dismissed, ignored, and labeled, especially from new nurses and doctors who aren't familiar with my health needs. I've become stubborn. I do my absolute best to tough things out, sometimes for too long.

Because of past experiences, I've learned to never underestimate the power and impact of having a compassionate, empathetic, and kind nurse and doctor. Whether in the physician's clinic, inpatient at a hospital, scurrying around the emergency department, or a part of one's medical team as a home health nurse, my medical team is an essential part to my patient experience and health journey. The past four years have been difficult for me. Having a health care team who I can depend on and trust as well as communicate with is definitely a valuable asset.

I'd love to say that every nurse and doctor I've ever had along my medical journey has been amazing. Unfortunately, that has definitely not always been the case. As I'm sure you already know, it can be difficult to find medical providers who are able to empathize, communicate, and create a trusting relationship with their patients. Having a chronic illness, one that is not well understood or even known, can be difficult for anyone. In my case, my digestive system became dysfunctional. Being unable to eat and process food normally has created severe symptoms of nausea, heaving, vomiting, intense abdominal pain, fatigue, dizziness, dehydration, and more. These illnesses have made me dependent on tube feeds, an ileostomy bag, and currently IV home hydration five times a week. Unfortunately, not all medical professionals are aware of or understand situations like mine. And sadly, when someone doesn't truly understand and does not know how to best treat the issue, it's easier for them to place blame on the patient or not believe the patient.

In 2016, I underwent surgery, a colectomy with ileostomy. What was supposed to keep me in the hospital for a few days, ended up keeping me there for two weeks due to complications of an ileus, dehydration, and difficulty receiving adequate nutrition through my feeding tube. I was extremely pleased with my surgeon, and surprised not to see my stoma as grotesque as I had originally imagined.

I was also surrounded by some amazing nurses who helped me navigate the learning process of how to manage my ileostomy without making me feel gross. They helped me communicate to my physicians the level of pain I was having physically, not only from surgery, but even moreso from trying to run my feeds. They knew something was not right with the severity of my symptoms, especially when trying to run my tube feeds. The kind nurses sympathized with me and kept my nausea medicines on point. They found heating pads for my abdomen, comforted me with cold wet rags on my forehead, and anything else they could think of to bring me some relief.

It was a horrific experience fueled by a dietician who wouldn't listen or believe what I was trying to say, but instead was more interested in following textbook guidelines. With the help of the nurses, and I'm not sure which doctors, we discovered that I had a postoperative ileus. In other words, my formula feeds were not moving anywhere. Instead they were just sitting there, because my small intestine was not awake and fully functioning from the surgery yet. This was a problem that could have been less excruciating and torturous if I were not forced to keep increasing the rate and volume of my tube feeds, regardless of how sick they were making me feel.

Eventually, I was discharged home with a peripherally inserted central catheter (PICC line), and home health nurse. Initially, I was frightened to have a home nurse as I had often heard horror stories online from other patients regarding their experiences. I was also fearful of having a PICC line due to possible infections. I was scared that my nurse would be judgmental and not properly take care of my health safety, such as not maintaining the sterilization necessary to decrease risk of infection. Many of my online friends had been hospitalized and some had even died from sepsis infections.

My main home nurse, Mike, was awesome! I knew I could depend on him to keep me as safe and as infection free as possible. I was impressed with how well he communicated not only with me, but also with my husband and even my GI when the need arose. He truly listened and was able to effectively communicate my needs (even if I was unsure of them myself) to whomever necessary. It takes a lot for me to trust new members on my medical team, but he demonstrated time and time again that I could trust him. He actually cared about my health and wanted to help me improve.

One time I was extremely dehydrated, lethargic, and weak. I was desperately not wanting to make a trip to the dreaded emergency room, even though I knew I was at that point. Mike worked alongside my husband in convincing me that it was time to seek assistance at the emergency room, while also working behind the scenes with my GI to get fluids back on board at home.

Another time, I began showing signs of an infection near my port. With increasing pain around my port, I eventually broke down and called Mike on a Sunday evening. He was very encouraging and made arrangements to come by and check out my port. Due to the pain and symptoms, he instantly removed my port's Huber needle and noticed that I had signs of infection near my surgical site. Calming my fears of not wanting to return to the emergency room, he was able to talk directly with my GI and get antibiotics on board immediately. Thankfully, the antibiotics eliminated the infection and saved me from having to have my port pulled and replaced. If it had not been for his calm but swift, caring actions and problem solving skills, I would likely have ended up in the hospital with a more severe infection.

My GI is phenomenal! I was nervous when my first regular GI moved to Florida, as I really liked him. I was extremely fortunate to have been assigned to my current one. My current GI's willingness to communicate between my family, home nurse, and me has been immensely appreciated. I strongly believe that he has taken a special interest in helping me find better treatments and relief. His personality helps me feel at ease communicating with him, though I do still hesitate as I don't want to be an inconvenience for him.

Even though I know I'm in great hands with him as my doctor, I can't help but get anxious prior to appointments with him. I'm not nervous of him. Instead, I'm nervous because I know that there are not many options for us to consider. There's no cure, and we're left doing the best we can with treating and monitoring symptoms. Sadly, he will be moving in July and I will have a new GI. Seeing a new doctor is always stressful for me. It makes me feel as if I have to prove myself as they are not familiar with my health experiences and struggles.

I know that it may be difficult to process at times, but I truly have been blessed with an amazing top-notch medical team. From my favorite hospitalist, previous GI, and extraordinary home nurse, to my phenomenal current GI and psychologist, I honestly do not know where I would be if these remarkable medical professionals had not been a part of my health journey. To be quite honest, I am nervous and literally scared about what my future health care team will be like, since there have been so many unexpected changes recently.

*

LISA COLANDREA

Lisa was diagnosed with gastroparesis in 2016 at age 42

Every doctor's appointment I go to is emotional for me. I always go with the hope that they'll do something else to give me some relief. Most of the time my needs are minimized, and I end up leaving really frustrated and unsupported. I don't think my doctors really understand what it's like living with gastroparesis every day. I never get to fully address all my concerns or medical needs in my appointments. I have so many symptoms and so many different medical needs, that it requires me to go to several different specialists. It's overwhelming trying to get the doctors to connect the dots on all my symptoms to be able to treat everything effectively. I've had a few of my doctors recently tell me that they've done all they can for me. I can't begin to tell you how painful it was to hear them say this.

*

TAMMY DOWNS

Tammy was diagnosed with Crohn's disease, irritable bowel syndrome, spastic colon, gastroesophageal reflux disease, and gastritis in 2006 at age 46, gastroparesis in 2015 at age 56, and motility dysfunction disorder of the rectum and pelvic floor in 2016 at age 58

I had stomach problems going back to the age of thirty-two years old. I had endometriosis and had five surgeries for this disease. It had attached itself to my uterus and bladder. It had also attached to my lower bowel, looped three times and pulled it all down into my vagina. I believe to this day, that was the start of a lot of my problems. I developed interstitial cystitis, plus I had kidney problems despite being born with three. I could not believe that endometriosis could cause so much trouble. Before having a hysterectomy, I wanted to make sure there were no other problems, so I started going to a gastro-enterologist to get answers.

As years went on, I started having further intestinal problems. I started out in Georgia, where I lived at the time, with a different doctor and that is when I found out I had irritable bowel syndrome, Crohn's disease, gastritis, and acid reflux. After six years in Georgia, I moved back to Florida. When I did, I started back with my old GI. When my Crohn's disease and stomach problems were getting worse, and my bloodwork was bad, I discovered that he was not listening to me regarding the problems I was having.

I was on a medication at that time that affected the blood, so my blood had to be checked. I was on mercaptopurine, a chemotherapy drug that interferes with the growth and spread of cancer cells in the body. It's an old medication that was used for certain types of leukemia, and they found it helped patients with ulcerative colitis and Crohn's disease. When my bloodwork started acting up, my doctor sent me to a cancer doctor who did blood tests to make sure I didn't have some form of cancer. I had been on the medication for twelve years and the most you should be on it is five years. When I went to the cancer doctor, he told me I needed a new GI doctor because the doctor I was going to was not listening or watching what was going on with me. He did a bone marrow test, and the test showed I had a damaged bone marrow which weakened my immune system.

After this, I was sent to a doctor in Gainesville, Florida, ninety minutes away. When I first went to my GI doctor, I was so excited I cried all the way home. He was supposed to know about the stomach and gastroparesis, gastritis, acid reflux, esophageal sphincter problems, and Crohn's disease, so I felt like he would be aware of everything. I felt like I had hope. I got bloodwork done, had a stomach emptying test, and had my gallbladder removed. I did everything and anything I needed in order for him to help me get rid of the nausea, pain, and the rock in my stomach that would cause me to throw up. He was very nice. He tried to make me laugh because I was serious about what was happening.

He gave me several prescriptions. One was a refill of a medication I was on. The second medication, pantoprazole, replaced Nexium for acid reflux. The third was an antibiotic, Xifaxan, for bacteria in my stomach, but I had a reaction and had to stop taking it. I was then given erythromycin to help contract the nerves and muscles in my stomach, to help push the food through. I had to stop taking that as well because it was way too strong, and I had a bad reaction. He put me on azithromycin to replace the erythromycin. I had a reaction to that as well, so he put me on amitriptyline, which is supposed to help relax the stomach to help pass food. Well, I had a bad reaction to that drug too. In the meantime, because I was having constipation, I had to go for a manometry anorectal test for motility disorders, which I was found to have.

I had medication prescribed by my GI doctor that my insurance refused to cover. The second time I went to Dr. Weiner, he was like a totally different doctor. He told me I had to fight my insurance, and to contact the prescription companies so I could get free medication. I felt like he attacked me in other ways, telling me I had to fight to help myself and that his hands were tied. He told me to have answers for him when I came back for my next visit, and that he hoped I had a different insurance policy that would cover the prescriptions he wanted me on.

Well, you bet I did my homework, but I hoped his attitude had changed. I told him I was so frustrated because I went to him for help and instead got one medication after another that did not work. I told him that I needed to feel better. After that, I started having problems with my blood pressure dropping low, getting lightheaded and dizzy. My medical doctor started running bloodwork, one test after another. I was dehydrated and malnourished. I started to drop more weight, and was down to ninety pounds. My wonderful nurse, Amy, told me to start drinking Propel mixed with water so my blood pressure would not jump real fast. She told me I needed protein, so I started drinking Boost, putting protein in my smoothies, and eating more baby food.

When I went to my next appointment with my GI, he started me on bethanechol, which helped make my stomach work and pushed food through. Plus I started Vitamin B_6 and probiotics, which helped my motility a lot and helped put good bacteria back in my body. In the meantime, they thought my adrenal gland had malfunctioned, so I was put on medication for that.

My medical doctor has been my backbone. He has helped me so much. I know it can be frustrating for doctors. Thank goodness my medical doctor keeps his cool, calm, collective self. That is what I like about him so much. As for my GI, we are working on our doctor-patient relationship, so we will see. My emotions are high because I'm in pain and can't eat without throwing everything up. Then I get to where I do not want to eat because I do not want to have constipation and motility problems. I do not want to put food in my stomach and have the feeling of a big, giant rock in my stomach. I just feel horrible. It's a feeling that I just want to go away. I want the doctors to help find a way to get rid of this problem.

*

SKYE FALCON

Skye was diagnosed with gastroparesis and other autoimmune diseases in 2006 at age 25

Doctor appointments are like round-trips to hell and back, each and every time. Except you're never sure how many extra demons you'll end up with every go-round. You are not really sure if you'll be allowed to come back alive, or if they'll keep you for being too deficient, too intense, or too weird. The demons are the new or morphed ailments, diagnoses, and issues.

The ladders of doctors and specialists that must be climbed for diagnosis and treatment is ridiculous. Dr. A listens, but then the next one, named Dr. Two, discredits and disagrees with Dr. A's diagnosis and plan. Specialist number three then says Dr. Two is whacked, but does not think Dr. A did the right tests. So, back to the drawing board we go. Then, mid-year your insurance changes suddenly, and all of the doctors and specialists disappear mid-testing. Finally, you have to re-establish in a new network, start over at the beginning, and go through the years of torture and hell you thought you crawled out of, and had been seated comfortably in the sun. Wrong! No rest or healing for the weary. The circle of the chronically awesome, I call it.

I have two main doctors: one general practitioner and one holistic doctor who are attentive. They have always listened, and know that if I am bringing it to them as a problem, it is indeed an issue. The holistic doctor, then obstetrician, was the one who listened and saved mine and my child's life during the uterine rupture years before. My general practitioner does not always have the answers and he is upfront about it. That said, he will research anything if there is a chance it could help, and is open for me to try what I need to try. He is honest about all possible outcomes and works with me regularly.

When my issues became too great for my general practitioner, I had to be referred to a large, well-known teaching hospital in Indiana. From there, it was a siphon of disasters, what seemed like millions of specialists, few answers, and poor patient care. Not only were the visible ailments ignored, my issues were brushed aside. This left me feeling beyond minimized, over and over again. I wasn't over or underweight at that point, so I was told just to deal with it until it became a problem either way. It was already a problem for me though, one that interfered with every aspect of my everyday life. These types of doctors do not help the minds of the chronically ill by making us question our own sanity because they essentially have no treatment plan to stick to, and might have to pretend to actually use smarts they might have retained from medical school.

For two years, I did everything they asked: all the tests, the diets, the trial medications. I made frequent weekly trips to the hospital that was hours away. I took poison treatments they said would fix it, or at least help. On multiple occasions, I swallowed a SmartPill only to have unreliable results because the thing got stuck in my stomach for a week instead of a day, and had to be forcefully removed. Tubes were crammed into my nostrils and down my throat, and through holes made in my belly. Nothing helped, no answers given or plans made, and then more weight fell off. Not enough for the big teaching hospital doctors to step in, but enough for my local doctors to pull me from that travesty of a place, and bring me back home to work on it locally.

I get incredibly burned out on everything medical. When the doctors do not listen, I don't want to go even when I know I should. I recently had some procedures done to ease the mouth issues caused by Sjogren's syndrome, and ended up canceling two months worth of other appointments. When I get burned out and finally make it back in, usually something has shifted again and I'm stuck on more medication or new regimens. It's more than stressful and unavoidable. Doctors and hospitals mean sickness and death. They mean I'm losing a bit of myself again, unwillingly. It is a constant fight between just wanting to feel like a semi-normal human, and wanting to live life. I know there is no real way to feel like a normal human again. If I were to try, that would involve stopping everything I do every day, and I will not do that. I can't stop now. I'm only thirty-five.

Feeling supported is touch and go. Not many of my closest family members really know about what is happening to me, inside of me, or what I deal with every day. And the same could be said about some of the gastrointestinal specialists I see. Some attend appointments with me regularly, but are often lost in detail and wandering around the cafeteria. I try to remind myself that even though they are distant, or have run away completely from the medical hell that is my life, they still care. Somehow, in their own way. Maybe?

My lifelong issues are compared to diets, my ailments dismissed or ignored, and I think I must wear a cloak of invisibility sometimes, because I am just not even seen. That said, life is busy for everyone, and everyone is going through something. Remembering that and helping others always helps ease the lonely feelings that sneak in, and re-grounds me. My children are great supporters, always in my corner, and always cheering me on. They bring me what I need, reminding me to sit. It's not a job I would ever have wished on them, but I am so grateful they are the wonderful humans they are.

I do not feel supported in the medical community, however. With gastroparesis, there is no set treatment plan. These days, thanks to new insurance laws and regulations, most doctors have no choice but to follow the protocol for such sicknesses. Trouble is, most all gastroparesis sufferers have ever-changing symptoms that differ from day to day, which can make lots of tests negative or inaccurate. No set diagnoses or a hundred percent positive test means no plan, missing out on medications that truly help, and not having services or necessary treatments covered by insurance.

Specialists who watch me closely, witness the issues I am having, and then send me on my way because there is just no treatment that will really work and they do not know what else to do hinder my ability to continue down the positive path with all of this medical hell. My fifteen minute stints once a month are barely enough time to cover the issues I am having, if I am brave enough to answer the question, "So, what brings you in today?" truthfully and honestly, which is rare. Answering truthfully with new doctors usually ends up with a psych evaluation, before they realize that this unfortunate deal is really my life. Once they determine I am not a pain medication patient, their whole demeanor changes, and once again they are willing to help me. This type of behavior disgusts me, but seems to happen everywhere.

*

ROBIN MCNAMARA
Robin was diagnosed with
gastroparesis in 2013 at age 55

With my former gastroenterologist, I wanted to physically shake the guy and say, "Wake up! I'm sick! I've lost twenty-five pounds! What is wrong with me?" as he stared at me with a soulless look. This is the guy who ignored my complaints, let chemical gastritis go on and on and on, and ignored me not only as a patient, but as a human being. Doctors are supposed to do no harm. I wonder how many more people from his practice are in the same boat as me. It's no surprise that his office is next to a funeral home either.

My current gastroenterologist is beyond amazing. He treats people with gastroparesis every day, and he cares. He even makes me laugh with his bigger-than-life personality. He cares about his patients and is a one-of-a-kind man. This guy took me in when the days were really bad. He had me go to his office or to outpatient for stomach and nausea drugs. Even the nurses who work for him are good. One time when I called saying I was really nauseated, they asked what I ate. I said fruit, and they barked at me, "You can't eat raw fruit!" I feel as though his entire office understands me, and like I'm his only patient.

*

TAMMY PITTMAN

Tammy was diagnosed with gastroparesis and irritable bowel syndrome in 2014 at age 34

I have learned that doctors only treat the symptoms of the complications associated with gastroparesis. There are only two medications to treat this disease and they have life-threatening side effects. Many doctors I've come in contact with have no idea what to do, from being uneducated to just giving up. My gastrointestinal motility specialist is at the point when there's nothing she can do until I get worse.

*

TAYLOR SCHMITZ

Taylor was diagnosed with idiopathic gastroparesis in 2014 at age 22

Every single doctor appointment felt like a waste of time. It's not that I wasn't optimistic, because I definitely was or I would never have gone in the first place. However, my doctors always gave me another drug, told me things I already knew, and never solved anything. In fact, I stopped filling prescriptions after the tenth one or so, because the side effects of all these drugs were far more terrible than any of the benefits, which was actually never anything.

This was my case up until I met Dr. Maleigha White of Toledo Naturopathic in Waterville, Ohio. She is a naturopathic doctor, but she also believes in incorporating a little bit of Western medicine in conjunction to natural treatment. She has been so loving, kind, and always concerned with my well-being. She always gets back to me so fast, no matter what my issue is. God led me to her, and He has blessed me with her in my life. Her remedies have been just that: remedies. Not a band-aid, no side effects, nothing. So now, except when I have to get a checkup for gastroparesis, I always look forward to my doctor appointments, because I know Dr. White will always help me, and even be a friend when I need her.

*

DEB SHRADER-TROTTER
Deb was diagnosed with
gastroparesis in 1999 at age 37

I feel very supported with my palliative care team, my motility specialist, and my primary doctor. It has not always been this way, but it is this way now.

*

JESSICA SPENCE
Jessica was diagnosed with
gastroparesis in 2016 at age 25

There once was a time when I would feel hopeful when I went to the doctor. When this first started I thought there would be answers. With every negative test my heart would sink. What was wrong with me? As time went on I started to become quite anxious before my appointments and tests. A million what ifs rushed through my mind.

What if they don't listen? What if they miss something? What if they're right? What if I am crazy? What if...?

After more than a decade, I was finally brave and angry enough with my doctor to switch to one who is far more supportive and understanding. I am trying to trust my new doctor, but those same what ifs—and more—still creep up in my mind. Some days I fight back the what ifs and manage to see those glimmers of hope that used to fill me. I want to have more appointments like that.

*

NICOLE STARZYNSKI
Nicole was diagnosed with
gastroparesis in 2016 at age 33

Where to start? There have been so many doctors, many of which the thought of makes me angry. I spent so many hours crying my eyes out because another test came back without any results. The doctors told me to deal with the never-ending nausea. They prescribed me medication that made me sicker. I was so sick, I would be on the bathroom floor wanting to die. When I called, they told me to come back in, and to continue to take the medicine. I had to put a stop so many times to the awful poison doctors just kept trying to shove down my throat because they didn't know what to do.

I have woken up from colonoscopies only to hear they didn't find anything besides a polyp, hemorrhoids and some inflammation, and broken into tears. The doctors looked at me like I was nuts. It had been eight years of going doctor to doctor, having test after test. When you are thirty-four years old, you should not have had more than four colonoscopies already. They are not normal and they suck. A colonoscopy and the radioactive egg test are two things I despise, despite being a proud member having just had my fourth test. I am tired of taking tests and I am tired of not hearing real answers. I have heard that a diet will solve all my problems, that gastroparesis doesn't cause pain, and gastroparesis isn't so serious that you would be feeling this awful. I wouldn't wish this disease on anyone but there are a few doctors who I wish could feel it for a few days, just so they could understand that everyday life is a struggle.

From 2009 to 2011, I was seeking help for the same symptoms I am battling today. While working on this book, I went through old medical records to bring back all the memories I had blocked out. I requested my records from everywhere I ever went last year just so I had my own medical records on hand at all times. I might not have ever gone back to look through everything if it wasn't for this book.

In 2010, I had an ultrasound which revealed a large mass in my stomach. They did an endoscopy and documented the results as a bezoar, a mass found trapped in the gastrointestinal system, with the diagnosis of gastroparesis. My doctor never gave me these results, nor did he tell me they found anything. Instead of that doctor investigating the bezoar more, he ignored it. He brushed me off with a diagnosis of irritable bowel syndrome, ulcerative colitis and celiac disease. For years, every time I ate food I had to drink a cola. If I didn't, I would throw up my food. It makes sense that the cola probably also took care of the bezoar. I am so angry that doctor ignored something that was so crucial in my diagnosis and prolonged my treatment by eight years.

What is wrong with these doctors? They are taking care of living, breathing humans! We aren't paper dolls or machines. We are people. I really hope any doctors reading this wake up. You can't continue to ignore your patients or overlook vital pieces of information. I understand you're busy, but your job is to take care of people. If you don't understand something then you need to educate yourself more! It is so frustrating that I am as sick as I am when I could have been better if it was treated years ago. I might not be better, but I still imagine how many other people are left out in the cold, not knowing why they are so sick all the time, just because some doctor was too busy or ignorant to spend the time to go over some results.

The doctor who diagnosed me with gastroparesis was not familiar with treating the disease. I was filled with so many different emotions after I received my diagnosis. My doctor was treating it like I had the flu or an ear infection. No big deal. I was already frustrated with the antacids she kept prescribing because I was convinced at the time they were going to kill me. I was told that a nutritionist would contact me but nobody ever did. I called my doctor's office and they scheduled me to come in and gave me the number for the nutritionist. That very same day I received a thick envelope in the mail. It contained a letter stating I had been diagnosed with gastroparesis, and a book of recipes for smoothies and meals to try. I burst into tears. How the heck was this supposed to solve my problem? I couldn't eat anything in this stupid Fodmap diet they sent me. How was some diet going to help me if I was sick when I wasn't even eating? Water had started to make me sick. I wasn't eating solid foods, everything was liquid.

I found that a lot of other people with gastroparesis were just as frustrated as me. Before I went into my next appointment at the doctor, I almost had a panic attack. I was angry because she had been blowing off every issue and concern I had with little or no guidance. I wanted to just flip out on her. I had all these things I wanted to go in and say. For some reason, once I was in there, I just didn't have a lot of words. She told me she signed me up for an irritable bowel syndrome clinic but the wait time was going to be a while. I was number fifty-three on the list.

At my next appointment, after another treatment failing, my doctor basically blew me off. She told me that the severe stomach pain I was experiencing had nothing to do with gastroparesis and that I shouldn't be experiencing nausea with the medications I was taking. Not only that, she kept trying to make me take MiraLax. She refused to accept the fact that a fiber filled laxative was making someone with gastroparesis sick, when fiber is one of the biggest things to avoid. She just made me very angry.

In my field of work, if I don't understand something, I research it so I can support people better. I work in technology not on human beings. I feel that it's the doctor's job to say, "You know what? I don't know how to help this person. What can I do to better help them?" It's very rare anymore to find a doctor who actually cares. When I was leaving, they gave me a breath kit to test for small intestinal bacterial overgrowth (SIBO). I never went back to her after that appointment. My insurance would not cover the test for SIBO so I spent three hundred fifty dollars and the test came back negative.

At that time, I was very close to getting in with Johns Hopkins and Cleveland Clinic. I was frustrated but still felt positive because I finally had a diagnosis. I requested my medical records from where I was diagnosed to be faxed to Cleveland Clinic. Getting the records there was such a hassle; it almost took two weeks. One of the biggest things Cleveland wanted was the results for the gastric emptying study. Once they received the results, they called me and told me something I was not expecting. My gastric emptying study had been documented incorrectly and could not be used to accept me into their clinic. I would need another four hour gastric emptying study. Within days, Johns Hopkins came back and said the same thing.

This news sent me into a total breakdown. I had a doctor who was totally ignoring me and basically giving me the brush off, and a useless test that wasn't going to get me in with any doctor who could help. To top it off, my doctor who diagnosed me was incorrectly documenting everything I told her. She reported no unwanted weight loss, but I had lost twenty-five pounds while I was seeing her! Hell, how is that not unwanted weight loss? Her notes made it sound like I was imagining being sick every day of my life and she just couldn't help someone who didn't want to be helped. No wonder I couldn't get in with another doctor.

I wasted three and a half months with a doctor who couldn't remember what I was telling her during my appointments. It was crazy. She would tell me, "Don't do this," but then the appointment notes said, "told patient to do this." AHHHHH! Doctors, we are human beings and when you treat us with less respect than a computer technician treats a computer, it's disgusting and you should be in another profession. It's hard enough getting help with this disease, let alone when your symptoms aren't even documented properly.

I was so angry and frustrated with the entire medical field. Why did I have some disease that nobody knew anything about? Why wouldn't anyone help me? I was depressed and exhausted with it all. I wanted to say, "Screw it, I will just deal with this on my own." I had myself so worked up I had a panic attack, and shortly after it felt like war had started inside my stomach. "Wake up Nicole, you can't continue to live this way. Your daughter needs you, your family needs you and you need you!" I kept saying this to myself, trying to convince myself that no matter how bad I felt, I needed to suck it up and put all that energy toward a solution.

I called Johns Hopkins. Since I was trying to be accepted into a clinical study there, they wrote an order for another gastric emptying study. Because I live in Pittsburgh and Johns Hopkins is in Baltimore, I booked a hotel and my boyfriend and I both took two days off to go down for my test. The day before my test we had the most wonderful day. We walked around the inner harbor of Baltimore, took a speedboat ride, and had a nice dinner. The next day we got up and I ate my second radioactive egg. This time I was given egg beaters, jelly toast and unlimited water until I was done eating. I was feeling good for the most part. I wasn't nauseous and I didn't have any stomach pain. It took me a while to eat everything; it was a lot of food.

Shortly after I finished eating, I puked it up and swallowed it. I didn't want the test to be ruined. I had already spent too much money on a hotel and driving down there. I couldn't afford to waste any more time. At the second picture, the lady told me I was finished. I held back the tears, I had no idea what this meant. Did I not have gastroparesis? I figured I wasn't going to get into the clinical study and I was back to the beginning. I cried hysterically for the first two hours in the car. My poor boyfriend had no idea what to say or do. He tried the best he could to try to calm me down and be positive. I wasn't hearing anything except that my test was finished at two hours. I eventually passed out while crying and didn't wake up until we got home.

I felt so defeated and upset. I decided to talk to some of the people on one of the Facebook gastroparesis support groups. Turns out having a normal gastric emptying study is quite common even for the most severe cases. All it takes is one good tummy day and bam, some doctor is trying to tell you that you don't have gastroparesis and you're basically left on your own. It made me so angry that a test that carried so much weight with doctors was so useless. What is the point if the variable isn't the same at each testing center, and if the test is dependent on how you feel that day? The emotions it puts people through is awful. It's not fair. What it does to people who are already sick—anxiety, panic attacks, questioning everything you're feeling—is awful. Trying to convince yourself you aren't that sick, it's no big deal, just suck it up and deal with it, only to be so sick you can barely move hours later. The realization that this cycle is your life and some stupid egg test was the brick wall blocking the help.

I called my regular doctor's office and scheduled an appointment. He saw me within the week. He was one doctor who always listened to me, was supportive and made me feel like I wasn't crazy. He even explained that over the years he has had this happen with severe gastroparesis patients. He said he would order another test and ask the nuclear medicine department to schedule it as soon as possible. I had an appointment a week later. The morning of my test I was so sick, I woke up dry heaving until I blew what felt like every blood vessel from my face. I puked up my breakfast from the day before. I felt absolutely awful; there was no way I could drive myself to that test. So I called and canceled. They rescheduled me for the next day.

The next day, I woke up and my day started the exact same way. What a nightmare. I took a Zofran and basically talked myself into getting dressed and driving to have the test. The test consisted of a quarter cup of scrambled eggs and a tiny bit of water. Again, there was no consistency with the variable of the test. The x-ray technician I had was wonderful. At each picture, she showed me where the food was in my stomach. I also told her about my first test being documented incorrectly and then what happened at Johns Hopkins, and she said she was familiar with that happening.

After the first hour, my stomach contents were barely moving. At the end of the second hour, there was still more than ninety-five percent left in my stomach. If you think about how much one quarter cup of eggs is, that isn't a lot after two hours. It's like a bite of food. So how was I finished at two hours three weeks prior, while this time I was nowhere close to being ready to leave? At the end of the four hours, the girl told me if we did the test longer, I would be staying. I still had sixty-five percent of that itty bitty bit of eggs retained. I received the results online the same day. I felt relieved that I had enough to get in with Cleveland and Johns Hopkins. That same day, I called my doctor and had his office send the test to Cleveland, and I sent the test to the contact I had at Johns Hopkins.

I was told not to expect a miracle to even get in with a doctor quickly to have surgery, even if I was losing five pounds a week and barely consuming liquids at that point. The next day, Johns Hopkins emailed me and scheduled me to see the doctor who was head of the clinical study for a gastric peroral endoscopic pyloromyotomy (G-POEM). Within days, Cleveland Clinic called me and scheduled me for the Friday before I would go to Hopkins. I was so excited! How could this be? How could I have almost given up? I had two of the best medical facilities finally agreeing to see me. I had watched so many interviews with both of the doctors I was meeting. They were some of the top doctors to see for gastroparesis. After all of these years, I was finally going to meet doctors who understood me.

The weeks leading up to my appointments felt like an eternity. The week before I started to get nervous, not only about meeting these doctors, but also making sure I had all of my notes, food diary, and medical records. I could barely make it out of the house, how was I going to make it to Cleveland and back, and a few days later to Baltimore and back? Almost fourteen hours total in the car.

The day of my appointment finally came. My mom was going with me and got to my house at 5 a.m. It stinks when you can't afford to stay in a hotel for a doctor's appointment. If we weren't worried about how many more appointments, we would have probably driven up the night before. We arrived early and were amazed at the size of Cleveland Clinic. The hospital itself was as big as eighteen city blocks. To me that's the size of South Side in Pittsburgh. There were all of these walkways connecting every building. Luckily a friend of mine warned me, so I had maps and knew where we were going.

Everything moved pretty quick. Once I met the doctor, I felt a little discouraged and kind of the way every other doctor has ever made me feel. Doctors always seem to look at me like they're thinking, "You're not skin and bones, you're not that sick." They don't realize the other part of me is gone. When you lose over seventy pounds, you don't even look like yourself. When a doctor looks at me and thinks I am healthy, not overweight and just right, it makes me want to snap. I haven't eaten in months without becoming so ill, I have just wanted to lay on the floor until I died. If I wasn't overweight to begin with, I would be skin and bones. I was happy I had the extra buffer, but I didn't want to be ignored because a doctor wants to be ignorant and not open to the fact that I have lost a significant amount of weight.

He sent me for a ton of blood work, x-rays, more tests, tests, tests. He also ordered a SmartPill test which I will talk more about later. My blood work came back with over fifteen different deficiencies, but not one of them came back for a reason why I had gastroparesis. Even the diabetes antibody test came back negative. My dad had diabetes and his father was a severe diabetic, who lost both of his legs and eventually died because he didn't take care of himself. I was relieved to hear I didn't have any new conditions but frustrated we had no idea what caused my gastroparesis. They don't really have a clue how to treat diabetic gastroparesis, and idiopathic is even worse. I had been so excited for this appointment and felt so let down.

A few days later, we were back in the car and on our way to Baltimore for my appointment at Johns Hopkins. We spent four and a half hours in the car for a thirty-minute appointment. I was still exhausted and upset from my appointment at Cleveland. We met with the doctor and he asked me many questions, since this was to get into a clinical study for a surgical procedure for idiopathic gastroparesis. I was a perfect candidate. They told me they would send me the information and someone would call me in a few days to schedule the surgery later in July. I was so excited. Finally some hope. My mom was excited that we had hope and that I wasn't going to be crying for the next few hundred miles. My boyfriend may be the only person I have ever met who stays so calm when I am having a complete meltdown.

Finally my hope was changing. I received a call from Johns Hopkins Medical Center. I was accepted for a gastric G-POEM. There was hope! There was no cure, but there was hope in remission of symptoms. I kept telling myself, "Don't give up. Hopefully I will be able to eat food again without being sick."

Weeks went by and I never heard back from Johns Hopkins. I called and emailed them but never heard back. Josh thought it was a blessing in disguise. He wasn't crazy about me having surgery to be treated like a lab rat. He was more concerned with the fact that after I had the surgery, besides monitoring how I was doing, they weren't going to be my regular gastrointestinal doctor. He felt that they didn't care and my best option for long-term care was Cleveland Clinic. He had a point, but I ignored it because I was so happy to have a chance at relief. I wasn't thinking about anything from a logical point of view. Josh listened and supported me, and if I really felt strong about having the procedure done at Johns Hopkins, he would have supported me.

The reason I discuss my health with Josh and my mom is to make a better rational decision. That way I won't jump to any choices that may not be the best choice, just because I am so fed up with how I feel that I will almost do anything if someone tells me I will feel better. This trio has been so important to helping me make the best decisions for me. Nobody is forcing their opinion on me, but I am not making the decisions alone. I also discuss most things with my daughter. I don't share things that may scare her but she likes to be a part of my care as well. We are family and this disease affects us all.

After I received the results of my SmartPill test, Cleveland called me to schedule an appointment with their surgeon and gastrologist who specialized in gastroparesis. The soonest they could get me in was September. A week before my appointment, they called to postpone my appointment until November. That was two months away. I couldn't believe I had to wait that long. They had scheduled me an appointment with four different doctors.

October 2016 marked more than a year since I had eaten real food without paying for it! After months and months of waiting, my big appointment day at Cleveland Clinic was finally here. I met with four doctors. My first appointment was with a neurologist, then a pain specialist, the surgeon, and then the gastroparesis doctor. I had been waiting for this appointment for so long, but now that it was right around the corner, I was so nervous. I knew this appointment was to schedule my surgery, which was freaking me out completely.

The neurologist was a doctor who also knew a great deal about what gastroparesis did to people mentally. It was basically like a psychological evaluation. But the doctor was very nice and was easy to talk to. He recommended staying on anxiety medication and possibly thinking about going to therapy to help deal with having a disease that was never going away.

The pain specialist also knew a lot about gastroparesis and for the first time I felt validated when I talked about the pain I was having. This guy knew his stuff. Everything I told him about the stabbing pain he understood. He suggested a few different things we could do. Just hearing a doctor validate that my pain was real, there were no words. Eight years of being ignored and someone finally knew what I was telling them was real and extremely painful. He prescribed me medicine for nerve pain that would take a month to work.

My next appointment was with the surgeon and then the gastrologist. We decided I was going to have a peroral pyloromyotomy. When my mom and I left that day, I was excited. After all the roadblocks, there was finally hope. My daughter cried when I told her I was having surgery. She was so excited I would be able to eat again. We had hope of finally being a normal family again.

I didn't take Nortriptyline, the nerve medicine. Since the surgery was less than a month away, it didn't make sense to start a medicine for pain a month before if it wouldn't have time to help me. A few days later, they called me with my surgery date: December 13, 2016. I had to fill out some questionnaires online, registration, all that good stuff. Then the reality of, "Oh, my. I'm having surgery two weeks before Christmas," set it. It was the week of Thanksgiving. I had to figure out how to get ready for Christmas and surgery in less than three weeks. Luckily I was able to do ninety percent of my shopping online and pushed myself so hard. Some days I was sick as a dog, eating Zofran like Tic Tacs and taking fifteen minute power naps every other hour. Somehow I was able to get it all done, I'll never let my baby down. Even with this disease, she is always my number one and no disease is going to keep her from a happy childhood, even if it takes everything out of me. It's amazing what love for your child can force you to do.

Remember that irritable bowel syndrome clinic the other doctor signed me up for? They called on the Thursday leading up to my surgery. They finally had an opening! Are you kidding me? Thanks Doctor, I appreciate all of your concern and hard work getting me into a clinic nine months later! I was so happy I didn't wait for her to take care of me, or obviously I would have been waiting a long time. It was more validation that when you have this disease, you have to be your own advocate.

On Friday, four days before my surgery, I had to go to Cleveland for my preoperative appointment. Nine hours of doctors, bloodwork, and electrocardiograms was incredibly exhausting. Two days leading up to my surgery, I was running around nonstop trying to finish up things around the house. I was on a crazy liquid and medicine diet. My daughter had a complete breakdown, screaming and crying. She was so scared something was going to happen to me. Even though I was scared, I had to be positive and tell her I was going to be fine and this was hope for me to get better. I can still hear that screaming and crying in my head.

By the time the night before my surgery came, I was beyond exhausted and I was scared. I was scared something was going to happen during the surgery, and scared it wouldn't work. Josh took me for my surgery so my mom could stay with Kirstin. I wanted to make sure she was comfortable while I was having surgery. Josh and I left at 4 a.m. the morning of my surgery. I thought because I was having surgery at Cleveland Clinic, the day would go well. Oh boy, was I wrong! I was told to be there by 9 a.m. that morning. I checked in at 8:30 a.m. At 9:45 a.m. they took me back to put my IV in. I was stuck in that room until 3 p.m. before they took me back to the operating room. After that, I got to lay in the operating room waiting for the doctor to get there. After my surgery, did he bother to talk to my family like he was supposed to? No, he did not. He didn't bother to tell me I wasn't allowed anything by mouth, not even water or ice chips, or that I would be having a scan the next day. I was not happy at all.

I wasn't allowed to drink anything until 1 p.m. the next day, after a barium x-ray cleared that I had no leaks. Then I was able to have a small liquid meal of beef broth, an icy and endless apple juice. I chugged four juices, some of the salty broth and the icy. I was so thirsty. It had been forty-five hours since I had a drink. I wanted to get out of there; I wanted to go home.

The following Monday, we had to go back to Cleveland for a checkup with the surgeons. I was feeling somewhat okay, but after the drive up there and then waiting for two and a half hours in the waiting room, I was extremely irritated and in pain from my surgery. When the surgeon, who I had never met, came in, I was a little rude. He said he was joining the gastroparesis clinic. I said, "Well, if you are joining the gastroparesis clinic, you better learn to be on time. I just had surgery, drove over two and a half hours to get here, and you left me in here for over two hours. That's rude and I would like to go home now." Some advice: don't do that. They marked that I wasn't in any pain and was recovering great from the surgery. I was in pain, I couldn't bend or sit for long periods, and I was still on a liquid diet. I was just annoyed and wanted to leave to go home. I wasn't really taking the pain medicine except for when the pain was so bad that I couldn't take it anymore. When you are only consuming a few hundred calories a day and weigh 113 pounds, Percocets can make you feel awful. I had felt like I wanted to puke long enough, so I just dealt with most of the pain.

I didn't talk to the doctor again until I started to become sick again in February shortly after I started eating soft food. They scheduled an appointment for me to see the surgeon and gastrologist at the beginning of April, so I had enough time to have my gastric emptying study at the three month mark. At the end of February, they called me to tell me the doctor was going on vacation and they needed to reschedule my appointment to May. I lost it on the phone with the scheduling guy, and cried. I had thrown my guts up that entire morning and the day before I had blown up like a blimp. I couldn't believe they were doing this to me. I ended up sending a few messages through the patient portal and never heard back from my doctor once! Not even when I wanted to confirm that he received the results of my gastric emptying study that showed that I still had a severe delay. Nothing.

I was so excited when the day of my appointment finally came. My mom and I drove up to Cleveland. We didn't wait long until we went into the waiting room. Then another doctor came in, not the surgeon I had just waited three months to meet with, but a doctor I had met at my postoperative appointment. He immediately started telling me I needed to have my stomach removed and the procedure that they would do. I was ready to lose my mind. I thought, "Are you serious right now? How are we going straight to this? Why did I just wait three months to meet with the other doctor? Why are you here telling me you want to take out my stomach?"

I flat out said, "No, I am not doing that. We are going to try the stimulator. I don't care if you don't think it will work. If it doesn't, then at least we will know. I am not going the other route unless I have no other choice. Life or death." Then the gastrologist came in with a nurse practitioner. He was not as attentive as the last appointment. He immediately pointed out I had gained weight so I couldn't be that sick, but that we would do the stimulator after we did some more tests to figure out why I was so constipated. I was no more constipated than I was before the surgery! I was experiencing extreme bloating, but he told me gastroparesis doesn't make you bloat. He mentioned that he wanted me to have another SmartPill but insurance probably wouldn't cover it because it hadn't been a year since my last. He also scheduled two tests. In one, they would stick a tube in my anus. In the second test, they would give me a barium enema and then x-ray me while on the toilet.

I had waited three months to meet with "I want to remove your stomach" guy and my doctor; it was a huge let down. What a waste of time. Do I have to be dying to get help? It will be December again before they schedule me for anything. I won't even be able to get an appointment for another few months. I am so outraged! I am also upset that I have to be violated to see if I have something called pelvic floor dysfunction, which has nothing to do with the fact that I throw up undigested food over twenty hours after I eat it. Sadly I will still be waiting when this book goes to press.

*

JENNIFER ZUBIK

Jennifer was diagnosed with idiopathic gastroparesis in 2010 at age 27

I experienced many emotions during each doctor appointment, with so many different doctors. I saw so many doctors at the beginning trying to get answers and relief that it was overwhelming. When I would first meet with a doctor, they showed concern and would want to help. However, after trying their recommendations without success, they would get frustrated with me and it would be time to look for another. I had many doctors tell me that there was nothing they could do to help me because they could not figure out what was wrong after there wasn't any positive results with their methods of help. Some would refer me elsewhere or would recommend a new doctor to try, others would just be cruel and blunt and turn me away. I had doctors insist nothing was wrong, that it was all in my head, and that I needed to see a psychiatrist for mental health. It was disappointing and heartbreaking to be treated that way.

When I was finally diagnosed with gastroparesis, the frustration increased immensely because now we knew what it was, but the doctors in my area didn't know enough about the disease or how to treat it. After seeing numerous doctors, I contacted the general surgeon who performed my gallbladder surgery. Out of all the doctors I had seen, he was the only one who acted genuinely concerned about making me better. We played the guessing game for a little while, but he never gave up and continued to treat through trial and error to give me some relief.

One procedure that began to work for me was Botox injections in my pylorus. Along with Compazine and Ativan, it allowed me to eat a little and gave me energy to be a mom and fiancée, feel comfortable enough to go outside of my home in general, go back to work, complete household chores, hang out with family and friends, and just begin to enjoy life again. During an endoscopy, the Botox was injected into my pylorus approximately every eight to twelve weeks. After receiving that treatment for three years with enough relief to begin living a somewhat normal life, my insurance provider decided to reject coverage for the Botox injections. Without insurance, the procedure would cost thousands of dollars out of pocket each time.

My doctor then stated he did not have any other solutions for me, and directed me to the Cleveland Clinic to explore the option of having a gastric neurostimulator implanted. I then began receiving treatment by several doctors and surgeons at the Cleveland Clinic. Most of the doctors at the Cleveland Clinic have done all that they can for me. They also made me feel they are genuinely concerned and care about my well-being and health, just as my previous doctor had.

Doctors are supposed to help and care for their patients, no matter what odds are against them. They aren't supposed to give up or turn you away. A real doctor will care for you and treat you the way they would want and expect to be treated if the tables were turned and they were in need of medical help.

*

When all you know is pain, you don't know
that is not normal. It is not our lot to suffer,
even if we've been raised that way.

SUSAN SARANDON

*

CHAPTER SIX

Juggling Treatments

> When I'm resting on a flare day, I need to remember that I am not wasting the entire day doing nothing. I am doing exactly what I need to do. I am recovering. -ANONYMOUS

Because the exact cause of dysmotility disorders remain unknown, treatment remedies run the gamut and are not an exact science. What works for one person may not work for another. What medical therapies have been offered? Which have you tried?

*

MELISSA ADAMS VANHOUTEN
Melissa was diagnosed with
gastroparesis in 2014 at age 47

I've lived with gastroparesis for only three years, so I am certain I have not tried as many therapies as others. I was initially offered no medications and attempted to lessen symptoms with dietary changes alone. This was completely unsuccessful for me, and that became clear within the first three weeks or so after diagnosis. I truly believe I would have died had I not agreed to try the medication I currently take, domperidone, a prokinetic which is thought to increase motility. I left the hospital with instructions to stay on a liquid/soft foods diet for a week or so and then begin adding safe foods that were low in fat and fiber. Well, even the liquids were intolerable, and it was mere days before my nonstop vomiting and unbearable pain returned. It got to the point where I couldn't keep down small sips of drinks. I was so weak and dehydrated that I knew I would be heading back to the hospital if my gastroenterologist did not intervene. Thankfully, and by the grace of God, he agreed to see me and prescribed domperidone.

It took a couple weeks before I could begin the medication, as it is approved for use only under the FDA's Investigational New Drug program and there are several requirements regarding its use. It comes with serious risks, such as sudden cardiac arrhythmia and cardiac arrest, but given my alternative—which was death, in my mind—I chose to try it. Reglan is often offered as an option, but due to the potentially serious and permanent side effects, my doctor advised against it, and I agreed it was not a good option for me.

Fortunately, domperidone has offered some relief, and I have not experienced any negative side effects. It has truly saved my life. It is no cure by any stretch of the imagination, and I worry about its long-term effects on my health, but it has almost completely ended my nausea and it has lessened my pain to the point where I can at least function. I will say that its impact has lessened somewhat over time, and my symptoms have worsened as of late, but my new specialist doubled my dose, and this seems to be helping. I am concerned that it will once again lose its effectiveness, but for now, it offers a measure of relief.

Domperidone is the only medication I take regularly now, but I have tried a few others. I was given erythromycin, an antibiotic which is also thought to act as a prokinetic, but I had a quite violent reaction to it (vomiting and severe stomach pain), so I discontinued it after a few days. I also tried Xifaxan (rifaximin), which is generally used as a treatment for small intestine bacterial overgrowth (SIBO), to help with my extreme abdominal bloating, but it offered no real relief, so I chose to discontinue it as well. I have, to date, refused antiemetics and pain medications. Many in the support groups must take these medications simply to get them through the day and lead any sort of functional life, but at this point, I am able to continue without them.

I fear what my future holds some days. An ever-increasing dosage of domperidone does not seem to be the solution, and the other medications of which I am aware would not be viable alternatives for me. Many opt for surgeries, such as pyloroplasty or placement of the gastric electrical stimulator, or must turn to enteral and parenteral nutrition. Perhaps that is what my future holds as well. I cannot say I welcome those treatments, but they are potentially lifesaving possibilities which I cannot rule out.

*

SAMANTHA ANDERSON
Samantha was diagnosed with idiopathic
gastroparesis in 2012 at age 26

I am going to be honest. I cannot remember all the different combinations of medications I was given. I started off with the antibiotic erythromycin. In small doses it's been shown to help some people with gastroparesis. I was told the effect of it can wear off, and they are short term, however I just couldn't keep it down to help me.

According to my consultant, I had all the different types of anti-sickness and antiemetic medications offered in the United Kingdom on the National Health Service. These anti-sickness medications didn't work for me. They often helped me keep food down for longer, but I still had nausea, early satiety and bloating, and eventually I'd vomit more violently. I know that may sound weird to many people, but the gagging seemed harsher. It felt like my body was really trying to keep the food down, yet my body wanted it to come up.

I had tablets and liquids to help with constipation even though I'd still go once a week (generally on a regular day). I had medication to try to line the stomach and help with pain but they didn't work; I wasn't keeping enough down.

I then went on to have Botox in the stomach via endoscopy to try to help. It's meant to help keep parts of the stomach open to aid digestion. However, I was sick as soon as I came out of this procedure and unfortunately didn't benefit from it. I had intravenous fluids, vitamins and pain relief every month or so. Somehow I'd cope. My nurse once said that many people get used to a lack of nutrition and will just get on with it. I think it was her way to trying to build me up.

I also had a nasojejunal feeding tube that surpasses the stomach and feeds into the intestines. I must say I truly respect people who have this as I found it hard to cope, to move, to breathe and so on. I managed a few days with it. My feeds were round-the-clock. Twenty-five milliliters per hour made me feel extremely full (I had no liquids with this, either). I think they took it up to forty milliliters per hour, but bloating and so on made this so hard. As I didn't want to vomit, I couldn't drink liquids either. However, it did give me some much needed nutrition.

Whenever a newly approved drug came up that could maybe help gastroparesis, my consultant offered me it. However, as you can tell, for everyone with this condition, the medication is just trial and error.

For pain, it was so hard to get medication especially as I couldn't keep things down. I had a nerve block in my back to help with the stomach pain. At the time, I wasn't sure it was helping much as I was still in pain. However, the effects of it started to wear off after a week and I realized the amount of pain I was actually in. Eventually, after being in pain with gastroparesis and a wisdom tooth, the doctor who really listened gave me pain patches. I used them for about six to ten months. They didn't take away the constant pain but took the edge off and made day-to-day living slightly easier. They were weekly patches, that contained four in a packet, but it was always a fight to get more. They were worried about me getting addicted to them and them not helping other gastroparesis symptoms. I stopped these after my surgery.

Finally the consultant referred me to the surgeon about getting the pacemaker. It took a long time for the surgeon to agree to the surgery, as like all other treatments it may have not helped at all. Once he said yes, we had to ask for funding. We couldn't just get it on the NHS. I suppose it's a bit like seeing if you can get it on your insurance, but I'm not positive so I hope I'm not offending my gastroparesis warriors in the United States. However, after three attempts and appeals, I was told I couldn't get the funding, so we had to raise the money for it (£20,000). We managed it and I got the pacemaker on March 2, 2016.

The pacemaker hasn't been a miracle. It hasn't stopped all symptoms. I still struggle daily, but it is so much easier and I'm happy I have it. I'm on and can keep down pregabalin, a tablet pain killer, most of the time. I'm working on diets that will help with it such as lactose-free, which I knew before I was ill, and gluten-free too. At the moment, puree is easier on the stomach than proper solids, and no more than half a cup of food at a time. I'm told I can try treatments I had before the pacer if I don't improve more over time. I can't do all things at once, as I need to know what treatment is helping.

My vitamins could also be low, even now, especially vitamin D. I have at times been given tablets to help with this deficiency. My iron can at times be borderline, but I seem to cope with it. It is definitely a journey.

*

JOLI ATKINS
Joli was diagnosed with
gastroparesis in 2015 at age 36

The doctors have tried giving me Reglan to try to speed up my motility but it does not seem to help. I have a bad reaction to it as well. It makes me very restless. The other medications they can give you for gastroparesis, the doctors do not want to try, because of the other side effects.

*

MEGAN BOGGS
Megan was diagnosed with
gastroparesis in 2017 at age 38

I have tried a gastric pacemaker, and numerous medications: Zofran, Benadryl, Reglan, domperidone, and Compazine.

*

TRISHA BUNDY
Trisha was diagnosed with
gastroparesis in 2013 at age 35

Initially, we attempted an all-liquid diet with the intention to slowly transition to soft solids that were low in fiber. Unfortunately, I was unable to receive an adequate amount of liquids orally. Boost, Ensure, Gatorade, and Powerade still caused pain and nausea. To improve my nutritional state, I received my GJ feeding tube in May 2013. This feeds directly in my small intestines. For a brief period of time, my health improved as long as I didn't eat and instead depended on my feeding tube for nutrition. However, during the summer of 2014, I began having difficulty with my formula feeds as well. In an attempt to decrease the severe pain that I was experiencing, my gallbladder was taken out in December 2014. We considered having a gastric stimulator placed, but after discussing my case with other physicians, I was told that I would not be a good candidate for it. Apparently, it is most effective for patients with diabetic gastroparesis (which I don't have) or patients without other gastrointestinal issues.

Though having my gallbladder removed was effective in eliminating a portion of my abdominal pain, and a feeding tube helped improve my nutritional intake, I still was having constant pain, nausea, and difficulties with receiving adequate nutrition. Therefore, we decided to administer the Sitzmarks study. During this study, I had to forfeit all laxatives for a week. For five days I consumed pills which had twenty-four markers within them. On day six, I had an x-ray to see where the markers were located. Ideally, they were supposed to be completely out of the digestive system. However, all the markers remained in the beginning of my large intestine. The result proved that I had colonic inertia—my colon did NOT work effectively.

As a result of the Sitzmarks study, I became impacted and had great difficulty resuming my bowel regimen. When trying to return to normalcy, I returned to using my daily Linzess, lactulose, MiraLax, senna, Colace, and enemas. In regards to treatment, we decided to use Mestinon to see if it would improve my intestinal motility, which unfortunately was not successful due to the severity of side effects without any recognizable improvements. After failing this treatment, in January 2016, I had a total colectomy with ileostomy pouch. My colon was removed and my small intestines empty waste into a bag located on my abdomen. Sometimes people with colonic inertia are able to have a resection, in which the colon is removed and the small intestine is connected to the rectum. However, this is not an option for me due to my pelvic floor dyssynergia, which did not improve with pelvic floor biofeedback or pelvic floor physical therapy.

In order to decrease dehydration symptoms, I receive lactated ringers IV infusions five times per week. These fluids, which I receive through my port at home, have helped me maintain my hydration levels. Along with IV fluids, we also continue to work on symptom management with medicinal trial and error attempts, making adjustments as needed. Iron infusions and specific vitamin supplements have successfully been administered when deficiencies have been noted.

Dealing with chronic illness can sometimes make me feel insufficient, sad, angry, frustrated, useless, guilty, and even scared. Psychotherapy has aided me in developing coping skills for times when I feel like I've lost my purpose and felt like a disappointment or burden to my family. Living with chronic illness is a difficult journey to accept; my old life is no longer the normal that I once knew. Instead I have a new normal that I have to learn to navigate.

Having a psychologist did not immediately solve all my problems or cure my physical illness, nor will it. Keeping my mindset and spirits positive can be a very demanding and troublesome task, especially when I feel so awful and miss out on special life events. Seeing my psychologist is helping me achieve inner peace and the ability to keep fighting with the mentality to never give up, no matter how difficult my health journey. Therapy is helping me rediscover how to live with my chronic illness, how to survive, and how to stay afloat during life's most tortuous storms.

Physical therapy is another treatment that my doctor suggested for me. Because of all the changes my body has gone through from weight loss, surgeries, malnutrition, dehydration, and inactivity from being so symptomatic, my muscles began losing their stamina. To retain strength, avoid additional muscle deterioration, and improve stability when on my feet, my doctor chose to have me treated by a physical therapist. My physical therapist is teaching me new exercises and stretches that I can safely do at home while sitting or lying down. She is also having me complete balance related exercises during our appointments.

*

LISA COLANDREA
Lisa was diagnosed with
gastroparesis in 2016 at age 42

Since my diagnosis, I've tried all the medications they typically prescribe to those with gastroparesis. The first was Reglan, which I and many others cannot take due to side effects such as shaking, tremors, and twitching. Nothing I took helped my motility. Zofran barely touched the surface of the debilitating nausea. Most of the medications actually made my stomach pain and bloating much worse.

I was never a candidate for the gastric stimulator because of previous stomach surgeries. The only other options I was given was to have a pyloroplasty surgery or have a feeding tube placed. A feeding tube for me was an absolute last resort. So I decided to have the pyloroplasty surgery in March 2017. The surgery didn't make any difference at all. I still continue to suffer from nausea, pain, vomiting and bloating. So I'm not sure putting my body through another surgery was worth it.

I spent just under a month in the hospital after the surgery due to some complications. I then returned home and ended up back in the emergency room twice and admitted into the hospital due to severe dehydration and malnutrition. During my last admit it was decided that I needed to go forward with the feeding tube or I would not be able to sustain any hydration, nor would I be able to become nutritionally healthy on my own. The feeding tube has just been placed within a few weeks of me writing this.

*

TAMMY DOWNS

Tammy was diagnosed with Crohn's disease, irritable bowel syndrome, spastic colon, gastroesophageal reflux disease, and gastritis in 2006 at age 46, gastroparesis in 2015 at age 56, and motility dysfunction disorder of the rectum and pelvic floor in 2016 at age 58

I have not been offered any medical therapies, except for my dyssynergic defecation dynamics (type II) motility problem. Probiotics seem to help me. I have no place to go for physical therapy that my insurance will cover, so I have to deal with my problems and do the best I can.

*

SKYE FALCON

Skye was diagnosed with gastroparesis and other autoimmune diseases in 2006 at age 25

Most of the medical therapies I've tried were pharmaceutical. From the time my symptoms first began over a decade ago, I was put on prednisone and a low dose chemotherapy cocktail to turn off my immune system. In the beginning it seemed to shut off and re-regulate whatever was happening inside of me reasonably quickly. At that time, it was only confirmed to be the scleroderma and scar tissue issues with celiac disease and a few minor secondary issues causing my troubles.

There came a point, however, when that medication cocktail tried to kill me, literally. After taking the prednisone and cycling up to my set dosage, I suffered a severe allergic reaction completely out of the blue. Spending some time in the hospital, flushing my system, and giving me medications to combat the effects seemed to put me back on track once again, and nixed steroids from my medication line-up. I have tried numerous medications for the issues that I face, and the majority of them cause those same kinds of catastrophic body reactions. The medications that I am currently on now, I have been taking for over six years. I have tried countless times to come off them, and try a newer, more effective drug, only to be met in the emergency room again, forcibly stopping another allergic reaction.

In the past few years, as things have shifted inside even more, some of the medications that were working well stopped. Reglan, one that works so well for many minus its own deadly side effects, began causing neurological damage, crazy nerve issues and more pain. The multiple proton pump inhibitors I've been on for over ten years have now caused some pretty serious esophageal issues, and I am dependent on them. Just like an addict needs their fix, I can no longer function without taking these medications. Except this fix has caused numerous cysts, lumps, and things that have been removed. The Plaquenil I have lived on for over a decade has begun to harm my eyes and sight. All the other medications have their own side effects, all of which I seem to be seriously affected by. There seems to be no effective pharmaceutical treatment for many of the big chronic illnesses, and treating them with drugs for other illnesses is not logical in my head.

*

ROBIN MCNAMARA
Robin was diagnosed with
gastroparesis in 2013 at age 55

My current doctor put me on Dexilant, Remeron, alprazolam, Zantac, and domperidone, which all worked their magic and got me feeling better. I also do acupuncture. When I fall off the acupuncture wagon, I feel it. The only side effect I can't handle is the nausea. It's beyond miserable, especially when it pops up out of nowhere.

*

TAMMY PITTMAN
Tammy was diagnosed with gastroparesis and
irritable bowel syndrome in 2014 at age 34

I was on Reglan with the side effect of severe dyskinesia (tremors, uncontrollable movements) and was taken off the medication. I take a laxative and stool softener daily. If I don't take it, my intestines go crazy and don't know what they're supposed to do.

*

TAYLOR SCHMITZ
Taylor was diagnosed with idiopathic
gastroparesis in 2014 at age 22

As far as western medicine, I've been on numerous medications. I honestly can't even remember them all, but I've been on nightmare medication after nightmare medication. None of the medications helped in any way, and they all had very scary and uncomfortable side effects. Reglan was the worst, and I highly advise people to not use this medication. Just because it's FDA approved, doesn't mean it won't be recalled for how dangerous it is later in life. I was also told that if I didn't gain any weight, I would have a feeding tube placed. I didn't go back to that doctor after that.

Natural therapies that have helped me are acupuncture, holistic remedies, natural diets like the specific carbohydrate diet, probiotics, vitamins and supplements, and various teas for different issues. I've also used Iberogast, sauerkraut juice, beet kvass, and bone broth for gut healing. Every natural remedy was worth it. Naturopathic doctors aren't covered by insurance where I live, so it's a bit more expensive, but in the long run it's so much cheaper and a much better investment. I don't visit the emergency room anymore. I don't go to the doctor and pay copays anymore. I visit Dr. White a couple of times a year and keep in contact via email.

*

DEB SHRADER-TROTTER
Deb was diagnosed with
gastroparesis in 1999 at age 37

I have tried many treatments. My gastric electrical stimulator had to be removed. I was offered the InterStim therapy but my gastric stimulator was shocking me and causing pain. It was not a good option for me because of the curvature of my scoliosis at my lower back. My peripherally inserted central catheter (PICC) was in until I was transitioned to my port. Oral medications do not work well due to the absorption issues I deal with as a result of the motility disorder.

While I have had all but seven inches of my large intestine removed, I still deal with my intestines backing up. The chronic intestinal pseudo-obstruction syndrome part of the motility disorder? It creates a constant battle of trying to move bile out of the intestine. My last obstruction in 2015, a piece of the upper small intestine was twisted and obstructed which required surgery to remove a small section and clean out as many adhesions as possible. I was then told my intestines were too twisted and there were too many adhesions to ever put a tube in for tube feedings. We had been discussing tube feedings as a possibility because of my nutritional stats at the time. They were doing TPN, total parenteral nutrition, in hospital but did not want to do it out of hospital and run up my chance of infection by doing it continuously.

*

JESSICA SPENCE
Jessica was diagnosed with
gastroparesis in 2016 at age 25

In the beginning, there were antacids and stool softeners that had zero impact on my symptoms. Next came what felt like dozens of different types of anxiety medications to help me calm down and sleep. Those helped me sleep but the side effects were an unbridled rage that cost me many friendships before I decided to stop taking them. I realized that the people who loved and supported me were worth more to me than a few extra hours of sleep.

After that I started taking Zofran which has been a lifeline in my worst moments, even if the relief is short-lived. I've been on and off Reglan a few times. It tends to work for a few weeks and then my body stops responding and I have to stop for a few months.

Last year I decided to ask about the gastric stimulator to see if that would help me vomit less. The success rate is better for diabetic gastroparesis, but I wanted to try it anyways. I had my Entera stimulator placed two days before my twenty-sixth birthday. It has been working really well for me so far, even though I do not have diabetes. There are still rough days, but I have gained fifteen pounds in the six months since my surgery, and am hoping to keep climbing.

*

NICOLE STARZYNSKI
Nicole was diagnosed with
gastroparesis in 2016 at age 33

Gastroparesis is pretty limiting when it comes to medication and surgical treatments. Unfortunately most people do not find relief with the treatments that are currently offered.

In March 2016, right after being diagnosed, I was put on Reglan. Reglan was probably one of the scariest medicines I ever took. When my doctor sat down with me and went over all the side effects, I was a little freaked out. I went home and looked at clinical studies and the FDA's website. What I found did not give me any reason to take it. So I decided to think about it for a few days. The script was sent directly to the pharmacy and they automatically filled it. When I went to pick up other prescriptions, my pharmacist gave me the Reglan. He also went over the side effects with me and told me to think it over. I talked it over with my boyfriend and my mom. Both of them were completely against me taking the medicine, so I decided I wasn't going to take it. From what I could find, the risk was usually after taking it long term, but if it worked I would be taking it long term. The statistics of people who had a side effect were a little alarming. I know sometimes this information is presented in a way to make people not want to take something, but everything I learned in my support groups, FDA website, and clinical studies, was just bad.

Two weeks went by. I was sick, and tired of feeling so sick. So I said, "The heck with it!" and took one. The first day I felt really weird and had the worst headache. By the end of the next day, my left eye started twitching a bit, kind of like an irritation. It was weird so I never took it again.

When I called my doctor's office, they said they submitted my name for the irritable bowel syndrome clinic and I was number fifty-seven on the list. They also prescribed me Linzess to help with the constipation, and finally stopped pushing the MiraLax. The Linzess worked but made every stool I had like water and gave me severe stomach cramps. I found if I took it a few times a week or once a week, it helped get things moving and didn't bother me as much. Sometimes it didn't help and that's when I felt like I was filled with concrete.

My first doctor would not give me any medicine for nausea. You would have thought I was asking for an illegal drug. I wanted something that wouldn't make me want to puke. My regular doctor prescribed me Zofran and even researched to see if there was anything else he could try, but at the time I had just got accepted into Cleveland Clinic and Johns Hopkins so we decided to hold off.

At my first appointment at Cleveland Clinic, the doctor prescribed the dissolving Zofran (I never leave my house without at least two with me) and started me on erythromycin, a prokinetic drug used as an antibiotic. As an antibiotic, people complained of having stomachaches when they took it. Researchers eventually determined that erythromycin stimulates motilin receptors in the GI tract, which in turn stimulate contractions and result in increased GI motility. However, erythromycin can also cause more stomach pain and slow down the small intestine transit. This leads to a total backup of your system and slows digestion. So I am not sure why they continue to try to use this drug. It did not help me; it made me constipated and made my stomach pain even worse. I only took this medicine for two months before I decided no more of this madness. Every medicine they have given me has had some awful, adverse effect. The exception is Zofran, although that does make me constipated.

The SmartPill test, which I had been waiting for insurance to cover since 2009, was one of the more interesting tests I have had. It involved a little, clear, Tylenol-shaped capsule that didn't look too big until I tried to swallow it. Man, oh man, when the lady handed it to me and I put it on my tongue, I had a few moments of thinking, "Oh, my god. This is going to get stuck in my throat!" But I was able to swallow it. I wore a black electronic box around my neck that looked like the first ever blackberry. It had a small LED screen that displayed pressure and PH. I kept my own notes the entire time. The PH did not go above one and the pressure stayed around negative nineteen to negative thirty for the first twenty-three hours. The day after swallowing the SmartPill, I felt so bloated and nauseous. I had to keep track of everything I ate and every time I took a bowel movement.

Sleeping was hard because I was so worried that the box around my neck would be too far from the SmartPill and the test would error out. Luckily that didn't happen and the SmartPill made its exit back into the world a few days after I swallowed it. I had a pretty good idea of what the results were based on the notes I took, but decided instead of making myself crazy, I would send the box back to Cleveland and wait for them to call me with the results.

The results of my SmartPill test revealed that it took twenty-two hours and fifty minutes for my stomach to empty. We already knew I had gastroparesis. The more important part my doctor had been worried about concerned my small intestines. Finally some good news: both my small and large intestines were normal, so I was finally cleared to have surgery! I still had to wait four weeks to see my doctor, but I was finally another step closer to beating this!

I had been experiencing blackouts. I puked and woke up two hours later on my bathroom floor, no idea that I had been out for two hours. That was scary. My kidneys started to have problems; I had infections, stones, and blood in my urine. The effects of this disease were starting to take their toll on my working organs.

Sadly, this is how this disease kills people. Since my immune system is so low, pretty much every time I leave my house it's almost guaranteed I will have some new virus or sickness. I am tired of waking up and vomiting like the exorcist. I want to eat food. I want to live to see my baby grow up. I am lucky to have such a strong support group in my parents, my daughter, Josh and friends. I also have gained some friends who have been so supportive through this journey and there are no words to express to these people for helping me find the strength to kick this disease's butt.

Like many people with severe gastroparesis, I am at grade three, gastric failure. I was told that I would never be one hundred percent, that my stomach is about eighty percent dead and they have no way of knowing if the nerves will still die or if it will stop. I was given three options for surgical treatments: peroral endoscopic pyloromyotomy, gastric stimulator or stomach removal. I went with option one, peroral endoscopic pyloromyotomy (G-POEM, POP), since I was told that most likely I will need other treatments, and even after this surgery I may need medication to help me digest. I started to freak out.

I was told that the surgery would be minimally invasive with no cuts on my stomach. They would use an endoscopy scope to perform the procedure. I was told only a few surgeons could do this procedure and it was very new. So far they had a great success. This was also the surgery that had me driving to Baltimore for their clinical study. During POP, the physician would cut the pylorus, a muscular valve that empties the stomach, without surgery. Using advanced endoscopic tools, the entire procedure would be performed through the mouth without the need for incisions. After the lining of the stomach was opened, only the pylorus would be divided under high-definition vision, improving the emptying ability of the stomach.

I knew the road ahead would be long. I was only thirty-four, a single mom, and just wanted to be able to eat and live a somewhat normal life. My daughter was only twelve and worried about me. She worried that this disease would take her mother from her.

My health had been on a steady decline over the past few years. I couldn't remember the last time I actually ate a real meal or anything that didn't make me sick. If it wasn't immediate, there was some awful aftermath. The doctors wouldn't let me wait to have the surgery. It was either that or nutrition tubes because my body was basically attacking itself at that point. I had kidney stones too many times to count since last summer. It seemed like one thing after the next.

During all of this I also had a cyst on the outside of my vulva that was so large I couldn't walk. They said it could be caused from numerous things, but considering what was going on with everything, they didn't think it was odd. I had to have that cut open while I was awake. The nurse started talking about Dr. Pimple Popper. Oddly enough, she had just been on TV a few days prior to that. She and the doctor mentioned that they couldn't believe I handled the pain as well as I did when they drained the giant cyst. When you are in pain almost every day, you learn ways to almost take yourself out of yourself. I use breathing techniques similar to lamaze for childbirth and sometimes I put myself somewhere far, far away. It doesn't make the pain stop but it might stop a panic attack which isn't going to help anything. It also helps to get through any extreme bursts of pain.

I wanted to have a successful surgery and thought this was the beginning of my road to recovery. T-minus twenty-four hours to surgery day! I was surprised at how calm I felt. I was excited to finally start my journey to living life again. The fourteen months leading up to that day had been long but it only made me a stronger, better person who appreciated the little things in life and learned to let so much go.

After eight months of visiting doctors to have this surgery, I couldn't believe the day was finally here! My daughter's Christmas wish was coming true. Kirstin wanted God and the Spirit of Christmas to bring us a Christmas miracle. She told me right before my surgery that she finally had hope and couldn't believe her wish came true. I knew the next few months would be long, but I believed it was my chance to beat this. I hoped I would be enjoying real food again by Easter. I was lucky that I had such wonderful doctors and it was very reassuring to have surgery at one of the best hospitals in the country.

Four days post-op, I hadn't been nauseous or puked since the morning of my surgery! That by itself was huge for me. I hadn't gone that long in over fourteen months. My surgery went very well. The hardest part was not being allowed to even have a drink of water for fifty hours. Right out of surgery, I almost went into cardiac arrest and woke up coughing with doctors all around me. That was pretty scary. They were afraid I may have ripped the stitches open, but did a contrast scan on Wednesday morning and said I was one hundred percent leak-free. So on Wednesday afternoon, I was finally allowed to start clear liquids and I tolerated them very well. They discharged me on Wednesday afternoon. I went home and took it easy. I was still very swollen and in pain, but already felt better than I had in a very long time! It looked like Kirstin's Christmas wish came true. I had to go back to Cleveland on the Monday following my surgery and hoped everything would continue to go well.

I was doing better each day. I ate puréed broccoli cream soup and was still nausea free! I was still very sore from the surgery and the trip to Cleveland was too much. The day after my appointment, I was in the most pain yet, but I couldn't complain. I still couldn't believe how great I felt, from only ten days prior being sick from drinking water to being nausea free. I had no words, except I really missed food. I couldn't wait to consume food instead of liquid. Luckily my mom was superwoman and made me new things every day.

It's really scary to have surgery that has been done on less than a hundred people, when they haven't done a procedure long enough to have any idea what will happen long-term. It comes down to taking a chance on something that could change your life, or not taking the chance on something because it's still too new. Only one person can make that decision and that's me. I decided to go with a procedure that was still very new instead of the stimulator because I wanted to start with the least invasive surgery first. I was overly confident the surgery was going to fix me completely.

Sadly it wasn't as successful as I had hoped. Hopefully next time I won't be so positive that something is going to work for me, but I don't want to be negative either. It's just that the let-down after that is not something you just get over or bounce back from. It's a daily struggle when you know you made the wrong decision, and have to wait another six months to have the next surgery. Plus, there's the fear of the next surgery not being your last, and of experimental surgeries not working long-term as planned. There is the constant dread that this is never going to end. The surgery wasn't a total loss. It wasn't as successful as I had hoped, but the next stop is a gastric stimulator and hopefully a more positive outcome.

*

JENNIFER ZUBIK
Jennifer was diagnosed with idiopathic gastroparesis in 2010 at age 27

I have experienced a wide variety of trial and error tests, treatments and medications due to having gastroparesis. Sonograms, ultrasounds, CT scans, MRIs, endoscopies, colonoscopies, Botox injections and gastric emptying studies are some of the tests and procedures I've had done. Medications included Pepcid, Nexium, Prilosec, Zantac, MiraLax, Zofran, Compazine, Phenergan, scopolamine patches, erythromycin, Reglan, domperidone, cisapride, Carafate, and Ativan, just to name a few.

Out of all those medications listed, the only ones that gave me any relief were Compazine, Ativan and Carafate. I ate Compazine like it was candy. At one point, I had to use Compazine suppositories because the pills were not effective since my body was not absorbing them from not being able to eat. Some of these medications were very costly, too. Zofran did not help me at all, which was lucky because when I was prescribed it, I did not have medical insurance and it cost almost two hundred dollars for only ten pills. Most of the medications were not effective for me and did not give me any relief.

I experienced side effects from some of the medications. Reglan was awful. It gave me migraines, muscle spasms, twitching, and made the nausea worse (I didn't think that was even possible). Phenergan actually made me drool; it was weird. Scopolamine patches worked well, but blurred my vision if I left the patch on for too long, so I had to limit my use of those. Most medications just made me extremely sleepy, especially when I would first start taking them, but then that would subside after being on them for a while.

Botox injections into my pylorus offered some relief and did help me function better. I had the injections every eight to twelve weeks for a few years until my insurance would not cover the procedure anymore. I was hospitalized numerous times due to malnourishment and dehydration and would spend days hooked up to IVs. I developed bile reflux gastritis, pancreatitis and my doctor also discovered I had dozens of ulcers in my stomach. Therefore, more medications and more treatments were needed.

My doctors kept telling me I needed feeding tubes and warned me it would happen, but I refused. At the time, the only other options available and offered to me were having gastric bypass surgery or implanting a gastric neurostimulator. However, I did not qualify to have the gastric bypass surgery because I only weighed eighty-seven pounds and the doctors feared I would lose additional weight. The stimulator had numerous side effects, as everything does, including the possibility of not working.

Despite the negative facts presented to me, in October 2013, I had a gastric neurostimulator implanted at the Cleveland Clinic. I was somewhat hesitant and anxious about having it done, but was also at the point of willing to try anything. What could it hurt? The recovery from the surgery was not as bad as I had expected it to be. The results were not immediate either, which I anticipated. After several follow ups at the clinic, which was over three hours one way from my house, I would go every two to three months depending on how nauseous I was, to get the stimulator adjusted. With each visit, my symptoms did improve and as time passed I began to introduce more food into my diet again. I began putting on weight, and had finally reached one hundred pounds.

It took about two years after the surgery, but I could enjoy food (still with a limited diet) and going out to eat with friends and family again. I had to slowly adjust and introduce different kinds of food and quantities. I had to retrain my mind and body to eat again, but I succeeded. To me, it was truly a miracle.

Then in February 2015, I began experiencing major pain at the location of the stimulator. The original surgeon who implanted the stimulator had left the Cleveland Clinic to open a clinic in Abu Dhabi. I had to be evaluated by the new surgeons who replaced him. I only met with one fellow surgeon first. To say the least, he was extremely disrespectful and ill-mannered. His nurse was as well. He insisted there was no reason to be experiencing the excruciating pain I was feeling and that it was all in my head. He told me pain management wouldn't help and that I needed to see a psychiatrist. Just to please me, he said I could see a doctor at home for pain management.

That same day, I met with my gastroenterologist at the clinic. He believed me and commented that it looked as if the stimulator was not in the original location where it was implanted. He believed something was wrong and was causing the pain. He said the next step would be to find out whether it was nerve pain. He sent me home with a prescription for lidocaine patches. He said to try those for a month over the area of where my stimulator was. If the pain went away, then he would know that it was not related to nerves and that the stimulator needed to be moved. However, when I went to get my patches at the pharmacy, my insurance would not cover them. The cost for a one month supply was three hundred dollars. Due to the cost, my gastroenterologist said to get a two week supply and hope that I got results.

Before that, because of the cost, I met with a doctor regarding pain management. Again, another rude and belittling doctor. The doctor stated that because I could walk, get dressed, drive, and push through the pain to work without any pain pills (I have never taken a pain pill during this entire gastroparesis experience because ibuprofen makes me sick so I feared anything else), that I was fine and it was a mental issue in my head. Again, I left another doctor's office in tears.

Therefore, I tried the lidocaine patches. I had almost immediate relief when I had a patch on; it was bewildering. I called my doctor who said that because the pain subsided with the patch, the placement of the stimulator was causing the pain. I went back to the clinic and met with the other surgeon this time. After evaluating me, he realized that the position of the stimulator had moved. He said that somehow, my stitches pulled and the stimulator had dropped and was now sitting on my pelvic bone, which was most likely causing all the pain. Therefore, the stimulator needed to be repositioned.

The nurse, the same rude one with the previous surgeon I met with, then had to meet with me to schedule my surgery to move the stimulator. She apologized for being inconsiderate and explained that in all the years they have researched and performed the implantation of the stimulator, they had never heard of that happening, or anything happening that would have caused that much pain at the site. My surgeon assumed that because I was so thin, which made the stimulator bump out of my stomach, and was so young and active, that anything I could have done may have caused the stitches to pull and make the stimulator fall.

Finally, in June 2015, one week after my thirty-third birthday, I had a second surgery to move the stimulator up higher. By May 2016, I had transformed. I gained all my weight back that I had lost in the beginning and was able to eat anything again. I was miraculously back to who I was before this terrible journey began, and had my life back. Fortunately, I was able to tolerate the stimulator and have recovered, which I thank god for every single day.

*

CHAPTER SEVEN

Toolbox of Relief

> Being able to walk pain-free is a blessing. Being able to walk without showing the pain is a skill. -KYLIE MCPHERSON

Many sufferers find traditional medical therapies aren't enough, and seek alternative and naturopathic remedies to augment the toolbox. Ranging from acupuncture to yoga and meditation to medicinal marijuana, herbal therapies and beyond, what each person keeps in her armory is whatever brings the most relief. Which remedies and self-management tools help you the most?

*

MELISSA ADAMS VANHOUTEN
Melissa was diagnosed with
gastroparesis in 2014 at age 47

I haven't tried many complementary or alternative therapies although I consider them options now when I once did not. I take probiotics and prebiotics regularly, but am not certain it helps. I want it to help, and I've been told by both my regular gastroenterologist and many in the support groups that it is beneficial for my health, that it will increase my good bacteria and aid in digestion, but I do not know that those benefits have materialized. It would be difficult to judge, I think. I continue the probiotic in the hope that it is doing something behind the scenes.

I've also tried a few natural remedies such as peppermint, ginger, chicory, turmeric, dandelion root, aloe vera, and apple cider vinegar. While they did no noticeable harm, they also offer no relief. I have also tried EnteraGam (a medical food designed for the management of enteropathy), IBgard (an over-the-counter irritable bowel syndrome medication essentially made up of purified peppermint oil), and FDgard (another over-the-counter medical food made up of largely caraway and peppermint oils), none of which showed any benefit.

The one natural product which has offered me a small measure of relief (by reducing nausea and the sensation of fullness) is Iberogast. Iberogast is a blend of herbs including bitter candytuft, caraway, peppermint, angelica, chamomile, St. Mary's thistle, lemon balm, celandine, and licorice. It is thought to help with gastrointestinal function. It is quite expensive and tastes worse than just about anything I have had, but it does have a minor beneficial effect. If I hide it in an ounce or so of coffee, it is tolerable. Spoken like a true caffeine addict, I know!

My heating pad is my current best friend. Mine is a homemade version: a pillowcase of sorts with cornfeed inside that can be heated to my preferred temperature in the microwave. The heat (and possibly the weight of it) on my stomach and abdomen relax me and dull the pain a bit—enough, most times, to allow me to avoid the emergency room. The downside is that this method of pain relief has left likely permanent burns and scars on my body—not pretty, but a small price to pay for the relief it offers. I am well past bikini years anyway.

I have never tried acupuncture, acupressure, hypnosis, massage, biofeedback, reflexology, or anything similar, but I am not opposed to exploring these therapies. I have heard from some of my support group members that they help with symptoms or at least provide a measure of comfort and relaxation. I believe this, and I believe they could reduce stress, if nothing else. It is simply a matter of one thing at a time for me, and I will gradually work my way through the list.

The tests and the treatments associated with the management of this cruel disease are time-consuming, burdensome, and financially straining. I often worry about how we will continue down this chronic illness path without going bankrupt both emotionally and financially. It weighs heavy on my mind, and I do not like the toll it takes on my family. I wonder what sacrifices they'll have to make to accommodate my ever-increasing needs. They have already given up so much. But my main concern is that all therapies, traditional medical and alternative, will eventually fail me. And that is the devastation I fear most for my daughter, my husband, and my many loved ones.

*

SAMANTHA ANDERSON
Samantha was diagnosed with idiopathic gastroparesis in 2012 at age 26

We (my family and I) decided to try a course of reflexology. The lady was lovely, but as someone who doesn't love pampering I didn't enjoy this. I'm not keen on my feet being touched anyway, but it wasn't comfortable. She brought a very comfortable chair, but it wasn't very pleasurable when she was touching parts of my feet. I was often glad she was moving on. After each session I felt awful. I know it sounds strange, but I felt worse. One time after a session, I got a stomach bug on top of feeling bad. I know I would have got the bug anyway, but I felt it wasn't helping.

In saying that, I do love a massage; I go for at least four massages a year. It doesn't particularly help with symptoms, and some parts of the massage can be uncomfortable, but it definitely helps to make me feel more relaxed and rejuvenated. Although I don't sleep well anymore, I do sleep better on nights when I have had a massage.

It was suggested I try acupuncture. I'm willing to try most things. I've spoken to people about it, and it being uncomfortable. The people I've spoken to were unsure about the procedure, and so I'm not sure I want to pay for this yet.

My best therapy, or one of the things that has helped me get through each day the most, is my dog. He wasn't bought for therapy. In fact, he wasn't bought at all. He was given to us by my sister. He was one of her dog's puppies. We, or mainly I, didn't want to have a dog. I thought it would be too much work. However, he helps me every day. Being with him and walking him every day, gives me a reason to get up and carry on. The love he gives me makes me smile and improves my day. He is definitely worth his weight in gold and I would recommend to anyone who is feeling poorly to get a dog if they have the ability to look after it.

When I first had the pacemaker I started taking Iberogast, an herbal liquid supplement that helps digestive issues and is meant to speed up gastric emptying. I only took it for a while and needed my pacemaker adjusted, so it didn't work too well but is definitely something I would try again in combination with other treatments. My only problem with it is that it can be costly.

*

JOLI ATKINS
Joli was diagnosed with
gastroparesis in 2015 at age 36

I have not tried any other therapies for this disease. I am hesitant to try any of these just because most of what I try doesn't seem to help. I have come to realize that as long as I keep on a mostly liquid diet, I do not have too many problems. At this point, I have to take my health in my own hands and do what works best for me because no one else seems to want to help me.

*

MEGAN BOGGS
Megan was diagnosed with
gastroparesis in 2017 at age 38

I've tried iridology, counseling, acupuncture, massage therapy, chiropractors, personal training, psychics and mediums.

*

TRISHA BUNDY
Trisha was diagnosed with
gastroparesis in 2013 at age 35

I have attempted ginger capsules and ginger chews to help with nausea, essential oils to place in the bath or rub on my skin in hopes of improving nausea, insomnia, and digestion, as well as probiotics. None of these therapies have proven to be of any benefit to me. I noted no improvement whatsoever.

Along with my current medical treatments, I use peppermint and cinnamon to decrease my nausea. I have found that hard candy and sometimes gum, along with my prescribed nausea medications can be helpful. They do not necessarily remove the nausea, but can help it be a little more tolerable. In addition, my heating pad, hot soaks in the bathtub, and listening to music can help decrease my pain levels. I have only had a professional massage once. It was a hot stone massage. It was very relaxing and definitely something that I would like to try again, but can't honestly say if it helped any symptoms that I've been dealing with.

My family physician has discussed the possibility of trying acupuncture for my chronic nausea and pain, which I was willing to try. However, upon consulting with the physician who specializes in acupuncture, they decided that it was unlikely to be beneficial in my situation. I will continue to keep my mind open to the possibility of trying acupuncture.

*

LISA COLANDREA
Lisa was diagnosed with
gastroparesis in 2016 at age 42

Alternatively, using medical cannabis has really been the only thing that has naturally helped my symptoms of gastroparesis. It helps with some of the pain, nausea and anxiety, and helps to increase my appetite. I've tried things like ginger, acupuncture and probiotics, as well as over-the-counter nausea treatments. None of these have helped. My doctors have been supportive of my alternative therapies. They feel that anything I can do to help the symptoms is worth trying.

*

TAMMY DOWNS

Tammy was diagnosed with Crohn's disease, irritable bowel syndrome, spastic colon, gastroesophageal reflux disease, and gastritis in 2006 at age 46, gastroparesis in 2015 at age 56, and motility dysfunction disorder of the rectum and pelvic floor in 2016 at age 58

I have used ginger root and made tea with honey to help with nausea. I have been taking Vitamin B_6, probiotics, and my medications that I am being given. I have started adding protein to my smoothies a little at a time. I have not tried homeopathy or acupuncture, and I cannot go to a chiropractor. My dietary supplements are Boost and protein powders added to my smoothies. I also add Propel to help with my electrolytes when I am dehydrated and becoming malnourished.

*

SKYE FALCON

Skye was diagnosed with gastroparesis and other autoimmune diseases in 2006 at age 25

I like to try anything if it is natural, and anything else at least once if there is proof there is a chance it will help. Twenty years ago, I was not as open and educated about the dangers of prescription medications. After my first year dealing with autoimmune issues, that mindset completely changed. Being educated about everything that went into my body was essential, because doing everything I could to avoid feeling as terrible as I always felt was a must.

One of the first therapies I tried was massage therapy. This was the main thing that kept my last pregnancy viable to thirty-four weeks. Not only calming, it was a good time to work through mental blocks that came with the diseases, shifts, and illnesses. During the massage, I was able to calm my mind and focus on other things. There came a point, however, when the massages all turned too painful to bear, and I could not lay on the table or sit comfortably for long periods of time. My back bones, which once cracked easily with stretching and twisting, now barely moved. I screamed at the slightest pressure. I was hardening internally, and massage therapy was no longer for me.

Biofeedback and meditation entered my life around the same time as my freshly built gardens at my then house, which was in the country. This was also around the time I made the dietary change to be free of gluten, dairy, and soy, and limit eggs to help ease the inflammation in my body. People thought I was losing my mind, and few took the time to understand what being gluten-free really meant. Meeting with a yoga master, I was taught how to be one with myself. That alone has helped me stay on track, continue to push forward even in the worst faces of adversity, and gives me the strength when no one else is around to help me out. Although these days, I can no longer do most of the yoga positions I was taught. I now focus on just the meditational aspects. With the outdoor meditation, often while gardening, came learning to breathe. Really, really inhale and exhale.

I had made some friends with respiratory therapists, and had a plan made for working my lungs and stretching tissues, since exercise was not on my high-end to do list. It is truly amazing what deep breathing, clearing your mind, and refocusing can do for illness.

Most recently I have begun trying essential oils. I do not play into the hype from any of the multi-level marketing rep companies out there, and choose to support any company that is natural, organic, and gives back to the community. My first experience with essential oil was horrible. I was sent to the emergency room with a severe respiratory reaction to lavender. Lavender! I was never told of possible side effects, or adverse reaction. The rep was more concerned with the sale than our friendship, or my health. It was just as much my fault for not researching first. From that point on I began researching, learning, attending classes, and teaching myself about oils. Now we use them for lots of things, although lavender is not welcome in our household. The oils help with nerves, muscle pains, bacteria around the house, nausea, and more. But that said, it is different for everyone, and how they help me might not be the same for someone else. We diffuse and use rollers, lotions, and creams, but we do not ingest. Due to the sensitivities in our gastrointestinal tracts, we have found by trial and error that is a bad idea.

I am also very open to trying and using cannabidiol (CBD) oil for nausea and pain. I've had the experience and joy of using it before and currently, and feels it would be most beneficial to so many others if it were available over the counter. Of all the alternative things I have tried, essential oils and meditation have helped me the most.

*

ROBIN MCNAMARA
Robin was diagnosed with
gastroparesis in 2013 at age 55

Acupuncture has worked well for me. With bad allergies, I recently got in with a Chinese woman's practice and she has been working miracles for me. The one thing that I'd love to get into more is yoga to keep things moving but their hours for beginner classes are not a good fit for when I can go.

Other than those two things, I use wellness chiropractic, which I was using long before having gastroparesis. I know if I can keep my physical structure in alignment, I will feel better. I'm not sure what else is out there, but thankfully I'm not a sucker for so-called cures.

*

TAYLOR SCHMITZ
Taylor was diagnosed with idiopathic
gastroparesis in 2014 at age 22

Ginger is seriously my go-to for everything. I put it in all my food, and drink ginger tea all day. It helps so much with pain and nausea, not to mention its effect on digestion. I eat dairy-free yogurt, drink kraut juice, and take probiotics and many supplements to support digestion, muscle health, vitamin retention, gut and colon health. I also use essential oils and Epsom salts.

I've benefited so much from acupuncture, it relaxes me so well. Being chronically ill creates so much anxiety and depression. The acupuncture really centers me and helps me calm down.

The main complementary therapy, and the biggest healer of my body, is Jesus Christ. I have grown so much in my faith since I've been sick, and I couldn't be more thankful for the Lord and all His wonderful blessings. He carries me through each day, and guides me with His words. I've been reading my Bible about once a night for a couple of years now, and it has completely changed my outlook on life and my illness. I cannot express enough how important it is to have faith. Faith in the Lord, faith in yourself, and faith that you WILL get through this. I've had some scary moments, moments when I didn't feel like I could go on, and moments when I believed my loved ones were so much better off without me. But my faith got me through. There is a time and reason for everything, and it is not my place to decide I quit, if it's not my time yet!

*

DEB SHRADER-TROTTER
Deb was diagnosed with
gastroparesis in 1999 at age 37

I find it helpful to use a high quality blender with organic herbs, which have been used to help inflammation, nausea, and neuropathy for centuries. Other things I have found helpful are Premier shakes, my Vitamixer, cardamom, organic ginger root extract drops, flax seed, coconut oil, and a little avocado. Using a base of Premier milk, coconut milk, or Lite almond milk helps. Whatever works for you. Taking in good protein and less sugar? You can actually feel your brain coming back to life from its attack from malnutrition and dehydration.

*

JESSICA SPENCE
Jessica was diagnosed with
gastroparesis in 2016 at age 25

In the support groups one of the first things anyone will tell you to try is ginger. I am so glad I listened! There is this spicy ginger soda that I like to drink when I need the carbonation to relieve the pressure in my Timmy (the Terrible Tummy). Some days, all I want is to sip on ginger tea in my bathtub. Heating pads never seemed to help me, and always made me itch. So my bathtub has always been my safe haven. Someday I would like to have one in my bedroom like those fancy hotel rooms.

I have switched up my diet to the gastroparesis-friendly one. I'm honestly still trying to figure this one out because some things on the list I just can't handle. Other things on the list that I'm not supposed to have will sit perfectly fine.

Someday I would like to try acupuncture and warm water therapy. I've heard wonderful things about acupuncture for gastroparesis, but we can't afford it until I can get back to work or get approved for disability. The warm water therapy will be a good way to exercise in a comfortable way. However, as with the acupuncture, we just aren't able to afford it right now.

*

NICOLE STARZYNSKI
Nicole was diagnosed with
gastroparesis in 2016 at age 33

Since the treatments and medications available for gastroparesis are limited, many of us try a holistic approach sometimes referred to as complementary or alternative therapies. First, as much as I wish there was some magic potion in a bottle that was going to fix everything, there isn't. There are some things that may help alleviate symptoms and take the edge off. I've done my own experiments at home to see if it was a placebo effect or if these things actually helped.

When I was first diagnosed, my mom and I researched smoothie recipes, recipes for mashed food that I could possibly tolerate to try to add some different things into my diet so I wasn't eating applesauce, chicken broth and sweet potatoes for the rest of my life. We searched online and a few things kept popping up: ginger, peppermint oil, probiotics, prebiotics and synbiotics (a combination of prebiotics and probiotics). I started shredding ginger into everything I was eating because we read it would help with nausea. I honestly can't say whether this helped or not because at the time I was nauseous no matter what, with the exception of Zofran giving some relief. I stopped doing it after a while, but it might be something to try again.

The doctor who diagnosed me, who refused to give me nausea medicine, was nice enough to prescribe peppermint oil. The only problem with peppermint is the smell of it. The smell made me want to vomit so that was a complete fail. Thanks Doc!

People say a diet can alleviate pain and nausea. For some people, it might help. I agree that there are foods that make me feel worse than others, but when I avoid everything that makes me feel sick, I am pretty much left with nothing. When I buy anything from chicken broth to protein drinks (most of which make me want to puke), I have to look at everything on the label before I buy it. I read the label to make sure it's not high in sodium or fiber, has no preservatives or antibiotics, is low protein, has a low-fat content but not actually low-fat, no added sugars, no ingredients I can't understand, no red meat, and no dairy.

I add Kefir to my daily smoothie. I think the smoothies help me go the bathroom, but sometimes I can't drink them so it's hard to know if it's helping. People watch a doctor on television and think they're an expert on digestion. There may be something to that gut to brain function, but if your gut is broken, not even Dr. Oz has a cure. If you find something that promotes nerve regeneration or has some magic ability to wake up a dead nerve, let me know. I would be interested in something that will actually make my stomach work again.

I have tried digestive enzymes since I don't produce enough of my own. I have tried Coca Cola to help digest food, and make up for some of the acids and enzymes I don't have. Sometimes the sodium is too much for me, however, and makes me bloat like the Goodyear Blimp.

I have read numerous studies about acupuncture. I just honestly haven't wanted to devote time away from home to something like that. Unless there was data that showed it would help, it's just not on my list of things to try. I am not dissing anyone who uses this; it's just not for me. It's too much like a medical test. I feel like it will stress me out more than it will do any good.

I have found a few things to help with some of the mental effects this disease can take on me. I consider them holistic because they aren't medications. One is a breathing technique I use when I am in extreme pain. I don't care if people are around. I sit down, put my head back, shut my eyes, and I take deep breaths in and out. When I am breathing out, my entire body is breathing out. I think of anything that makes me happy. Sometimes it can be the most random thing. Other times I imagine I'm on a bikeride or at the beach. Anywhere except in extreme pain. It's really mind over matter. You can't give into the pain. No, this is not going to make your pain go away. It's a way to deal with the pain. Sometimes it's excruciating, and your eyes fill with tears and you feel like you are being stabbed to death. To me, it has worked get me through those bad times so I don't have a complete panic attack, which triggers me to get nauseous and then sick as a dog. No thanks. If I can avoid a panic attack with a breathing exercise, I am going for it.

Another thing I do every day will sound weird, but it works so I am sharing it. I try to pick a time when nobody is home because I just want peace for ten minutes. I don't want the dog licking my face, so I make sure she is outside. I set a timer for ten minutes and I lie down on my bed, on my back. I start to hang my head off the bed with my arms reaching toward the floor. I stretch my entire body. I keep my eyes shut and I just breathe in and out. I clear my head of all thoughts. I push bad thoughts out, until there are no thoughts. Once the timer goes off, I normally feel a little better, especially if I was having a bad day, stressed or frustrated with this stupid disease. It's not going to cure anything, but it keeps me from having panic attacks every day. The key is that every activity you do cannot contribute to stress. This is why it is key to stay away from news, social media or individuals that promote stress. Completely unplug yourself.

Nature is another thing that helps calm the mind. A nice walk through a park or a bike ride on a trail. If you can, visit a body of water. All these things are great if you feel well enough to actually do them. We used to do so much stuff outside, but the past two years we have become hermits because I have been sick. There's just something about being outside and seeing all that the world has to offer. Maybe it's a reminder of why life is so precious. My next mission is to make my own retreat in my backyard with flowers, a mini fairy garden, and a vegetable garden. Something pretty I can look at while I am home. Then I can go in my backyard and feel like I am on a retreat.

*

JENNIFER ZUBIK
Jennifer was diagnosed with idiopathic gastroparesis in 2010 at age 27

Most people are skeptical of using alternative therapies—I was one of those people before I became sick. After suffering with the symptoms of gastroparesis, I was willing and have tried many alternative therapies. I have tried acupuncture, chiropractic care, massage therapy, medication studies, reflexology, ginger, peppermint, garlic, vinegar, all-natural herbal supplements and vitamins. Every alternative method I tried only worked momentarily or temporarily, if at all, or made me sick. And, of course, I prayed every day and every wish I made (on a star, when throwing a coin in a well or fountain, or while blowing out my birthday candles) was to feel better. Everyone has their own beliefs of remedies and therapies that may or may not work. However, you won't know if you don't try.

*

CHAPTER EIGHT

Social Challenges

> Remember, you don't need a certain number of friends, just a number of friends you can be certain of. -UNKNOWN

Chronic health conditions, especially invisible ones, affect many areas of our life. Unpredictable symptoms and flares create social challenges that can be difficult to manage—and explain. How has the disorder limited your social life?

*

MELISSA ADAMS VANHOUTEN
Melissa was diagnosed with
gastroparesis in 2014 at age 47

I have written two stories I would like to share which describe the impact gastroparesis has had on my life in terms of social engagement. My world is ever-changing, ever-shrinking, and I do what I can to slow this process. I would like to live as close to normal as I can, for as long as I am able. That is getting more difficult. The first story, I believe, addresses my feelings about loss and details all that has disappeared, and yet all that still remains of my beautiful, tiny world.

IT'S A SMALL, SMALL WORLD

I wrote in a post yesterday morning: "A few days ago, my doctor asked me what I eat in a typical day, and I had no answer. I just sat there because the answer really is, 'Nothing.' I am so tired of starving. I am so tired of the pain and of seeing my friends go through this. I want a normal day, just one, just a break—but it is never there. And it likely never will be again." That is a difficult truth to face, but one that I must if I am to cope with this illness. My world is contracting, and I can choose to either hold tightly to the things I still have, appreciate them, and spend every precious moment cherishing them, or I can elect to feel like I did yesterday—embrace the pain, loss, heartache, and grief and allow them to steal away the moments that remain.

I am not normally one to dwell on how I wish things were or how they used to be. But yesterday? Yesterday was a rare exception. I am not sure what set me off. I think perhaps it was a picture of my daughter and me together at an event from a couple of years ago. Or maybe it was watching her play basketball in our driveway and realizing that she was not the same small child I had once observed. I am not positive, but what I am certain of is that something put me in a reflective and brooding mood, and things went downhill from there.

I permitted myself, for a moment, to think about the friends I have lost, the family members who no longer call, the many times I have sat alone while others have gathered together, the isolation that being homebound has brought, and the immense world who moves on around me and without me. I allowed myself to experience all the physical pain and the sheer agony of trying to get through each day without food. I chose to feel, really feel, the loss I have endured. I did not distract myself. I did not pursue alternate actions or thoughts, and I did not change my perspective as I usually will myself to do. I practiced none of the techniques I know to be beneficial. Instead, I sulked, pitied myself, and mourned the passing of my old life.

Since the day of my diagnosis with gastroparesis, I have tried to accept and make the best of my circumstances. I am not an optimist nor a pessimist. I am a realist, and I believe in doing what I can with what I have. No point in dwelling on what might have been, right? Further, I have, for the most part, come to understand that though my life will not be exactly what I once envisioned, it still has value and meaning. I am an advocate and an administrator in several online support groups, and I find that helping others aids me in shifting my focus away from my own problems and maladies. It helps me to feel that I am making a difference, albeit small, in the lives of others and in bringing awareness to this cruel disease. My efforts in this area have given me purpose, and that is generally enough to get me through the roughest of the long days. But yesterday it struck me just how small my world has become, and it made me wonder how much more it can and will diminish.

As I looked at the photo of my daughter and I visiting with the survivors of the USS Indianapolis who had graced us with their presence in downtown Indianapolis, I remembered how it felt to be there that day. It was a good day. I used to relish book signings, trips to museums, watching movies at the theater, dining in restaurants, visiting relatives, attending concerts and sporting events, and a whole host of other happenings. I used to have a life outside the walls of my home. But those days are long gone and are likely not coming back. Nowadays, I am fortunate if I make it to my medical appointments.

As my daughter made basket after basket while I watched through the window, clinging to the heating pad covering my stomach and abdomen, I recalled how I used to play Horse with her when she was smaller and was reminded of the leisurely walks we once took through the neighborhood. I thought of our trip to the ocean from several years back, the ocean that I love more than any place in the world, the ocean that I will likely never see again. I remembered the times we visited the zoo and sat by the pond eating a picnic meal, and I reflected on how much I miss not just those outings but the food itself. It has been more than two years since I have consumed anything close to a meal, and it has been many months since I have been able to take more than a couple of bites of even soft foods.

As I sipped my Ensure, I thought of sitting with my husband at an ice cream shop shortly before my child was born and experiencing the strange realization that it would likely be the last time we would make such an outing without our child. I thought of our many vacations, visits to festivals and fairs, walks alone, anniversary dinners, and holiday gatherings with family. I recalled the elaborate desserts I used to make him when I was trying to perfect my newly-found baking skills just a few years ago—a hobby that holds not quite so much delight for me now. I recollected the ballroom dancing classes I forced him to take and the joy they ended up bringing us. I permitted myself to reminisce about every single moment, and I grieved over the fact that I failed to realize then that I would never get these times back. I guess that all this time I have held out hope that these things would someday happen again. But yesterday, when I took a good hard look at how this disease has already progressed, I suppose it hit me that this will surely never be.

As a family, we have made the necessary adjustments. We do what we can to enjoy our time together at home, and my husband attends (solo) the events that require an appearance. We have learned to cherish the small moments and to be thankful that we can rely on each other for love and support. On rare occasions, we still manage to delight in a brief excursion (although I pay for such outings in pain for many days afterward), and we relish those times. But yesterday, there was the nagging… the memories flooding my mind.

I was reminded of my child's conversation with a relative a short while ago: "Today was such a good day! Mommy took me shopping and we were able to stay out a whole two hours!" I thought of the many times she has stood behind me, gently caressing my back, whispering, "Are you okay, Mommy? Is this a bad day?" I heard the echoes of her sweet voice comforting me, her graceful and compassionate response to being told that I would have to miss yet another choir performance, play, Tae Kwon Do tournament, or birthday party: "It's okay, Mommy. I understand. You can't help it if you don't feel well. Daddy will videotape it." I replayed in my mind all the moments when I have heard her patiently explain to teachers, friends, and everyone else who has inquired a thousand times, that her mother has gastroparesis and this means her mother cannot do the things that many parents do.

I further recalled how this beautiful, precious little being has participated in every Go Green event and campaign we have ever held, and has done so with enthusiasm. All the nights I have heard her pray for healing and comfort for me and for all of those in my gastroparesis community came to mind as well. I considered how difficult it has likely been for her over the past couple of years to hold her tongue when I have screamed at her for no reason at all other than my pain getting the best of me. I contemplated how significantly this illness must be impacting her well-being and happiness, and while I admire her fortitude, I mourned her loss of a normal life.

I thought of my husband who comes home exhausted every night from work and still must help care for this beautiful child and attend to the chores that have piled up during the day, tasks that I could easily complete a year ago. I remembered the many episodes where I have watched him hide while eating so that he will not intensify my torture. I played over the moments in my mind—him patiently enduring my screaming fits of anger and apologizing even when he has done nothing wrong, him holding onto me when I am crying and on the verge of throwing in the towel, despite the fact that I have likely just scolded him, pushed him away, and blamed him for every horrible thing that has ever happened to me. Him telling me that I am beautiful, though anyone can clearly see the truth in the dark circles under my eyes and in the skeletal reflection in my mirror. I was reminded of the many evenings he has rubbed my shoulders and feet, despite his own fatigue, so that I can relax and sleep well. I thought of how often I have heard him whisper a prayer with our child in the other room, for my healing, strength, and peace.

Yesterday, I dwelled on all we have lost, all we have borne, the abnormality and horror of it all, the smallness of my world, and it was nearly unbearable. I tried to focus on the good that has come out of all of this, and there is much: friendships, compassion, understanding, wisdom, passion, spiritual blessings, and more, but there was still the nagging. What if my world, our world, diminishes even more? What will happen when my daughter graduates or gets married, and I am left alone? How can I endure her absence when I have so few treasures left? I often wonder if I will be around to witness the significant events in her life, given my current deteriorating state of health, but I rarely think about what will happen if I do survive that long.

And then truly awful thoughts came. What if my husband gets sick or decides this burden is too much and abandons us? What if he passes away? Who will care for us? Who will be my support system then? What if I am truly on my own one day? What if, instead of dying early, I actually live to see those days? Yesterday, those uncertainties and fears were too much, too much.

But today I am in a different state of mind. Today, I grasp that I cannot remain in my dark thoughts. Today, I am focusing on other truths and approaching the moments with a fresh perspective. I have a devoted husband; an affectionate, trusting child who admires and adores me; compassionate, supportive friends and loved ones; groups and projects that give my life meaning and purpose; and a loving God who still watches over me and directs my path for good. I have beautiful, precious memories that no one can ever take from me. I have a family who knows the true meaning of love and appreciates every moment we have been granted. Most days, I have hope, however dim, for a brighter future—if not for me, then for the millions who follow me and share in this cruel diagnosis.

Today, I choose this life, whatever bit of it I still have left. I choose purpose and willpower. I choose faith and hope, and the struggle to overcome the hardships and obstacles. I choose to advocate and to support others on this same difficult path, and I choose the fight that goes along with this journey. I choose to pursue the thoughts, feelings, techniques, and actions that I know will get me through the day. I will embrace the good for as long as I can and recede deeper into the center of the shrinking circle of my life until I can retreat no more. It has been a good life. It is still a good life, if I choose for it to be.

* * *

The second story I would like to share was written a couple of years ago. I hope it provides some insight into how difficult it can be to have any sort of meaningful social life with this beastly illness. Since the time of this writing, it has become even more burdensome to participate in evenings out. It is always my goal to accompany my family on events and outings such as the ones we used to enjoy together, but these moments are far less frequent than before, slipping away. It saddens me to the core. We need a cure.

BEHIND THE SCENES AT THE MR. ROB THOMAS CONCERT

I absolutely loved the Mr. Rob Thomas concert in Indy this past Tuesday evening. I counted down to it on my Facebook wall and in my Twitter feed for sixty-seven days. It was one of the most exciting events I have ever attended, and I described it to my friends as perfect. I am, if you can't tell by now, a HUGE Mr. Rob Thomas and Matchbox Twenty fan. Always have been. The first concert I ever attended in my life was a Matchbox Twenty concert in Fort Wayne a couple of years ago, at the age of forty-six! I got to meet the band and had pictures taken with all of them. Beyond exciting! So, needless to say, I was highly motivated to attend this concert and looked forward to it from the day I heard about it. Couldn't wait to show off my pictures after it was over. Almost everyone has seen them by now. But what they haven't seen, and what I haven't let them see, is what it took for me to get to that concert—and the consequences for someone like me, living with gastroparesis or maybe another chronic illness, of undertaking an outing such as this. They aren't privy to what happened behind the scenes of the concert.

It started the day I heard Mr. Thomas would be touring—the worry, the fear, and the hope that despite the effects of my illness I might be able to attend. You see, because of my gastroparesis, I cannot eat, and this causes all sorts of issues that most other people never have to experience. Every time I consider going to an event, I fear I'll be too sick to actually attend. I don't like dealing with that disappointment, but what I like even less is disillusioning the friends with whom I have looked forward to enjoying the evening. I have let them down so many times already that I am surprised they agree to include me in anything. But I have good friends, friends who understand and are sympathetic to my plight. They tolerate my shortcomings.

When I was sixty-seven days away from the concert, I could pretty successfully ignore my worries and fears, but as the days flew by, it became more difficult. I knew that during the week or two before the concert, I would have to eat less. If there was any chance of making it there, I had to eat as little as possible to reduce the likelihood of nausea and pain on the actual concert day. Food equals pain and nausea, and that equals missed events. So, I limited my already meager intake of sustenance even further. By concert week, I was pretty run down.

The night before the concert, I ate and drank practically nothing, and on concert day, I ate nothing at all, not a single bite, and drank only what was necessary to keep me from being dehydrated. I couldn't chance missing Mr. Thomas and disappointing my friends. I was drained from days of food deprivation, and this day was almost unbearable. I was shaky, dizzy, and weak. Every time I walked into the kitchen and saw the food, I longed to take just a bite. I made my family lunch, and I could smell the food. I wanted so badly to sit down with them and eat just a little. If I did, though, I would have been in agony. I would get nauseous, be in excruciating pain, and likely bloat up to the size of a nine-month pregnant woman. I was miserable, but I was determined. I hardly ever went out, and I knew I wouldn't get this chance again anytime soon. I sucked it up and moved on.

I picked out an outfit and started getting ready to go. As I combed my hair (which continues to thin due to malnutrition), I took a good look in the mirror. I thought I was hideous. I looked like a skeleton. I barely recognized the person staring back at me, and I hated what I had become. I could comb her hair, put a nice outfit and makeup on her, but I couldn't make her what she was a year ago. I couldn't change this. It saddened me, but I did the best I could and tried to convince myself that I wouldn't scare small children with my appearance.

My husband and I decided to arrive at the venue a little early because I really wanted to get a picture with Mr. Thomas. There was a slim chance of this, but I was willing to give it a go. It was scorching outside, and that added to my misery. Hot, weak, and shaky—not a good combination. My husband helped steady me. The security guards at the venue were incredibly friendly and helpful (really!). They pointed to a spot where I could wait for Mr. Thomas, and I stood there for a bit until he finally arrived. Yep, I got sunburn, too! He was such a gentleman, so friendly, and he let us take a picture. Yay! Success! Despite my hunger and weakness, the day had been wonderful so far! We met up with our friends and prepared for the concert.

As I stood outside the closed doors to the auditorium, my legs shook with weakness. My husband held onto me and reassured me that we would be able to sit soon and that I WOULD make it. I could smell popcorn in the lobby, and I longed to have some. I love popcorn, but I haven't been able to eat it (not even a bite) in more than a year. People passed by enjoying this delicious, buttery treat, but I could only watch and savor the smells. I was thankful when the doors finally opened so that I could focus on something else. We had front-row center seats that evening, and I was able to concentrate on only what was in front of me—the stage and the band! No crowd-watching from that point on, and I was glad.

I concentrated on appearing as and behaving like a normal person. I did not want anyone to know I was sick. I didn't want my friends to worry. I didn't want to take away from their enjoyment of the evening. I didn't want to cause a scene. I silently prayed that I would not vomit or faint or reveal in any way that I believed I was at the end of my rope. I smiled, laughed, and joked as if nothing at all was wrong. I was happy, and I wanted it to be that way, so I pretended, and sheer willpower got me through.

I enjoyed the opening acts (Vinyl Station, which is a fantastic group, and the Plain White Ts), but I was actually thankful when their portion of the show ended because I was wearing down quickly, and I wanted to see Mr. Thomas perform. When Mr. Thomas took the stage, I disregarded all the difficulties it took to get there. I ignored my weak, shaky legs, which I could no longer really feel and which could barely hold me at that point. I grabbed onto the stage floor in front of me and I thoroughly enjoyed the next two hours. I had to sit a couple of times, but, for the most part, I made it! For just a brief spell, I forgot all the agony and worries in my life. I delighted in the time I had with my friends and spouse. I relaxed and let go of my pain for a bit. I knew I would pay for this later, but at that moment, I did not care. It had been months since I had been out for anything other than a medical appointment or mundane errand, and I was having fun. Fun—not something we experienced in our house very frequently anymore. I was ecstatic.

All too soon, and yet way too late, the concert ended. As I made my way back to the car, leaning heavily on my husband to steady myself, I began to think about the consequences of this evening out. I would pay for this dearly the next day. I had spent weeks preparing for this and many days depriving myself of even the basics, knowing that when this was all over, I would be in worse shape because of it. I knew that night I would collapse, and the next day I would have to begin to try to erase the ill effects of the evening and the rough days leading up to it. I would eat what little I could the next day, and it would be harder than usual to tolerate it. I would begin to try to make up for the calories I had lost, but I knew I would never be able to. It didn't work like that. I would suffer from exhaustion and pain from pushing myself considerably beyond my limits. But most of all, I would face the mental anguish of knowing that my life had to return to this new normal—to the place where I was homebound, where I had to spend every day trying to balance my physical need for food against the pain it caused me, where I had to deny myself the basic needs everyone else takes for granted because I couldn't live with the agony it caused me when I partook, and where I spent all my days online advocating for others who must live with this disease.

But that night? That night, I was "Overjoyed."

* * *

The take-away from all of this, I hope, is that my life has changed dramatically since being diagnosed. It is not the life I envisioned, but that does not mean it is not worth living.

I miss most family gathering, outings with family and friends, school events, and holiday celebrations. Many of my old friends have dropped out of my social circle these days as well. But I have new friends and closer bonds with those loved ones who have remained by my side through thick and thin. I have learned to alter my activities to fit the limitations of my illness and to live one day at a time, taking advantage of the rare moments when I feel well enough to engage and making the occasional sacrifices required to participate when the importance of the event dictates this.

Having any sort of social life with this illness is problematic, to be certain, but with adjustments in both attitude and expectations, I have learned I can still have a meaningful, fulfilling life—however small my world becomes.

*

SAMANTHA ANDERSON
Samantha was diagnosed with idiopathic gastroparesis in 2012 at age 26

What social life? Before I got ill, which was six years ago, I used to have a very active social life. I would go to the gym five to six times a week; I loved it. I would go out with my family and friends often to restaurants, pubs, and nightclubs. I ate food, had drinks and good times with friends, and so on. But as soon as I got ill, it all stopped. A lot of social life revolves around food and drink. I tried to go to some social functions and events. However, friends and family often felt uncomfortable and embarrassed that I was not drinking and eating, especially as they knew what I was going through. Soon, invitations stopped coming and I found myself watching from the sidelines, wishing I could join in more. I wanted to do all the stuff I used to do. Not doing much was driving me crazy but at the same time I was too exhausted to enjoy joining in.

I would go to special occasions like birthdays, maybe a wedding every so often, and a christening. I wouldn't drink or eat to make sure I could attend and enjoy it slightly more. Since getting ill, I have had to come to the realization that I can enjoy many things, but not the same as before. I suppose to keep going, you have to find the positives out of the smallest of things, which isn't a bad thing really.

Even now things are easier with the pacemaker. I sometimes see my closest of friends, but when we are out, I still won't really drink and definitely won't eat. I'm still very tired and in pain, but love it for what it is. I try to make the big occasions. The people closest to me understand. I'm close to my family. Without them, coping would have been much harder, but even family gatherings are different for me. I still try not to eat or drink around them, not because they are embarrassed or that it bothers them, but because they don't like me being ill. They would rather me be around them. They also need a little education on lactose and gluten-free recipes

I really want more of a social life, I miss it and want so much more.

*

JOLI ATKINS
Joli was diagnosed with
gastroparesis in 2015 at age 36

I have lost friends thanks to this horrible disease. I no longer plan events around food or go to restaurants that I used to love, because of this horrible disease. If we do decide to go out to eat, we have to plan it around the very few things that I can eat. I am scared to go out to eat sometimes because I am scared that I will get sick. There are many days when I have to cancel plans because even though I want to go, I don't have the energy to go. It takes so much energy to get up and get ready that by the time I have done all of that, I do not have the energy to actually go to the event. I have to put my personal health first.

*

TRISHA BUNDY
Trisha was diagnosed with
gastroparesis in 2013 at age 35

I definitely feel like the quality of my social life has drastically been impacted by illness. Fatigue, nausea, and pain all limit the way I interact with others and to what degree. Less vacations, more passive lifestyle, having to make plans with the understanding that I may have to either cancel or shorten at a moment's notice all make a social life more difficult. I also often have to deal with guilt and regrets, as I struggle to figure out what are the best actions for me, physically and emotionally. These decisions are usually not easy, as respecting what I need in one area may interfere or be counterproductive for the other.

Living with any illness, especially an invisible one, is tough. I never know what kind of day it's going to be until I wake up. Even then, things can change immediately, for no apparent reason. A couple bites of fruit, a little bit of my favorite flavored milkshake, or sliver of whatever my taste buds desire, on a day when I actually feel more normal can cause me dire consequences. In just a couple of moments a great low-symptom day can become one of my absolute worst.

Similarly, a nice walk in a park, an essential grocery run, or even a child's ballgame can drain me. The majority of the time my family's and my day is determined by the day-to-day symptoms and the severity that I am dealing with in the moment.

Prayers, faith, blogging, and listening to music all help me deal with more troublesome days. Prior to any social activities, I try to be proactive. I create plans for how to remove myself if my symptoms become too problematic for me, and play it safe by not trying anything by mouth prior to the upcoming experience. In addition, I rest to save up energy days before, and try to prepare time to rest and refresh afterwards, which often also requires multiple days.

Constant nausea, abdominal pain, and fatigue keep me from being able to actively engage or enjoy my once valued hobbies. As much as I love the idea of going outside and playing ball with my kids, I just don't have enough energy, not to mention the challenges my symptoms create. Knowing how important it is to relax my mind and focus on other things besides my body, I have searched and searched for new hobbies. I love watching my daughter play softball; she makes me so proud. Yet, sometimes it takes all of my energy just to get there. It would be nice if I could say that going to her ballgames help hide my symptoms, but sadly that's not the case. While enjoying being out and attending her games, I still have to battle the abdominal pain and nausea, which is increased by the heat. I also have to be extra careful not to become more dehydrated than I already am. Yes, I enjoy the time and will continue to push myself to attend the games, I just have to remain mindful of the likely consequences.

Not only have activities that I participate in on the home front changed, but so have family vacations. In July 2013, just a few months after gastroparesis made an impact on my life, I witnessed the impact that illness could have on an exciting New York City vacation. I was just beginning to learn how to live with not only my day-to-day symptoms, but also a feeding tube that I had received during my second hospitalization in May 2013. I was most definitely sore but extremely strong-willed. I was determined that my illness and having a feeding tube would not define my life. I had been looking forward to visiting New York City for many years, and now my family and I were actually going to be there. I was eager to take in some sightseeing!

Overall, we had a nice time. Due to my low energy, we depended on subways, taxis, and tour buses to move us around. We were unable to have a true New York City experience, since I was unable to physically walk around and explore, but we were okay with that. We had a lot of fun even if I was exhausted. At times, I didn't even think I would be able to make it to the subway or back to the hotel, but I did and it was definitely worthwhile. I returned home very sore and fatigued, but felt strong mentally, and loved the time I had with my family. I looked forward to returning with more energy. Little did I know that my level of energy would continue to dwindle as days, weeks, months, and even years passed by.

In spring 2014, my family decided to take an extended weekend trip to the mountains, just a few hours away. We had reserved a cabin and planned on it being a low-key, relaxing with each other, kind of trip. Overall, we enjoyed our time at the cabin. My husband cooked the majority of the meals outside on the grill, we had a s'more cookout one night, and enjoyed time in the jacuzzi. I swear if I had a jacuzzi, I would live in it. I'm not sure if it was from trying a little bit of a biscuit, from eating a graham cracker, or just me, but that night my husband almost had to take me to the emergency room for intense pain that my regular medicines would not even begin to touch. The next day, we spent the entire day at the cabin, mostly watching TV and playing on technology devices. Once again, I was fighting as hard as I could to stay away from the emergency room due the intense pain that I was experiencing. I was extremely thankful that my kids didn't seem to be irritated about how our trip ended. I honestly believe it bothered me much more than them. I was so upset and hurt that they were worried and frightened. Yes, all in all I appreciated the time with my family, but was frustrated with my body's lack of cooperation.

As a result of imperfect vacations and increasingly bad symptoms, I began to be even more cautious. During summer 2014, my husband and kids took a few small vacations, involving just one or two nights, away without me. My gastroparesis symptoms and the side effects from my medications were too much for me to handle and I did not want to hinder their fun and enjoyment. I wanted my kids to have a great time! I didn't want to be a burden to them. They went deep sea fishing a few times and to Kings Dominion, all of which I wished I could have been a part of. It was extremely difficult for me to stay home. I desired to be with them so much. I felt increasingly isolated. But how could I have gone? I could barely do anything at home. At least I was able to stay busy by spending the majority of my days with my dear grandmother, Mama.

In October 2014, I decided to attempt a vacation with my husband and kids once again. Now this was a magical trip for me! God really blessed me here. I had just lost my grandmother a few weeks earlier. My kids and I were hurting emotionally from letting her go, even though we knew that she was in a better place. To ease our pain, my husband and I decided to embark on a family trip to the Nascar Race in Charlotte. I didn't know how this would work out, but I pleaded with God to please help me be able to enjoy this time with my kids.

God truly answered my prayers. My nausea, pain, and fatigue remained present, but at least they remained tolerable (with medications) and I was able to hide them from the family. We were even able to meet a few of the race car drivers, including my all-time favorite, Martin Truex, Jr. Memories were definitely made on this trip that will be treasured for a lifetime.

Since then, I have had to miss out on many family vacations. If I do choose to attempt a vacation, it has been sparingly, maybe once or twice a year, and low-key such as a weekend trip to the beach with family. As my kids enjoyed the pool and beach, I tried to relax in the cabana and hotel room. Unfortunately, I was often attempting to hide the severity of my symptoms so they wouldn't worry too much. Yes, sickness still occurs when on vacation. The vacations, while nice and needed, still left me feeling extremely fatigued with increased dehydration, taking a week or two to recuperate.

Simple things like going out to eat with family and friends to enjoy time together and celebrate special occasions or holidays, are no longer the same. I did not realize how much our culture revolves around food until I became sick. Now going to restaurants and gatherings can be awkward for me and the people I am surrounded by. Many times they feel uncomfortable eating around me when they see that I am just sitting there watching, or if it's a good day, sipping on liquids or attempting a scoop of ice cream. My social life has been through a dramatic change since becoming ill. I carefully consider the options before me, think about the choices I have and analyze the possible benefits and consequences before being selective over which activities I choose to participate in. I consider all opportunities and then determine which ones are most important to my family and me.

*

LISA COLANDREA
Lisa was diagnosed with
gastroparesis in 2016 at age 42

Since my diagnosis, gastroparesis has affected many aspects of my life. I can't find the energy most days to even get dressed, never mind leave the house. My family and I moved to a new state a few years ago, and I've been hesitant to put myself out there and make new friends because of my illness. Being sick has been very isolating. Nobody can possibly understand what it's like unless they are going through it themselves. If I know there is somewhere I need to be or a social engagement that I've committed to, then I make sure I do not go out or overexert myself for several days prior to the engagement. Anything I do takes everything out of me, so I need to prepare in advance when making plans.

*

TAMMY DOWNS
Tammy was diagnosed with Crohn's disease, irritable bowel syndrome, spastic colon, gastroesophageal reflux disease, and gastritis in 2006 at age 46, gastroparesis in 2015 at age 56, and motility dysfunction disorder of the rectum and pelvic floor in 2016 at age 58

Gastroparesis has affected my life with motility dyssynergic defecation dynamics (type II) due to how embarrassing it can be. It affects me when my stomach is in so much pain and I am nauseous from trying to eat solid food that does not agree with me or that's heavier than I am used to. The food can take days to pass through my stomach, and then causes major bathroom problems that can last at least three to four days. I have no choice but to be on a liquid diet. Eating out can be a problem. Gastroparesis is the stomach from hell. There has to be something that can cause it to work properly so I can eat. Along with all the other stomach problems, I experience burning like I have a fire in my gut, and then I have issues swallowing. It just gets ridiculous. Something has to be done.

*

SKYE FALCON

Skye was diagnosed with gastroparesis and other autoimmune diseases in 2006 at age 25

My medical issues, illnesses and life traumas have essentially squelched my social life. It began as a casual demise, and now is an uncontrollable monster. I am isolated, though sometimes on purpose, and sometimes by accident. As an entrepreneur and business professional, my business meetings are geared around lunch or dinner dates, or even worse, group luncheons. Events are torture. Not only is there food, but long hours of standing and talking for hours and hours upon end. I am all but ostracized from most friendly social events and family parties, mainly because I cannot attend due to one of many reasons. Sun allergies, food allergies and intolerances, a non-functioning gastrointestinal tract, hardening internal organs, and the blue fingertips from Raynaud's and I am more of a side show act than party guest. Being treated like a circus freak-show act is not fun or exciting, and sort of degrading. And the exhaustion, wow. It is so heavy and intense. A healthy, functioning human really has no idea how much energy is used by just simply listening, and responding in a standard conversation.

Because of my issues, I pay close attention to my children's schedules, work schedules, and life happenings. With three kids, some teenagers, it can be complex and difficult. I only sign up for what I know I can handle, and spend weeks before planning it out and making decisions for ease through whatever it is. Even being proactive, I end up backing out of some things just because I physically cannot do it when the time comes. Dinners out mean menu reading, studying and planning a week before. Although most of the time I still cannot eat out because they do not have broths or softs without gluten and dairy. Holidays are depressing because there is nothing I can really turn to, except whatever I bring for myself. Sometimes I purposely avoid events and parties because I know the physical demands will take me out for a week or more, and it is not worth it. I spend my free energy on my passions and children, all of which I happen to love.

Thankfully I am the boss at my out-of-the-house job, and am in charge of the scheduling. I travel constantly with heated vests, heating pads, vomit bags and buckets, and a whole pharmacy of prescriptions to ease whatever ailment may show up. My children are well-versed in the art of CPR and medical aid just in case. I carry information with me at all times regarding my issues. I limit my traveling for author events to the surrounding states, or locations within two to three hours away. If it is any farther than that, I normally have to leave an extra day ahead of time to allow my body time to relax before the event. I do not like to be out of the house when I am in a flare, or when I am struggling. Hotel staff are kind, but do not have the patience to deal with strange medical issues, tubes, or dietary needs.

What makes things a million times harder in public are people's reactions, whether it be strangers, friends or family. When I am grilled by strangers about why I am not eating but yet am so skinny, it hurts me in ways you will never understand. I know what they are implying. When I am at my local sports club watching my kids swim, and I hear the side chatter about why I never get in, why I am so pale, and what all the bruises are all over my legs and arms, I retreat to where I am safe because I know what the back-chatter can do. In those gossipy situations, they would not believe what I have to tell them anyway, so why should I bother?

When wait staff at restaurants berate me about not ordering anything but an iced tea. When my friend compares my inability to digest food to the difficulty they are having avoiding sugary candy in their diet. When someone I just discussed my liquid diet with brings me a treat, fully knowing it will literally tear my intestines apart with one bite. I die a little inside each time. Or when I am in the middle of a business meeting and have to smash my hand over my mouth mid-sentence to hold in the vomit and run away embarrassed. All the while knowing I have to come back to those people and finish the meeting. I have to finish my sentence about how the newest project is going, with flushed cheeks and sweat droplets looming across my forehead. The constant reminders about how I no longer fit into this perfect-seeking society even with basic things like eating is extremely mentally challenging, and the reminders are everywhere. It hurts a little more sometimes knowing even those closest to me cannot relate.

*

ROBIN MCNAMARA
Robin was diagnosed with
gastroparesis in 2013 at age 55

I'm a crippled foodie. I used to love to go out to eat and try anything and everything at the drop of a hat. I've traveled for food! Now if there are cookouts and other gatherings, many people seem to have forgotten that I exist. They were never true friends to begin with. I decline weddings and other gatherings because I need to make sure I have food and need to eat on time. If it's a family event, I make sure I keep up with sleep and good nutrition, as well as keeping stress down which will, on most days work pretty well. I now pay more attention to my needs versus the needs of others

*

TAMMY PITTMAN
Tammy was diagnosed with gastroparesis and
irritable bowel syndrome in 2014 at age 34

Gastroparesis is very difficult for others to understand, and a lot of people want to tell me what I need to do to get better. This gets irritating and depressing. Therefore, I have stopped going around those people. This has shown me who is willing to understand. Family gatherings and holidays with food are not something I can do anymore, because there are few types of food I can actually eat. Then there's ridicule if I only eat a few bites or if I have to vomit. I no longer have the energy to play sports with my kids. About an hour drive is all I can handle.

*

TAYLOR SCHMITZ
Taylor was diagnosed with idiopathic gastroparesis in 2014 at age 22

Gastroparesis can be devastating to not only the patient, but to their loved ones as well. My social life has changed so very much, but I am so blessed to have the support system that I do. I have a small group of amazingly wonderful friends, and a tight group of supportive family members. My husband and daughter are my biggest supporters, as they help me day in and day out, and my beautiful daughter defends me when people question my illness. She's only four! It hurts so bad always letting my friends down, having to miss events and not being able to be there when my friends need me the most. I don't think it will ever get any better in this aspect, because I'm the type of person who lets guilt eat me alive. I love my friends and family, and I always want to be there for them and help them in any way possible.

As far as social events go, it's a very difficult subject. Not only can I not eat "normal" foods (I use quotes, because our world has turned unhealthy foods into normal foods), but I can't walk for extended periods, I can't miss meals, I have to take medication, and I physically just can't do a lot of things. Going to dinners is very awkward for me. I always get the stares, the questions, and the disgusted looks like I'm anorexic and don't want to eat (who wouldn't want to eat that chocolate cake?). I was such a foodie before my disease!

My family doesn't go on vacations, because I can't leave home for long periods of time. We get a lot of scrutiny from family members, because they never try to understand how difficult it is for me to function in the world without all my devices. In order to travel, I have to be able to take that amount of time's worth of my homemade foods with me, all of my remedies, supplements, drinks, and so on. Not to mention, I can't go hiking, swimming, canoeing, scuba diving, or anything that is strenuous, or else I'll be dragging everyone down, and slowing down the group.

Being understood is the hardest part of this disease. It's such a mental strain, trying to figure out what's wrong with you, when you've had test after test, doctor after doctor, all saying nothing's wrong when you know something is wrong, let alone having your own family question and snuff every move you make. Also, there are people who comment, "You need to eat more," or "Why can't you just force it down?" And the age-old, "If you don't eat, you'll die." Thank you, educated scholars, for your phenomenal input. I feel like I am so enlightened now, I'll just go force down that salad I've been craving and go get bezoars and blockages! Thank you!

*

NICOLE STARZYNSKI
Nicole was diagnosed with
gastroparesis in 2016 at age 33

Gastroparesis has affected my entire life. I pretty much do not have a social life. I have referenced living in a snow globe and that my house is like a homebound prison. Just like prisoners, I don't get out too much and I don't see anyone unless they visit. Not too many people come by to visit. Prisoners essentially live a much better life than me. I spend a lot of time alone. Well, I do have my pug, Zoey. I'm not sure what I would do without her. I talk to her more than I talk to any humans. Somedays it feels like I'm the only human alive. I stare out my window and see other people living their lives. I've gotten to the point I am afraid to go anywhere. What if I have to go the bathroom because I am on this new poop medicine? I am tired of pooping my pants in public. I try to joke when it happens, but if I never pooped my pants another day, hallelujah! I would not shed a tear. I also dread going anywhere because if I am feeling sick and I have to go somewhere, I need to make sure I have enough Zofran.

What if I want to eat something, what am I going to eat? Fast food is completely out, so for any doctor's appointment I have my mom make special food. All the chicken has to be special chicken, cooked a certain way. If I am not going to be at home long enough, that requires me to eat out, which sucks because everything has to be thought out. Not to mention everything I can eat is four times as expensive as everything else because of all the food whackos out there. I am not eating this stuff by choice; I have no choice.

Anything centered around food sucks. I don't go to parties, I don't go to restaurants. In the event I do have to go somewhere, I just pray I don't have to cancel. I have canceled so many times for different things. When my daughter has softball or softball tournaments that last days, I go into no food mode and pray that I can keep it together long enough to get through the next few days. I don't eat any food. I bring food for Kirstin to eat at the games, and sometimes even have to sit far away from any concession stand fumes. I've been lucky that I haven't puked or pooped my pants at the softball field yet. I think

Kirstin would want to die. But who knows? This year just started; anything is possible. People ask me when we are at softball tournaments why I never eat. Sometimes I explain it to them, others I just say I am not hungry. Sometimes I don't want to share that I have a disease, simply because I didn't want a chicken wing.

Every holiday, it is always, "What can Nick eat?" Sometimes I want to avoid the question altogether, because even what I say I can eat, most likely is still going to make me sick. So for the past two years, I have forced my entire family to have all the holidays at my house. If I am going to be sick, at least I am in my own house, in my own bathroom—no car traveling required. This makes the chances of pooping my pants less. It's not completely impossible, but at least I would be at home.

I know my family is annoyed by it. My mom has to cook everything at her house and drag it to my house. Nobody can trust me to cook dinner because if I end up sick, dinner won't get started. I would love to be able to cook and host the entire holiday, instead of my family doing everything for me.

I found this journal entry from this past Thanksgiving.

"Happy Thanksgiving! Today is a day to recognize everything we are thankful for. So many people are less fortunate. Despite some of the challenges that we are faced with, I am very thankful for my family who has been so supportive, my mom who is there by my side for every test and doctor's appointment, my daughter who has taught me to be strong no matter what you are faced with (my littlest biggest supporter), and my boyfriend for staying by my side, especially this past year. We have been through so much and we are the closest we have ever been. Not too many guys will watch a Gilmore Girls marathon for a week straight because it makes you happy! Ha ha. This year has had its challenges but I wouldn't trade my life for anything. I am thankful to have such wonderful people in my life. I am thankful that I finally have hope for beating gastroparesis, and this time next year I will be able to eat Thanksgiving dinner. Happy Thanksgiving to all and I hope everyone has a wonderful day! Remember to eat a huge dinner today and take a bite for me!"

I've turned into the Home Shopping Network lady. I have found a way to buy almost everything I need online. I pretty much buy everything from Amazon. As soon as I can find a place to deliver cold grocery items, I will be set.

Just going to the grocery store gives me anxiety. It's a reminder of all the food I can't eat. It's an hour of reading labels or being disappointed because that one thing I can eat they didn't have, because the workout nut who lives on protein shakes just took the last one, and I'm stuck with nothing. Leaving my house is scary because the chance of getting sick is so great and I would rather be home.

*

JENNIFER ZUBIK

Jennifer was diagnosed with idiopathic gastroparesis in 2010 at age 27

Gastroparesis was literally controlling every aspect of my life. I was unable to have much of a social life at the beginning. Most of the time I was too sick or in too much pain to even leave my house.

Getting ready was exhausting and sometimes by the time I was done, I no longer felt well enough to even go. If I could actually go somewhere or attend anything, I would make sure I had a supply of my nausea medication with me and had something I could eat and drink, if tolerable that day. Once I would arrive, I would first analyze where the restrooms and exits were. If I was at an event with row seating or large crowds of people, I would only sit on the end or an aisle seat if available, or stand in the back by an exit just in case I needed to run outside or to the bathroom. I was always so tired too, and would usually have to leave early.

Family events were not too big of a deal, as long as I could get there if it was a long car ride. Being in the car for too long made me nervous because I feared I would get sick and we wouldn't be able to pull over because of traffic. Most of the holidays were held at our house anyway. That worked out well for me, except for needing a lot of help for preparation with cleaning and cooking. If I needed to miss a family function, everyone was very understanding.

My anxiety wasn't as bad if at someone's house, but was much worse when out in public. I started to experience high anxiety when going in public because of the fear of getting sick. I also felt very insecure about how people viewed me. I thought they were thinking and talking bad about me. "She looks sick, I wonder what is wrong with her." Or, "Oh, my. Look how skinny she is. She must be anorexic or bulimic."

I was very self-conscious about the way I looked. I knew I had transformed drastically. I felt horrible for the life my fiancé and daughter had to live at home with me being sick and my needs, so if there was any kind of function for my daughter at school, sports or birthdays, I did everything I possibly could to make sure I made it. I would sometimes have to begin preparing days or a week ahead by not eating so that I would have less of a chance of getting sick while there. I would have to take my anxiety medication to leave my house and be wherever we were going, but I did my best and tried my hardest to be there for her. It wasn't fair; we used to take her to the movies or to a park or shopping almost every weekend and would try to always have fun and keep her entertained, but that became limited. Most of the time Lou would have to take her by himself, if at all. But she was wonderful and so understanding, saying, "It's okay, Mommy. Maybe next time. You need to rest and make yourself better." It was heartbreaking how understanding she was. She was only nine when I became sick and wasn't supposed to be worrying about me.

After two years of being sick, I could manage better and had gone back to work part-time. I was functioning better socially, just with limitations. If we went out, I still couldn't enjoy foods and drinks, but enjoyed the company. Lou and I began planning our wedding at last, which was very difficult because I couldn't participate in every aspect of it. It was depressing when Lou and his aunt had to handle the food taste-testing because I, of course, could not ingest anything we wanted to have served. At least I got to be involved by helping to choose what to have, and then they would taste it and tell me if it was good.

On the day of our wedding, I tried so hard not to panic or let my anxiety overtake me, which is difficult in general for anyone who isn't sick. I was still only ninety-three pounds, but I felt like a princess in my dress, with my hair and makeup done. That was the first day in almost three years I could look at myself and feel pretty. There were so many appetizers and cocktails at the reception I could not enjoy; it was infuriating. Dinner was awkward because our table was displayed up on stage, so everyone could see that I wasn't able to eat. Although, every person who attended our wedding knew about my situation so it probably wasn't awkward to them.

Despite not being able to eat that day, I did everything in my power to endure the entire day and night. I do have to say that special day of ours was perfect. I had waited for that day to come for so long, and had waited even longer because of this disease. Regardless of what was hindered or why, it was exceptional and I couldn't have asked for anything more. Everyone had a great time with us.

It was a day I feared would never come when I became sick two weeks after our engagement. December 1, 2012, was both our nine-year anniversary of being together, and the day Lou and I tied the knot with hopes of many more anniversaries to come. I am fortunate that I could have that kind of experience with this disease. I know many are not, which saddens me, but I do have hope for all and continue to pray every day for strength and wellness—for myself and every person living with gastroparesis.

*

My mom can't eat meals with
my family or go places with us
anymore. We used to go to the zoo
and McDonald's all the time. Now
we're lucky if we go twice a year.
She's on the computer often, helping
find a cure, and can't watch movies
or stay up late with us. Not even on
New Year's Eve. :(

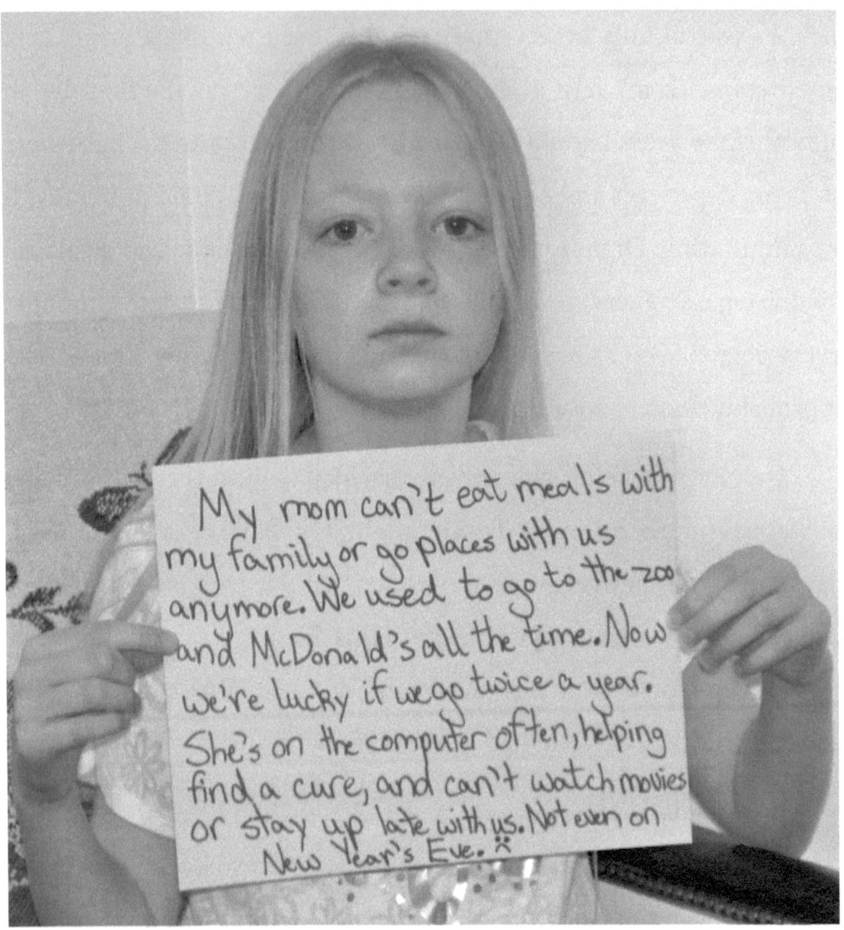

Melissa's daughter.

CHAPTER NINE

Impact on Relationships

> The worst thing you can do to a person with an invisible illness is make them feel like they need to prove how sick they are. -ANONYMOUS

When we suffer from an invisible condition involving chronic pain, it has a ripple effect on other areas of our life including relationships. Some of our relationships are understanding and supportive while others bear the brunt of the disorder. What relationships have been impacted the most by your motility disorder?

*

MELISSA ADAMS VANHOUTEN
Melissa was diagnosed with
gastroparesis in 2014 at age 47

It is not easy for friends and family members to stick by those of us with ongoing, serious illnesses. Our illnesses change our circumstances, for certain, but they change us as well. I am not the same person I used to be. I am often tired and weak, unable to enjoy gatherings with friends, even in my own home. I do not see my loved ones nearly as much as I would prefer, and I am largely confined to my home. Those are the unfortunate limitations of this illness, but there are other, more positive changes, as well. I'm more understanding, more compassionate, more forgiving, and more accepting of others. At times, it is difficult for others, especially for those who have known me for many years, to know how to react to these changes. It is only the heartiest of souls who have been able to bear with me.

My husband and daughter have undergone tremendous lifestyle changes since my diagnosis. They have given up so much, and yet they rarely complain, and seldom break down. My husband has become not simply my spouse, but to a large extent, my caretaker as well. I am certain he must miss our old life, but he has not allowed this to alter his love for me. He continues to stand by my side despite the truly horrendous trials I have put him through. He rises every day, performs the household chores that I can no longer complete, and takes care of our child's many needs, acting as chauffeur, maid, butler and general caretaker. He shops for me, searching an ungodly number of stores, trying to find that one perfect, organic, gluten-free, non-genetically modified food that I am just sure I will be able to eat this time, and then watches silently when I cannot tolerate it and throw it across the room in frustration.

He stands strong on the days I decide "I am not going to eat or drink another thing because it only prolongs my agony," and he knows that I do not really mean this. He listens to endless rants about incompetent doctors, the evil politicians and media members who will not help us, the lack of research and treatments, and the details of the many projects I want to undertake for my gastroparesis community.

He comforts me, despite my bad behavior, because he understands that pain and lack of nutrition make me crazy and irrational, and he believes I still love him even when I tell him I despise the world and everything in it, including him. He accompanies me to every doctor appointment so that they might take my illness (and my description of its effects) seriously. He counsels our child, "You have to try to understand and forgive Mommy. She's just tired and sick. She doesn't mean it." And most of all, day after tedious day, he exhibits never-wavering confidence that we can continue to get up every morning and do what is necessary to get through the day. He never fails me, and our bond is stronger for having endured this illness.

Likewise, my daughter has been forced to endure upheaval, but she has faced it with grace and wisdom beyond her years. I know it must break her heart to give up the many little things other children take for granted. I almost never make it to any of the school or extracurricular events which are so important to her. Though her father is in the crowd, I am almost always at home. I listen to her stories and often watch video of her performances after the fact, but I am sure that is not the same as being there. She also takes on extra chores and responsibilities at home that I do not believe any child should. She has become a mini-caretaker of sorts to me as well, and she frets. She worries so much about my future and about what will happen to her if I am no longer able to function or if I die.

It is impossible for me to fathom how she manages to hold me in such high esteem despite my many shortcomings. But she does. She cherishes any bit of time I can spend with her and finds enjoyment in any outing we undertake together, no matter how mundane. We remain close in the face of hardships.

While some family members have stepped back from their interactions with me, many have stayed faithful. My parents, siblings, and many of my in-laws have done their best to maintain relationships since my diagnosis. I am not sure they love the changes, but they have done their best to accommodate my needs and be sensitive to my plight, nonetheless. They strive to support me from afar in the ways I ask rather than in the ways they think support should be offered. My father and stepmother actually refrain from visiting, even though they want to see me, because I find it too difficult to entertain visitors these days. They sacrifice financially to help me with my ever-mounting medical bills. They travel to see their grandchild because I cannot bring her to them. My dad leaves messages on my answering machine: "I know you don't feel like talking, but I wanted you to know that I love you, and I am praying for you. I pray for you all the time." My stepfather never fails to call to tell me, "We are going to get through this, kid. We are all going to be alright."

My brother and sister-in-law pick up my child from school on the days my husband cannot, because they know it is a significant burden on me to get to the school in the late afternoon when I am generally feeling my worst. And that same sister-in-law stays for my child's birthday party when I cannot attend and helps serve the children there, monitor their activities, and clean up afterward. She takes pictures and videos at such events so that I can see what I would otherwise have missed.

My sister and brother-in-law sit out in the rain at a concert in which they have little interest, so that I can enjoy a very rare evening out. They travel over an hour, pick me up to take me to that concert because I cannot safely drive, and then try to refrain from eating dinner in front of me because they do not want to hurt me by consuming foods that I can longer have. They go out of their way to make every moment I am out feel like the best moment in the world, to treat me as if I am the center of attention and the most significant person in the room. They focus on meeting my needs, making me comfortable, and pushing aside their own desires to accommodate my wishes. They spend far too much money—money they could have used for events of their own choosing—on overpriced tickets, knowing full well they may have to leave that high-priced concert at the drop of a hat should I start to feel bad.

Many of my old friends have faded away since my diagnosis. While true, it's also expected. After all, we now have little in common, and I rarely see them. The ones who have remained are quite dear to me. My neighbors, whom I consider friends of the highest value, sometimes cook dinner and make treats for my family because I am too sick and too tired to provide this. One neighbor plants flowers for me and delivers homemade hard candies for Christmas because she knows they are one of the few treats I can still enjoy without pain. Another takes my child swimming because I can no longer get her to the pool, and watches our pets when I must be away for medical appointments or brief outings. Still others ask about me frequently and send countless offers to assist in any way they are needed. In addition, I have all sorts of online friends who call, play online games with me, comment on my posts, share coffee memes, write notes for no particular reason, and tell me every day that I matter and that the things I do make a difference in their lives and the lives of others. They offer endless encouragement and brighten even the darkest days.

I am fortunate to have so many kind, caring people in my life. Though I know many others in my community have experienced devastating relationship losses and have been scorned, mocked, and injured beyond reason, my core group has remained by my side. In fact, I've gained more friends, dearer friends than I could ever have imagined. If chronic illness has taught me anything, it has taught me that love is the day-to-day thoughtfulness one displays and the commitment to enduring anything life throws your way. It is standing by each other, offering support and comfort in difficult times, and placing the wants and needs of your loved one before your own. I am eternally grateful for the love I am shown by those around me on a daily basis, and I value the friendships and support from those who have stayed the course more than they might ever know.

*

SAMANTHA ANDERSON

Samantha was diagnosed with idiopathic gastroparesis in 2012 at age 26

I don't see many friends now, just a select few, but will chat to anyone I know and will spend time with them if the situation arises. It is always a pleasure to see and spend time with friends no matter how difficult it is and how bad I feel.

My mum in particular is always on edge, calling to check up on me when we are not together. Even though things are slightly better, she still worries. I feel many in my family, like my parents, siblings and my eldest niece, have been affected by it even if they don't always talk about it to me as they don't want me to feel bad. However, I'm still close to all of them.

But from my perspective, even though I've got some amazing family and friends, they don't truly know what I'm going through. I've felt incredibly lonely at times. I really hate admitting to that because the people I've had around me are amazing. Online groups, especially those on Facebook, help with this. Being able to chat to someone who really understands, even if it's virtual, has helped.

*

JOLI ATKINS
Joli was diagnosed with
gastroparesis in 2015 at age 36

I have lost friendships because of this disease. My friends do not understand that I just cannot do the things I used to do. They don't understand that I cannot just pick up and go whenever I want. Even my family members have backed off from me and do not invite me to family events because of it. My boyfriend has been the most supportive person in my life. He never questions me when I say I don't feel good. He just does his best to make me feel better and comfort me. I have one very understanding and compassionate friend, Melanie, that I would be so lost without. If not for her, I don't know what I would do. She is always there for me whenever I need to vent or cry, or just need a friend to listen.

It is very hard to hear people imply that I don't look sick. I have learned to just let it roll off my back. They don't walk in my shoes and don't have any idea what I am going through, so they can't have any idea what it is like.

*

TRISHA BUNDY
Trisha was diagnosed with
gastroparesis in 2013 at age 35

Like it or not, when dealing day in and day out with being sick from a chronic illness, one learns very quickly what the people around them are truly like. People who I looked at as friends are nowhere to be found. Very few of them care to contact me, even by Facebook messaging. Very few choose to like, or more importantly read, what I post. Cute pictures or jokes are seen and shared by many, but serious articles and awareness videos are ignored. If it's not the cheery, happy me, my normal friends seem to disappear. I try to persuade myself that it's because they don't want to bother me or because they don't know what to say, but a simple little, "How are you?" or "Thinking of you," message or email goes a long way. The truth is, they are not necessarily my truest friends; they are nice, friendly people I came to know across my life journey.

My truest friends are very limited, and that's okay with me. It's better to have a few close, true friends, than many that are just there when times are good. Having a chronic illness has definitely made me rethink and ponder over the relationships and friendships that I have. I honestly have found out the true colors of so many. Now that I see the real them, I don't have to pretend anymore. I don't have to worry about offending or hurting anyone's feelings, as they will probably never read my postings anyway.

I am very appreciative of the new friends I've met along this crazy ride. We are connected by fate, possibly. I know I can say anything and they are there to support me. If I am quiet and not posting during the day, they are checking on me to make sure I'm okay. If I need someone to vent to, they are always there for me, as I am for them. These connections, these friendships, are more meaningful than most will ever realize. We can truly see each other's invisible battles and help each other fight through them. We don't have to hide. We don't have to put on a mask. We don't have to pretend to be feeling well. We don't have to pretend to have control over our condition.

We can be real again. We can openly share our troubles and gain strength from others while at the same time giving hope to one another. We can be honest about what is bothering us (medically, physically, and emotionally) because we know someone is truly listening, someone who can relate. We can cry and laugh together over situations that others can't even imagine. We can share and receive the best possible advice. We can work together to bring awareness publicly. What's ironic is that I am closer with a few friends I met online, than I am with some of my friends who I've spent years and years of my life with.

During my childhood and early adult years, I did not put a lot of thought into characterizing nurses and doctors. Basically, if I needed a flu shot, had an injury that needed to be looked at, was dealing with a cold, or sick with a common virus that was being passed around, I could simply find a doctor to visit. It really didn't matter to me which nurse or doctor I saw. There was a blanket trust that they would know what was wrong, share with me how to treat it, and then send me home to recover and feel better. I did not understand the importance or value of remaining with a specific doctor or taking the time to create a bond. During this time, any nurse and any doctor could meet my needs, whether they had seen me before or not. But now, that's not true. When plagued with a chronic illness, you learn really fast how important it is to actually create a medical team. A team that knows you and understands you. A team that will work with you to devise a game plan. Communication, empathy, and compassionate care all become necessary, along with their medical knowledge and expertise. It's no longer a quick in and out, routine, easy fix. The relationship with my physicians and nurses matter now. I can no longer survive with just any doctor. The type of relationship formed can be extremely powerful, possibly even a game changer or lifesaver.

Being sick has also altered the relationships that I have with my family. Prior to being sick, I was close with my parents. Since being sick, I have experienced an even deeper and closer relationship. I already felt that I had a supportive family. But being chronically ill, being in and out of the hospital, and traveling to and from medical appointments (most of which are out of town) have proven without a doubt how fortunate I am to have them. Without complaining, they take me where I need to be and endlessly provide me with the emotional support that I need as well.

Before becoming sick, and even in the midst of being ill, I tried to handle how I felt independently. I did not want my family, especially my parents, to be aware of how awful I felt. I did not want them to perceive me as being weak or sick. I did not want them to worry. Seeing them hurt or worried would make me feel worse, or so I thought. I was sure that they would not understand my ailments or the severity of my symptoms. Even today, I catch myself trying to prevent them from witnessing bad days. However, I have learned that being honest about how I'm feeling physically and emotionally has valuable benefits. If they see or hear that I'm having a difficult time, they do their best to help me out in whatever way they can. During some of my most troubling times, they worked together to convince me to reach out for medical help from my doctors or hospital.

The relationship with my husband has been affected as well. Being sick to the point of being unable to work and unable to actively participate in life puts a damper on our relationship. I know it has to be challenging for him to helplessly watch someone he loves suffer in pain and unable to join in normal family activities. In some instances, he has had to take on the role of being a caretaker as well as a husband. Worrying about me and my future health has added additional stress and strains on our marriage. Learning how to better cope with the emotions of chronic illness and communicating our fears to one another has become not only important but also essential in order to have an effective and loving marriage.

My role as a mother has not decreased due to illness. Instead, it has been altered in ways that I never expected. Worries, concerns, visions, participation, protecting, teaching, and loving my children are still very present, yet how I perceive the effectiveness of my parenting skills varies greatly, depending on my health situation and how I feel. I have dealt with feeling lots of guilt for not being the type of mother I envisioned for myself. Sadly, I have had to miss out on so many special events, activities, and experiences with my children. My kids have always been patient and understanding with me, aware that I couldn't always do everything that we wanted, because sometimes I was too sick or it was just too demanding on my unhealthy body. I could not have asked for stronger or more loving children.

Even though they understand, I know that it is hard on them. It's only natural for them (as well as myself) to feel disappointed and hurt when plans change or I'm unable to meet our expectations. The important thing is that they are aware that I have and will continue to do my very best to be there in any and all ways that I can. Regardless of my illness and my lack of being as active as I desire, my children will still receive everything they need and more from me as their mother. For every example of what they are missing as a result of my illness, there's a replacement of something else they have learned or experienced about life instead.

I admit, motherhood has altered for me. Doesn't it for everyone? My fears and guilt are senseless. I've not become weak, just different. I continue to teach my children how to be strong and independent adults. I continue to teach my children how to love. I continue to teach them what unconditional love between a mother and child looks like. And I continue to teach them about God's love and blessings.

Coincidentally, the very things that made me feel guilty as a result of my illness, have actually been new lessons for my kids. They are now being taught that everything in life is not always perfect, and that's alright. Deeper conversations replace the backyard playing and practice sessions. They are learning how a family support system works. They are learning to never give up and how to always keep hope alive. They are learning how to advocate for themselves and others. They are learning that God works in mysterious ways. They are learning that prayers are answered in God's time.

Additionally, being chronically ill has impacted the relationship that I have with myself. There are times when I don't feel like I really know who I am anymore, and sometimes I'm not even sure if I like who I've become. It's not uncommon for me to feel worthless and like a burden due to the impact that gastroparesis and other illness related issues have had on my body, mind, and spirit. Sadly, there are days when I'm embarrassed and ashamed of how my symptoms limit what I can and cannot do. It's affected my ability to teach (at least currently) and has altered my parenting style. I am no longer as independent as I once was and have to rely on others more.

I have to remind myself that not all the changes have been negative. While I miss out on some activities and am unable to do everything I want, having to say no or "not this time" more often than I desire, helps me to authentically appreciate moments much more and not take time for granted. The type of lessons taught and activities enjoyed together with family may be different, however, there are still various new meaningful experiences available.

I have also learned a lot about myself along this medical journey. I have realized the importance of self-reflection. I have recognized how blogging and advocating, help with self-healing and feeling as if I'm living with a purpose. And I have come to understand that in order to help others, I must first take care of myself.

*

LISA COLANDREA
Lisa was diagnosed with
gastroparesis in 2016 at age 42

I feel as though gastroparesis has had the biggest impact on my marriage and my family. Although my wife and kids have been very supportive, me having gastroparesis affects their everyday lives. My biggest support is my wife. She has been by my side through my whole journey—mentally, physically and emotionally. She comes to just about every doctor's appointment with me. She makes a lot of my appointments, takes time off from work to take care of the kids when I'm too sick at home or in the hospital, and makes sure I'm always taking my medication. She also does most of the shopping and cooking to make sure I'm eating the foods that I am able to.

Some of my friends and family who I expected to be there for me have been the least supportive. I've spent the past year in and out of the hospital, and trying to educate others on my condition so they know what I'm going through. I've posted information for them on social media only to be ignored. Even though I do have support from certain people, this illness takes such a toll on me physically and emotionally that I still feel very alone and isolated. I have no choice but to cope with those who don't understand. I don't have any coping mechanism. I guess I just ignore them and try to focus on the people who do understand and who are there for me.

*

TAMMY DOWNS

Tammy was diagnosed with Crohn's disease, irritable bowel syndrome, spastic colon, gastroesophageal reflux disease, and gastritis in 2006 at age 46, gastroparesis in 2015 at age 56, and motility dysfunction disorder of the rectum and pelvic floor in 2016 at age 58

Well, thank goodness Jim has been very good. He has learned a lot. At times, he still has a hard time understanding it all, but he is doing good in trying. I learned I had no choice but to make decisions that were going to affect me when it came to bathroom problems, nausea, pain, and my blood pressure lowering. I enjoyed seeing and getting my grandsons, and sometimes helping out, but I had to decide not to help for now. I did not want my grandsons put into a situation that was of my control. So I will see them at family gatherings, and when I feel good. I feel horrible because that is what kept me going, but my energy would be gone by afternoon. My anemia and blood problem affected me also. I would get so worn out so quickly, and be passed out for hours. It was horrible.

*

SKYE FALCON

Skye was diagnosed with gastroparesis and other autoimmune diseases in 2006 at age 25

All my relationships have been impacted by my illnesses, and not just by the gastroparesis. There are few people who truly understand or have taken the time to learn about my illnesses. Most people do a lot of generalizing, guessing, or just blatantly ignore my issues. People have stopped asking how I am, because my answers are never positive enough, as my medical issues are a permanent part of my being. Just as with most invisible illnesses, many people just choose that it is easier to ignore it because they cannot see it, thus making me invisible too. I think they get tired of hearing that nothing is getting better, and only worsening. I know it depresses some, and leaves others feeling helpless and stuck. But I cannot help but wonder if they have ever stopped to think of how I feel being stuck with this every single day?

I have lost many friends simply because I cancel too much, and according to a few, I just have too much going on, or am too sad and heavy. Like I have a choice in the matter. I think I am supposed to be thankful that one person was able to speak those truthful words to me. Better off for me to know who not to waste my precious time and energy with, I suppose, in the grand scheme of these illnesses. I do not even hear from some of my closest people anymore, because their own lives do not allow time to slow for their sick friends. I really do not deal with people who refuse to understand, constantly compare my issues to dieting, or treat my issues with any sort of disrespect. Dealing with these types of friends just adds another level of difficulty to trudge through. I also think if they are truly your supporter, they would take the initiative and learn the basics.

Gastroparesis is a loud illness, which means that it is always in your face. Always demanding attention. Always causing problems. The vomiting, the intense pain, the constant and permanent residence taken up in the bathroom is life-stopping. The symptoms, ailments, and issues that come from gastroparesis are also visible. The weight loss, protruding bones, shrinking body, and sunken eyes do not allow me to hide how I am really feeling.

My marriage has struggled in the past few years since my gastroparesis diagnosis more than it ever has in the past, and we have been at it for almost two decades. The third wheel in our marriage now seems to reside directly between us, keeping us at an arm's length more than it should. I often find myself trying to step into my husband's shoes, and the terror that he must feel going through this with me. As an empath, it is easier for me to empathize with how he feels observing all of this, than it is for him to convey how he is feeling. But the silence kills me. Being left to my own devices to cope and deal is unimaginably difficult, and makes hanging on to my ever-changing mental state that much harder.

Hearing that I have stressed him out and made our relationship so complicated adds unexpected and unrelenting levels of stress which just restarts the sickness cycle. This screaming, yelling and squeaking third wheel sits in between us, dictates our conversation topics, tells us what we can do with our free time, and now shows us where all the tough spots are in our relationship. This man though, is my rock. The absolute love of my life, however long that life may be. There are no rule books, or directions, for navigating marriage through chronic, terminal illnesses. So every day we do our best, trying to keep ourselves together as we both promised, with our bond that has been there since the first minutes we met.

All that said, I find myself wondering if any of these disappearing friends and family ever stop and think just how all of these changes have directly impacted me individually and altered my everyday life. If they ever think about how hard this must be for me, and how much I must hate being limited in such ways. Every day when you wake up, you face the possibility of losing yet another ability, or being unable to do something that just two days before you had successfully completed. I am not sure I can, or could, ever put into words what losing little pieces of yourself as you're walking down life's path is really like with this chronic, lifelong issue. You just watch the little pieces fall away: the ability to eat, the ability to function, and the ability to be out of the house for more than an hour at a time. There is nothing you can do. Many times, on top of that, we are then left wondering where our friends and family went because we were there to support them when they needed it. And when no one comes around, still, we are just reminded where we stand.

I do not need or want pity. No special treatment or favors. I just want to be acknowledged for the badass woman, hard-working entrepreneur, dedicated mom, and giving human that I am. I wish my limitations were not the focus of conversations, but my goals, accomplishments, and future plans. I wish, when my illnesses arise in conversation, that those engaging me and asking are truly vested, and not furthering their own gossipy game. Most of all, I wish people would still treat me like a person. My human needs did not change, although everyone seems to have reacted as if they did.

*

ROBIN MCNAMARA
Robin was diagnosed with
gastroparesis in 2013 at age 55

My work relationships remain in place. Work family is okay with a couple of exceptions, which is fine. I have a couple of really special friends who have been the most supportive, along with a sister who has been there through my nightmare. I still get angry at those who don't understand, don't ask questions, and just go on with their agenda and journey. I try not to get angry, but I just can't help myself.

*

TAMMY PITTMAN
Tammy was diagnosed with gastroparesis and
irritable bowel syndrome in 2014 at age 34

I've lost many friends because they can't understand. My parents are absolutely no support; they only ridicule. My ex-husband is very supportive. He helps me with so much. My kid's father says I'm faking it because I don't want to take care of my kids. He has my daughter convinced of this. My son helps—he's held my hair while I vomit, helps with housework, helps me walk on bad days, cooks, and makes sure I take my medication. I try to ignore those who are not supportive.

*

TAYLOR SCHMITZ
Taylor was diagnosed with idiopathic
gastroparesis in 2014 at age 22

Since the beginning of my journey with gastroparesis, I have lost friends, and I've even lost family members. I've stopped talking to family members, because they just don't understand, nor do they try to understand. I've learned that people will always judge you, no matter what you do. They always think they know better than you, which makes it difficult to maintain those relationships, because they will never understand why you can't do certain things.

My marriage has been the ultimate test. My husband has been through hell and back with this. He supports me financially, but he also helps me physically and emotionally. Whenever I'm scared, he always makes me laugh. He is always up for a crazy new alternative remedy, and he always has faith that I will get better. The same can be said about my dad. He doesn't ever let me whine, or freak out, but when I need to cry, he always has a soft heart and the most comforting words. He always has a fix for everything, and is positive things will get better. They never lose faith.

Faith is the most important thing in life, especially with a chronic illness. Another thing necessary is compassion. If more people could just put themselves in our shoes, they would be able to see why we can't go on that fancy trip, or go grab a drink, or get to that party.

*

NICOLE STARZYNSKI
Nicole was diagnosed with
gastroparesis in 2016 at age 33

Kirstin has had a hard time dealing with me being sick, but has been my biggest supporter. She is a tough kid with a huge heart. This year, even after all the wonderful gifts she received, she said the best gift was that her mom wasn't going to be sick anymore. Made me cry.

My boyfriend has stood by me. He has dropped everything to help me at home, with everyday tasks around the house. Being sick every day, things start to get unorganized. He doesn't live here, but he always makes time to help me. The past year hasn't been easy. We have had to travel to Baltimore numerous times, and to Cleveland Clinic too many time to count. Overnight stays, leaving the house at 4 a.m. to get to an appointment by 8 a.m. All day tests. Tests that spanned multiple days. Between my mom and Josh, I had someone with me for every single appointment. I never had to go through it alone.

Josh's ex-wife told their daughter I made up the disease and I wasn't sick at all. That caused kids at school to give my daughter a hard time. Recently, since my surgery and the fact that I weigh 116 pounds, all of a sudden my disease is real. It's those heartless people who add to the stress of a chronic disease. My daughter has been through enough without having to validate the fact that her mom has been sick for over a year. My point is that Josh and I have been through more in less than four years than most relationships ever go through. From the nasty ex-wife with no soul or heart, to endless doctor visits and never-ending tests, to finding a doctor who could help me. I've been pricked and poked more than a pin cushion. Hearing that one day I may lose my stomach completely and would receive nutrition from tubes was the hardest thing I was ever told from a doctor.

In the past year I've gone through things with a positive attitude and I attribute that to the support of my boyfriend, family and the few friends who have never stopped being there for me. Plus, there have been a few people who have been very important in helping me find my own strength to fight against this disease. The past year has been one of the hardest years of my life and I know I couldn't have done it without my support system. I pray for a future that is gastroparesis system free. I know the battle is not over, but knowing I don't have to fight it alone is worth more than anyone could ever know.

One thing I have learned over the past year is that some people will run as far away from you as they can when they find out you have a chronic illness. With the exception of a few people, all of my friends have kind of nixed me because I have been sick for so long, they just gave up on me completely.

It hurt when some of my best friends I grew up with didn't even bother to call me after I had surgery. Most haven't even called me to see how I've been at all. Sometimes it frustrates me and makes me angry at them, and other times I say, "Oh, well." The people who care are still here. This disease creates enough mental anxiety and exhaustion. I've learned with everything else, to just let it go. Sometimes it's harder when it actually hurts, like when people who have been in your life for over twenty years leave you when you need them the most. I have also been reacquainted, however, with some wonderful, supportive people.

*

JENNIFER ZUBIK

Jennifer was diagnosed with idiopathic gastroparesis in 2010 at age 27

I can honestly say that every person in my life has been supportive, thankfully. I am fortunate to not have this disease ruin any friendships or relationships. Even though I struggled and felt like an inconvenience, guilty, ugly, rude, and depressing to myself and others, my family and friends supported me and accommodated all my needs.

Lou and I struggled financially and intimately, but he stood by my side regardless of the difficulties. He took days off to take me to every doctor appointment or to just take care of me. He would take me to the hospital emergency room if needed, at any time of night or day, and never left my side. He worked extra hard when he could to take care of our financial needs. Lou and my daughter helped around the house and took care of themselves when I couldn't do it. It was unfortunate how much our lives had changed, and that they had to experience the hardships too. I felt guilty for what I was putting them and our family through.

My daughter, my angel, struggled a lot, but she too adapted and did her best to overcome. Having to explain to her friends and teachers my illness and why she didn't have that assignment done or couldn't have a sleepover that night was difficult for her because nobody understood. One day, she told her teacher I had gastroparesis and about my symptoms and what was wrong, and her teacher told her, "What is that? I have never heard of such of thing? That is not the problem, that can't be a real disease." My daughter was angry at her teacher after that.

Friends who I hadn't seen in a long time would comment on my weight loss and would ask how I did it. "You look great, you don't look sick." My response would always be, "I did want to lose weight, but not this much. And you may think I look great, but I feel horrible.

Thanks, though." Then they would ask questions and I would explain my disease and they would feel terrible and apologize. Although, they would then commend me for still fighting, having hope and being in good spirits.

Overall, I had an ultimate support system. I thank god for all of them every day. As angry as I had been to have to suffer with this disease and make those around me suffer as well, my family and friends have helped me survive and have given me the will to continue to fight each day.

*

CHAPTER TEN

Engaging in Intimacy

Being able to feel good having sex is what makes me feel like a woman. Having that pleasure taken away and replaced with pain is a feeling that can't quite be put into words. -ANONYMOUS

For many, the painful symptoms of gastroparesis affect our intimacy resulting in rejection and hurt feelings. For others, it's an opportunity to indulge in creative pleasure. How often does your gastroparesis interfere with your ability to experience pleasure instead of pain?

*

MELISSA ADAMS VANHOUTEN
Melissa was diagnosed with
gastroparesis in 2014 at age 47

I decline to answer this question, as I believe some aspects of relationships must remain private. I don't feel comfortable discussing physically intimate details. A personal hang-up? Perhaps. Nonetheless, I hope you can gather from all I've written and from the feelings and tone I have expressed that intimacy, indeed, still exists. This is a difficult life, one fraught with pain and weariness, but love remains. The bonds are strong and the feelings are deep.

*

SAMANTHA ANDERSON
Samantha was diagnosed with idiopathic gastroparesis in 2012 at age 26

Ha ha, that is how I feel about this. Being single at the time I got ill didn't leave much room for finding a relationship. Who wants to be with someone who is vomiting? I'm embarrassed about my condition, which I shouldn't be, but just can't help it. To be fair, it is disgusting. I don't feel that way about others who have it, but it seems to be different when it is yourself. I'm always very hard on myself anyway and do still need to learn to be less self-critical.

I often feel a little jealous of those getting in new relationships or moving to the next level. It's not that I'm not happy for these people, I am. But I would like to be doing similar myself. I'm not blaming the condition solely for it. I'm to blame for a lot of it. I'm lazy in this way and not sure where to start. I'm a person who gives my all to those around me and I'm always so tired, so wonder how I would get on trying to do it for extra people. Doing that and all the other things you do when fresh in a relationship is very difficult. When do you approach being ill, and maybe not eating or drinking around them for a while? Not seeing a future with someone, and the possibility of having children shrinking is often how I see things, I think more as a defense mechanism. I look to the future and don't see it changing, but hope it will change.

I'm not a negative person so I'm sure the future will be brighter. It has to be. I know people who have gastroparesis do it. I would love to know how and need to get some advice from them on this matter.

I must admit that I've written blogs in the past when raising money, but writing for this book has been very hard. I have written about and admitted things I haven't admitted before. Sometimes it was because I felt guilty about it, or because I try not to be negative about everything that is going on, otherwise life would just be a complete drag. It's bad enough as it is having gastroparesis without being completely miserable.

*

JOLI ATKINS
Joli was diagnosed with
gastroparesis in 2015 at age 36

It is very difficult to please my boyfriend and myself. There is an eighteen-year age difference between us, so it can be difficult. He can be a very sexual man and I want to please him, however, my disease has other ideas. There are nights when I feel great, and then I go to bed and I start to feel bad. I have to sometimes do a mind over matter approach and allow myself some pleasure, and worry about the consequences later.

*

LISA COLANDREA
Lisa was diagnosed with
gastroparesis in 2016 at age 42

My gastroparesis interferes with many things including personal, intimate relationships. When you're sick and tired all the time, your body doesn't have the drive nor energy. I have a partner who understands what I go through and all the emotion that comes with it.

*

TAMMY DOWNS

Tammy was diagnosed with Crohn's disease, irritable bowel syndrome, spastic colon, gastroesophageal reflux disease, and gastritis in 2006 at age 46, gastroparesis in 2015 at age 56, and motility dysfunction disorder of the rectum and pelvic floor in 2016 at age 58

It has a way of causing issues at times. Thank goodness Jim is very understanding. I do my best to make sure this area of my life is not destroyed. We talk and I keep him updated on what is happening with me, and how I'm feeling. He works with me very well. That is important.

*

SKYE FALCON

Skye was diagnosed with gastroparesis and other autoimmune diseases in 2006 at age 25

Gastroparesis has almost become an extra individual in the bedroom. Every day it tells me when I should or should not touch my partner, when I should try lying flat, if my body can tolerate any pleasure, or when I should just give up. If I adhere to my liquid and softs meal plan, then there's a chance I can tolerate being touched. Sometimes the pain is so great, the only relief comes from some high level of BDSM (bondage, domination, submission, and masochism) interaction where one pain counteracts the other pain. My illnesses have opened a whole new world of intimacy and pleasure-seeking methods in my life, so much so, that it is my beloved profession. In a life without intimacy, there is a certain piece of our humanity missing that helps keep us internally calm, so intimacy during any illness is extremely important.

As a degree-holding adult educator, I work with cancer patients and the chronically ill on this issue. Intimacy is such a huge, important part of life and our well being. Without intimacy, we cannot be whole. That said, intimacy is not just intercourse. Even knowing all of this and being a sexpert, I still have moments of pure madness and struggle. Gastroparesis is a constant battle, every day, and it is relentless. The pain and discomfort alone are enough to turn away any sort of touch. Add in the constant trips to the bathroom, vomiting, and general malaise from those things, and what is really left over for that? Just what is left for intimacy? Relationships and marriages take a ton of work and effort, so which do I choose to deal with? Do I heal myself enough to get through the day and be human? Or do I use my energy to work through things with my partner, and hope for a few moments of intimacy? These are questions I cannot seem to find a happy balance with. I am a very sexual, physical person and this is one of the biggest issues that arises in my life.

In my work and studies on these topics, and in my personal experience, I have learned that we must be okay and comfortable with ourselves to settle into any type of intimacy. We have to be okay with having our illnesses, and be at peace with whatever is happening. That doesn't mean we have to accept it. We have to live with our scars and embrace them as fought and won battles within ourselves. If we have not yet won the battle or conquered the scar, then it is one we are still comfortably working on. The less comfortable we are with ourselves and those scars, the less we will ever want to interact with another intimately, or believe that they want to be that close with us.

The same can be said about body types, and feeling too fat, or too skinny. People often forget that those who are super thin often do not choose that path, and they too, just want a taco. We have to be comfortable with ourselves before we can share ourselves fully with another. We have to love ourselves enough before we can love someone else. Communication is a huge factor in being comfortable in even attempting intimacy with these types of illnesses, and one at the forefront of my marriage. I do not think I ever stop talking about anything and everything. My poor husband. This is where we differ; he works best with silence.

I am extremely in touch with myself, my needs and wants. I have found that most types of intimate release do offer pain reducing and muscle calming moments. While some of the standard positions are no longer achievable due to the internal hardening of joints and tissues, there are still a myriad of intimate things that can happen. Heating pads and going with the flow are really the key, and not being set to only be intimate at night, as many are. I find I am livelier in the morning, and my body is calmer after a nap or rest period. That said, as my body has changed, become weaker and unlike anything I have ever seen, I feel him pulling away more than ever. Only time will tell if it is my frailty, the illness, or how things will pan out in the end.

My partner struggles to know how to handle me from one day to the next. My level of fragility seems to change depending on how my body is functioning, and it can be hard to read, even for myself. Some days I need the intense touch to balance out the body pains that are holding me back, and other days I can't tolerate the touch of a feather.

Even on those rough days, there are still numerous possibilities for intimacy. Cuddling, deep conversations, discussing memories, and even role playing can help ease tensions, and bring us back together again. There are times when I can tell he is afraid he is hurting me, and in those moments, I do my best to reassure, and press on.

We have discussed these things so often, and so much, that it helps us to navigate the tough days. Discussion and communication help see us through the gross issues that arise too, like sudden bathroom breaks for vomiting or exploding. Because intimacy means so much to both of us, it is something we push to the front of our marriage at any cost or difficulty. These days, as we struggle to find the balance and common ground, our discussions are more focused on what the point of everything is if I am just going to die. Morbid, heavy, and just another real part of a chronically awesome life with gastroparesis.

*

TAMMY PITTMAN

Tammy was diagnosed with gastroparesis and irritable bowel syndrome in 2014 at age 34

I don't have a sexual partner.

*

TAYLOR SCHMITZ

Taylor was diagnosed with idiopathic gastroparesis in 2014 at age 22

Being intimate is so hard when you feel like you are going to throw up at any given moment. It's like feeling hung over constantly.

I love my husband so much, and I know he loves me. But I'm sick all the time, and he's exhausted from dealing with me being sick all the time, so it's very difficult for us to show how we feel about each other. We have gotten much better about showing our feelings without having to be physical, though. You really need to focus on little things you can do to show your significant other you are thinking about them, and genuinely want them to be happy.

I have to build up the strength, and force myself to think about him and my daughter instead of focusing on my disease one hundred percent of the time. If our spouses focused on something else one hundred percent of the time, we would call them cheaters! So why is it okay to feed into my illness all the time? It is very difficult at times, even though my husband is so supportive of me. It causes depression and frustration, and we do our best to combat these by talking about everything we possibly can, although this is something my husband really needs to work on still! I use essential oils and ginger tea for the pain, which greatly help, even if we are just trying to cuddle or give massages, as they even help sometimes. But having patience for each other and communicating how you feel are the keys to a healthy relationship, even if you aren't ill.

*

NICOLE STARZYNSKI
Nicole was diagnosed with
gastroparesis in 2016 at age 33

I'm very lucky that Josh is so easy going. He's my best friend first. We talk about everything, which is very important when you are fighting a chronic disease. Especially with intimacy, you have to talk to your partner. That is key. They aren't a mind reader, and even though they know you are battling a disease, they can't be expected to know when is a good time and when isn't a good time. Some days when I feel very bloated and haven't pooped in a few days or a week, I'm not in any mood to be touched. I don't feel very attractive, and my stomach sometimes hurts because the skin feels like it's going to rip. So we talk about it. This way he knows it's nothing he has done or that I am not attracted to him. This way he knows it is simply because I don't feel well.

Since being diagnosed, we talk all the time about how this disease affects me, my daughter and our relationship. He is one hundred percent supportive in every way. He never makes me feel bad, he doesn't put me down. Instead, he reassures me we will get through this together. There have been many times that a doctor's appointment or procedure makes it a few weeks before we can be intimate. It's frustrating, but as long as we continue to talk about it and stay open, I believe that we will only continue to grow closer.

*

JENNIFER ZUBIK
Jennifer was diagnosed with idiopathic
gastroparesis in 2010 at age 27

My husband and I struggled quite a bit with this disease. These years have been like a rollercoaster ride, up and down and all around. Lou has been wonderful, though. I wouldn't be here today if it wasn't for him staying by my side and getting us through the turmoil we faced. Emotionally, he was there for me, but there were many moments of frustration. Physically, intimacy became difficult for us. We would attempt to go to bed together, but the majority of the time we were unsuccessful. I would get out of bed, and grab my pillow, electric blanket, and my bear. He would say, "I guess you are going to sleep in the bathroom again? Just stay here, lay with me, you will be fine." Or he would get close and kiss me and attempt to be intimate, but I wouldn't feel well enough to continue.

I feared getting started and getting sick, and having to stop during the heat of the moment. It became a major battle for us at one point in time. He was experiencing a lot of frustration with it. I didn't want him to feel like I didn't want to or I didn't love him as much or wasn't attracted to him anymore, but I know he did feel that way at times. I also struggled with not feeling confident in myself and not being attractive to him anymore, but he would reassure me I was still beautiful.

We learned to talk and improvise and compromise. I normally felt better in the morning than I did at night, so we made more attempts of intimacy then. We had more spontaneity throughout the day when I would be having a better one. Or we would even just lay on the couch or in bed and cuddle, hold each other and tell one another, "I love you." As time passed, we learned that an act as simple as holding each other's hand or giving a hug or a kiss was more than enough for us to show affection, and get by during this difficult time.

*

CHAPTER ELEVEN

Coping with a Career

It's not what you achieve. It's what you overcome.
That's what defines your career. -CARLTON FISK

Chronic health conditions can play a significant role in our ability to be gainfully employed. How has gastroparesis affected your ability to work and advance in your career?

*

MELISSA ADAMS VANHOUTEN
Melissa was diagnosed with
gastroparesis in 2014 at age 47

I have not worked outside the home in any significant fashion since the birth of my daughter thirteen years ago, so I cannot say that gastroparesis is the reason I dropped out of the workforce. However, I can say that it is largely the reason I have not returned to work outside the home. The severity and unpredictability of my pain, nausea, and bloating would make it difficult to advance in any sort of meaningful career, I believe. I am unable to travel much at this point and am largely homebound due to the effects of gastroparesis.

This does not mean I have given up on finding meaningful work, though. Besides caring for my daughter, my husband, and our household affairs in whatever fashion I still can given my limitations, I now spend my days working from home in the service of the gastroparesis community. I consider myself an online patient and gastroparesis awareness advocate, and I also act as administrator in a number of gastroparesis support and advocacy groups.

I volunteer for a nonprofit which assists those living with motility disorders. My volunteer work involves writing articles and awareness materials, hosting calls and chats, and offering other assistance with short-term projects when needed. It keeps me quite busy, but it also allows me to set my own schedule and work only when I feel well enough to work. It adds meaning and purpose to my life and makes me feel as if I am doing something significant to help others who struggle with this same cruel illness. In short, it makes me feel as if I am making a difference. The downside? No income, of course.

I have considered looking into working from home, but am not certain my skill set matches available opportunities, and, quite frankly, I enjoy advocating for and assisting my community. How could I neglect the people I have grown to love? It may not be the flashy career I once dreamed of, but I am fulfilling a need in my community and following what I believe to be a purpose, a calling. I am more at peace with the path I am pursuing now than I have ever been in the past, and it is an amazing feeling to sense I am on my intended path. I am blessed to be able to function well enough to contribute (albeit online) to a cause so dear to my heart and so significant to my community.

In addition, my new, unexpected position has given me the opportunity to spread my wings a bit and pursue creative projects and tasks I once believed impossible for me. I pen essays and poems, generate memes and visual aids, produce videos, and maintain a website and blog. I've spoken at local events and even a digestive disorders conference. I continue to work to create materials designed to assist and educate the gastroparesis community. This has opened up a new world to me in terms of self-expression and imagination, one I would most surely have continued to neglect had I remained in the business world.

Though I miss aspects of the real work world, I have found ways to compensate for my loss and still manage to find fulfillment in my online world. It has required an adjustment in perspective and attitude on my part, but the blessings it has brought are unmatched by anything I have known to date. I am thankful for the many opportunities I have been afforded both outside and inside my home.

*

SAMANTHA ANDERSON
Samantha was diagnosed with idiopathic
gastroparesis in 2012 at age 26

When I first got ill in 2011, I was working as a primary school teacher with a year four class. I went from not having time off work, to at first having a few days off thinking I had a bug, to going back and every couple of weeks having time off for a few days to a week. I had been to the doctors and the hospital. Doctors diagnosed me with everything from indigestion to constipation to having a urinary tract infection. I continued working, feeling weak and very rough for ten months, but it was taking its toll on me.

I'm a person who gives one hundred percent to what I do. I was getting into work for 7:30 a.m., working through the breaks, and then leaving when the school building closed at about 6 to 6:30 p.m. I worried how it could be affecting my students. After all, I was living in a constant daze and, to be fair, it isn't much better now. I felt like I was an awful teacher and was terrible at my job. Having observations on top of that often pushed me over the edge. In the end, I could do it no more and went off sick long-term, until I realized that I wasn't going to get better anytime soon—then I left.

I really didn't want to have to give up work. It left a sour taste in my mouth (excuse the pun). Even though I was feeling so ill, I was walking the walls because I was bored and wanted to be doing something. I still wanted to be as active physically and mentally as I could. I am one to definitely push my limits, but I needed something.

A few months after not working, we got a dog. It actually wasn't out of choice. I really didn't want him at the time, but now I know he was my little lifesaver. Taking him for walks became the highlight of my day. No matter how ill I felt, it would help clear my mind. He is one of my best buddies now. I love him and couldn't be without him. He has made having this awful illness a little bit easier to deal with.

At heart I am a foodie which, with this condition, is a nightmare. Luckily, I don't really get hungry, but I do miss being able to eat and enjoy proper food without comebacks. However, I still took up baking for everyone else to enjoy. It gave me little things to do.

In 2016, eight months after having the gastric pacemaker, I decided to go back to work. My health was far from great, but I had no money and no other way of getting money. I knew that I couldn't go back full-time as I would have ended up feeling very poorly, so part-time was the only way I could go back. Still not being able to eat properly and having to really watch the times I ate, I needed to be selective.

I thought what I had been trained in was wasted. I couldn't yet go back into a school and was very unsure (even now) if I would be able to go back properly, however, upon looking online I found tuition centers that were more suited and would work around my illness. I thought that maybe I could do some midday (lunchtime) supervisor's work in a school, just so I was in that environment. I went about writing my resume and applications and it wasn't long before I got a job in tuition centers.

The hours are actually longer than I believed and it's very difficult, but I am doing it. I wanted to get more of a life back, but I haven't really managed this yet. Now I work, and I deal with my health when I am not working. I like the fact that I feel like I am doing something and trying to move in the right direction. I probably could do with working more hours. However, I know that although I could do that for a while, I don't think my body would be able to cope with my issues surrounding my gastroparesis, and I would end up off work again.

I'd like to think I will work in a school, teaching again in the future. It may not quite work out that way. I'm not sure if doing it full-time would work, even if I would like to believe it will happen. I am positive enough to believe things will get better, and I will be able to do the things I want, so I will not rule it out!

*

JOLI ATKINS
Joli was diagnosed with
gastroparesis in 2015 at age 36

I am one of the fortunate ones who is still able to work, but my gastroparesis has hindered my ability to work at a normal pace and normal hours. I am very fortunate to work for a great place that is very understanding when I am sick. I also suffer from migraines, so I have times when I will be out for weeks. It can be very draining on my morale and even on my relationship. I do my best to make it to work as much as possible because I have a lot of responsibility at my job. I want to do the best that I can for everyone.

*

TRISHA BUNDY
Trisha was diagnosed with
gastroparesis in 2013 at age 35

I'm not going to lie. Illness has caused me to experience a myriad of emotions as it has interfered with my life more than I ever could have imagined. Besides interfering with family activities, it has also restricted me from continuing my teaching career. I became heart-broken because I honestly felt as if I was being forced to give up everything that I had worked so hard for and more. I had dedicated my life to achieve my long-time ambition of being an inspirational teacher. I had pushed myself through sickness and pain, spent endless hours searching and planning for meaningful classroom lessons and experiences, laid my heart out to reach and connect with students who didn't see the potential that resided within. But now, unexpectedly, illness was robbing me of my livelihood.

I loved teaching with a passion. Without a doubt, it was a dream come true. It was a career I enjoyed, a career that made me feel full of pride. I honestly felt like I was making a positive impact on the lives of others and thought I was using the talents I was blessed with to live a life full of purpose. I was sure that I was taking the path God intended me to follow.

When I became sick, I admittedly didn't listen to my body's personal needs. My body and my health were not my priority. Teaching and being an active parent were much more important to me. I literally continued teaching, working, and staying on the go with my kids with every ounce of energy I had. While feeling worn down and sick I continued to stay busy with all of their school related and extracurricular activities, as well as all the motherly duties I expected of myself. I even took classes online at night for a few years so I could earn my master's degree in 2012, and better provide for my family.

Regardless of what my body was trying to tell me, I was strong-minded, strong-willed, and gave everything I had to live the life that I envisioned as a mother and teacher. I was determined to not let anyone or anything (including my own body) destroy my desire for teaching. I did not bother to consider or listen to the advice that my family kept expressing. Instead, I kept fighting and kept pursuing my dreams until my body ultimately crashed. I did not value my needs, because to me that felt as if it would be selfish, expressing weakness, and simply did not see me as being a priority.

In retrospect, and as an outsider looking in, I realize that to give my best, I need to be at my best. And that can only happen when I fulfill my personal needs, namely my health. Ignoring my health needs and symptoms will not make them disappear. I've tried that thinking over and over again, and all it does is lead me to more issues. Unfortunately, some of that ideology came from medical professionals such as doctors and nurses who minimized my concerns and the impact it was having on my personal life, when I did finally reach the point to actually ask for help and assistance. My dreams of making a difference in the classroom have ended, at least for now. In the beginning, I was persistent that illness was not going to interfere with my personal life. Wow! That was a joke. The harder I fought for normalcy, the worse my health declined.

The largest and one of the most difficult decisions in my life revolved around working. For a long time, too long according to my family, I continued to teach while trying to figure out my health. Trying to managing both my illness and my career, I wasn't as effective as I wanted to be and should have been. However, I did the absolute best I could under the circumstances. I missed a lot of work due to health and health-related appointments, and found myself prioritizing my students' class experiences before my personal well-being. After being out on short-term disability with the school system for almost a year, I was forced to decide if I would be able to return to work or if I needed to apply for extended short-term with the school system.

Hesitantly, I made the difficult choice (even though my health was not truly giving me a choice) to give up my position at my school. I loved being the fifth grade science teacher there, but going on extended sick leave to achieve better health was requiring me to not only lose my fifth grade position, but also my school. I was told that when I was able to return to work, Central Office for my school system would determine which school I would be assigned to based on vacancy needs. Due to my health, pain, energy, and upcoming surgery at the time, I bit my pride and tearfully cleared out my classroom. As difficult as the decision was, looking back I know for a fact that it was the best option for me, as the surgery did occur and recovery was, well, quite a challenge physically and mentally. As heartbreaking as it was, closing that chapter of my life and putting my health first was a necessary and worthwhile choice.

My extended sick leave expired months later, and once again I was left with a difficult choice. A choice that was dependent on not only myself but also my medical team. The choice left me torn and fearful. I had to decide if my medical team and I believed that I should apply for long-term disability from the school system, which would heartbreakingly require me to resign from my dream career at the age of thirty-eight, or attempt to return to work before December 2016.

Honestly, as hard as it was for me to admit, I understand that long-term disability, at least for now, is the best and only reasonable option for me. I am still struggling with my health, energy, and at times emotional state. I currently require IV hydration five times a week, which requires home health to visit weekly to manage my port.

In addition, I have medical appointments that are necessary for monitoring my health status, managing my medical devices, and maintaining mental stability. All of which would require a lot of time away from the classroom and prevent me from being able to work.

*

LISA COLANDREA
Lisa was diagnosed with
gastroparesis in 2016 at age 42

Gastroparesis, along with a few other medical conditions, have prevented me from working, so I don't have a job on the line or other employees getting upset with me for having to cover work shifts. However, my wife is my biggest support and help, and she's had to work from home and miss work more times than I can count. She's also had to take leaves of absence to be home to help me. Her job has definitely been on the line, and because of that, it fills me with even more anxiety than I already have. I feel horrible my family has had to go through this with me.

*

TAMMY DOWNS
Tammy was diagnosed with Crohn's disease, irritable bowel syndrome, spastic colon, gastroesophageal reflux disease, and gastritis in 2006 at age 46, gastroparesis in 2015 at age 56, and motility dysfunction disorder of the rectum and pelvic floor in 2016 at age 58

Crohn's disease put me out of work in 2005. Since then, I've had multiple illnesses that compounded my inability to work. I would think, "I can do this," but my body had a different idea. Employers look at people with certain diseases not always in a good way. They do not feel we can do our job properly. I even had doubts in myself because of situations when my disease caused problems that made it difficult and embarrassing. I tried working, but had to give it up when I found out I had fibromyalgia, osteoarthritis, Crohn's disease, irritable bowel syndrome, gastritis, acid reflux, and other illnesses. As years went on, other illnesses came into play, including gastroparesis.

Gastroparesis and motility issues are big problems for me. I often get flares and wouldn't even attempt to try to work. Since I do a lot of eating through smoothies and soups, it's not easy to be in a workplace where you have to set up the supplies you need for nutrition. I cannot just eat out all the time, and restaurants don't have what I can eat or drink. It does put me in a spot with what to do at times.

*

SKYE FALCON

Skye was diagnosed with gastroparesis and other autoimmune diseases in 2006 at age 25

My gastroparesis and other illnesses have indeed changed the way I am able to work, how often, and what jobs I can do. In the beginning of my autoimmune journey, I was in public teaching. I absolutely loved teaching, and loved the kiddos even more, but I did not love their germs! There came a point when I could no longer tolerate being exposed to any of them, and every time that I was, I was admitted into the hospital with a debilitating sickness. It just so happened that at the same time, certain issues arose in the school system we were in, and suddenly home schooling was on the table for our family.

It was then when I opened my own private home school out of my house, that I had for close to three years. This allowed me to continue doing what I loved, gave me time to be sick, and let my children excel at their own pace, work ahead, and stay away from the heavy germs public school offered. This also became a very beneficial set-up, as my youngest daughter had to have major heart surgeries, and this allowed for her to be germ-free, rested, and in her own environment to heal as long as she needed. There was a definite point in our private homeschool adventures where things shifted. Our extra friends and their parents were completely checked out, and making it a chore for my own children to learn. At that time, I made the decision to shut it down.

It was around that time when I began to focus more on my other teaching job, which is teaching adults about everything and anything intimate and sexually related. I also began writing more, sharing my special recipes I was crafting for myself and my celiac daughter, and really thinking about how I wanted to further my businesses in the future. Being my own boss really helped with scheduling and ensuring that I did not overbook myself, or take on too much. These in-home jobs help me maintain a busy level that I am comfortable with, and allow me to help support our family. I can grow at my own pace, and be a part of just the things that I want to. I am hopeful that I can really grow these businesses into something to be proud of over the next decade, body willing.

I do still work some out of the house too, as an adult sexual education and intimacy specialist. My work staff are very supportive, and know about most of my medical issues. They allow me to work how I need to, when I need to, and support me when I cannot. I am so grateful for this job and the people there. They are open, welcoming, and not judgmental in the slightest. In our industry, we see it all, hear it all, and help all different kinds of people and situations. One of the main reasons we branched into dealing with the medical side of intimacy and issues was because of my own situations, personal experiences, and growing knowledge of the chronically ill.

I do not worry about promotions as I am already in management, and was promoted to this job while I was incredibly ill! I am excited to work and to help people regain their own intimacy needs, even when chronic and terminal illness reign. Knowing that the work I do benefits others, helps others find happiness and pleasure, and keeps other humans feeling just that: human, is more reward than I ever imagined, and keeps me looking toward the future. This job is indeed one of my greatest passions, and I am told and reminded regularly, just how much good, support, and calm I provide.

There are times within my job where my illnesses do step in and prevent the work from being done. I have had to cancel presentations and classes last minute because I did not have the level of calories or nutritional buildup to suffice. There have been times my gut just stops working minutes before a class or event, and I am forced to continue, pale, sick, and with a sub-par energy level. Not being able to complete or follow through with my obligations is one of the worst things I have to deal with due to the gastroparesis, and other chronic illnesses.

*

ROBIN MCNAMARA
Robin was diagnosed with
gastroparesis in 2013 at age 55

The longest amount of time I've missed work was when I was first diagnosed. I went back to work after ten days. When allergy season hit, I had severe daily nausea. I left work one day, and called in sick the next. I'm truly blessed that I can work and remain productive. I have not had any promotion opportunities, so I cannot answer that question. Being older than mid-thirties to mid-forties, I'm not in line for any promotion based on succession planning.

*

TAMMY PITTMAN
Tammy was diagnosed with gastroparesis and
irritable bowel syndrome in 2014 at age 34

My gastroparesis has hindered my ability to work for over ten years, but I pushed until I just couldn't physically do it anymore. Being in nursing, management is supportive of me and understands my conditions, but at the end of the day, they have to have employees who are dependable and well enough to do the job. I haven't been able to work the past seven years, and it's been a real strain on me and my family, both mentally and financially.

*

TAYLOR SCHMITZ
Taylor was diagnosed with idiopathic
gastroparesis in 2014 at age 22

Since I have had gastroparesis, it has limited me in many ways. I was a soldier before I got sick, but unfortunately, I lost my ability to perform at my best. I became weak, and was always ill. Therefore, the army deemed me as unfit for service, and sent me out of the military. I lost my health insurance, and the love of my life (the army). It was a difficult time for me, because I had always wanted to be a soldier, and I wanted to make up for how sluggish and slow I had been during and shortly after my pregnancy. I wanted to do the best I could, and help as much as I could.

After this happened, I tried to keep a small job, but was also unable to do that. Constantly having to take care of myself was a job on its own, alongside being a mother. Ever since, I haven't been physically able to work, but unfortunately, the government won't grant me any type of disability to help pay for my medical expenses. My wonderful husband works his hardest to support our family, and all of my medical costs.

*

NICOLE STARZYNSKI
Nicole was diagnosed with
gastroparesis in 2016 at age 33

Gastroparesis has screwed lots of things up in my life, including my career. I have always been an extremely hard-working and driven professional. I work in technology and when I first started in this field there were not a lot of women. I became the first woman to do several things at a few different places. My achievements over the past sixteen years are quite significant and I take a lot of pride in my work. I have always busted my butt and gone above and beyond, working well past the required forty-hour mark.

Prior to the job I am at now, I worked in kindergarten through grade 12 (K-12), higher education, and sports. When I worked in K-12, I was sick for a few years. Luckily, I had forty days to use every year for sick, vacation and personal days. So most of those days went to doctor appointments and being sick. I also had several accidents where I pooped my pants, puked or was sick as a dog and had to leave work. My original boss there was very understanding, and knew I would make the work up. I was working sixty to eighty hours every week, but only getting paid for forty. I won awards there for many different things I had done. So it's not like I was slacking off. Even sick, I don't slack off ever, even if my life becomes sick, work, sleep, puke, work, and so on.

Once the lady I actually hired became my boss, everything changed. She didn't understand technology and didn't understand that I could do ninety percent of my job from home. Even though that issue got resolved, I decided it was time to move on. For the next eighteen months, I was somewhat okay but not great. I wasn't eating much so that I could start a new job. Which is where I am at now. I've been there two and a half years. I have been working from home pretty consistently since October 2015.

A few months before I had surgery, we were hiring a contractor to help people with their broken computers and software. It was a position I had been fighting for since I got there, because a one-person information technology department is just insane. Even sick, I was still putting in over sixty hours a week. I would build out computers and take them into work. If I got sick, I would end up finishing my day from home. I felt like I was going to get fired every day I put a work-from-home day in, but my work never suffered.

At times, all my life consisted of was being sick and working. I am a single mom and I can't lose our only source of income and health insurance. I worked so hard to get where I am today and had so many dreams of what my future was going to look like. It certainly did not look like me working from my living room with my cube buddy being a twenty-pound pug named Zoey. I love my dog but I do miss humans.

It makes me sad to think about what I could be if I wasn't sick. I have been waiting for a promotion at work for almost two years. Because of the insurance increases, I actually make less money now than I did two years ago. I feel like when I bring it up, I can't push it, even though I make thirty thousand less than someone in a similar position who has less experience than me and no direct reports. But I can't push it because I still have a job, and they allow me to work from home. It doesn't matter how much money I have saved them, or how much I have fixed, or the hundreds of unpaid hours I have put it. I still feel like I can't push for what I deserve because I feel lucky to even have a job. I have never been put on a performance plan. I always complete work. I can still work on projects with people, and I am in constant communication with everyone I work with. I feel like if I was at work every day, I would be making the salary I deserve, and be respected more when I try to enforce policies and new initiatives.

Work has really stressed me out because I feel like I am constantly letting people down. I hate telling my boss I am not coming in because of my stomach. When other stuff comes up that normal people have, like your kid's sick, a pipe in your basement burst, you have kidney stones or a cold, your car won't start, they don't think, "This is it. Today they are firing me." I am constantly apologizing to my boss for not coming in, and have had to share with him more than he wants to hear. Poor guy doesn't even have kids yet and is newly married. I've gotten desensitized to sharing with someone, "Hey, just pooped my pants." My mom told me to give a girl at work a bag with underwear and pants in it so every time that happened, I didn't have to go around commando. Nothing like a hot day, pooping your pants and having to throw your underwear out. That's also the day you will need gas on your way home and probably have somewhere else you have to stop.

While we were conducting interviews last October, I was so sick, nothing was staying in me, not even water. I remember the one morning, I puked on my way to work. I had spent my entire morning puking, but we had interviews and I could not miss them. While we were conducting the interviews, I puked during one and swallowed it because who wants to throw up in front of a bunch of people. Not me.

The smell of food at work would sometimes make me sick, and would send me running to the bathroom. I still go into the office when I can or if I absolutely have to. I've pooped my pants at work several times. Nothing like pooping your pants and a server breaking. I was stuck in a small room with five guys working on a server issue and I had just pooped my pants. Instead of being able to go home and shower, I was stuck with no underwear on, in the most uncomfortable situation. I had so much anxiety about going to work. It took me three weeks to be able to leave the house without having a panic attack.

*

JENNIFER ZUBIK
Jennifer was diagnosed with idiopathic gastroparesis in 2010 at age 27

Gastroparesis has caused restrictions for me in the work force. When I became sick, I had my own house cleaning business and I also worked part-time as a paralegal for an attorney. I was unable to work almost immediately. Fortunately, the attorney I worked for was completely understanding and let me work around my illness. He was kind enough to continue paying me for the full twenty-five hours per week I was scheduled to be there, even if I was unable to be present. My customers I would clean for were very understanding as well. They would be alright with rescheduling around my needs and my good days.

However, I eventually had to shut down my cleaning service because of being too sick and weak to perform the duties. I had eleven houses I would clean, sometimes two per day, and I could no longer handle it physically. I had a difficult time going to the office with the attorney too, so I was seldom there. It was frustrating not being able to work and help with providing for my family. I felt like I was letting Lou and my daughter down. Lou had to work extra to compensate for the time and money I lost. It was extremely difficult and stressful and caused a lot of financial debt. With support of both of our employers and our family, we fortunately could make it work and were able to get by.

After two and a half years, I was able to manage going back to work part-time again. It was very helpful, yet still stressful because of the fear of making it through my shifts. My employer during that time was very understanding and would let me go home early if I didn't feel well, thankfully. Then, in December 2014, I was healthy enough to begin working full-time again. I got a new job, which is extremely stressful at times, but it feels good being successful both financially and physically.

*

CHAPTER TWELVE

Support in the workforce

Surround yourself with people who provide you with support and love and remember to give back as much as you can in return. -KAREN KAIN

Support can play a significant role in our ability to manage the challenges of chronic pain while being gainfully employed. The people and organizations who understand the journey, and offer compassion and care, can become true lifelines. If you work, how supported do you feel by coworkers?

*

MELISSA ADAMS VANHOUTEN
Melissa was diagnosed with
gastroparesis in 2014 at age 47

Since my work nowadays consists of administering online gastroparesis support and advocacy groups, I consider my coworkers to be other administrators and group members, as well as the members of the gastroparesis community at large, and other patient groups and their members, to some extent. I am amazed at the support I have received from the vast majority of those I have encountered. I am praised and thanked far more than I deserve, and many people go out of their way to show their appreciation with kind comments, likes, and private messages expressing their gratitude. Most people are gentle and supportive, understand that the limitations of my illness keep me from accomplishing as much as I would sometimes like, and encourage me when I am feeling lost or struggling to continue.

Of course, I have also encountered my fair share of problems and obstacles. Rather than outright personal attacks, I have generally been met with outsiders who are apathetic toward our cause. Only a few times have people been downright hostile. Most people have never heard of gastroparesis, and the ones who have do not fully understand it or decide to ignore it and dismiss it as if it is a stomachache. It is difficult to get them to comprehend that we are not griping about minor issues. They do not see what I see: tremendous physical suffering due to pain, nausea, the inability to eat, seemingly endless doctor visits, emergency room trips, surgeries, and procedures, isolation, loneliness, depression, resignation, financial distress and ruin. And because they have little knowledge of the impact of this illness, they largely ignore my pleas and our plight. I continue to press our cause, despite their resistance, and try not to get discouraged.

I have also come across a few administrators and group members who do not appreciate my approach or dislike the decisions I am sometimes forced to make. I frequently must make difficult choices based on group rules and what is best for the group as a whole, and the losing side does not always take kindly to this. I have been accused of ignoring and dismissing people, treating them unfairly, behaving egotistically, acting as a dictator, and all manner of other egregious sins. None of this is due to my illness though. These are typical reactions one would find in any workplace, although perhaps exacerbated by illness.

For the most part, I feel supported and loved. I am overwhelmed by the encouragement and generosity of spirit that all who are around me offer. I know this is not always the case for those in the gastroparesis community who work outside the home. Many face resentment from coworkers and supervisors who believe they are not doing their fair share or are using their illness as an excuse to miss work or exert less effort in their tasks. My heart goes out to those in this community who must face this situation in order to keep from financial ruin. This is a misunderstood illness, to be sure. I can only hope that someday everyone will comprehend the limits it places upon us and the hardships we must endure.

*

SAMANTHA ANDERSON
Samantha was diagnosed with idiopathic
gastroparesis in 2012 at age 26

When I worked, before having to leave and before my diagnosis, I didn't feel supported. I did by some colleagues, but not all of them. I did not know what was going on and what was wrong with me. I didn't really understand, so how could others? It would've made my life easier though. Saying that, I feel that most people don't understand the condition, so it is difficult. There is, however, a difference between understanding something and being able to support someone.

Now I feel my coworkers—well, generally my bosses who really know about it—try to understand and support as much as they can. I have to explain how I am feeling often, so they know, but don't want to do it too much either. Just because we are working our hardest, doesn't mean we are fine and feeling great. Sometimes because you are doing like everyone else, people just think you are okay. Two coworkers in particular ask me questions about my condition, know I work hard and noticed I have managed despite having gastroparesis and shingles.

*

JOLI ATKINS
Joli was diagnosed with
gastroparesis in 2015 at age 36

My boss is the only one who I feel supports me, and that's because he is a good friend of mine. Most of my coworkers do not understand how I can be absent so much and still keep my job. They do not understand the pain and nausea that I go through on a daily basis or how important it is for me to keep to a strict diet. They bring in food and taunt me with it and make jokes about how I cannot eat it. It gets frustrating but I try my best to laugh it off because it's better than letting them see how upset it makes me.

*

TRISHA BUNDY
Trisha was diagnosed with
gastroparesis in 2013 at age 35

At the beginning of my health journey, prior to having my feeding tube and during my first year after having it, I was able to continue teaching. This was prior to my cholecystectomy, colectomy, ileostomy, and IV home hydration needs. Teaching was an important part of my life and identity. Overall, I felt supported by my coworkers and administration. I was required to be absent on days when I was extremely symptomatic, had doctor appointments, needed diagnostic tests, or needed to have my feeding tube replaced. For the most part, my administration and fellow teachers were understanding and empathetic, even though nobody, including me, could grasp the magnitude of my illness.

To minimize my symptoms and continue to appear fine, I avoided taking anything orally and tried to hide my nausea and pain as much as possible. My fellow teachers, especially the fifth grade team, stepped in to help with planning on days when symptoms became too harsh or when I had to call in sick. My principal was supportive and always tried to schedule one of the routine substitutes who were familiar with my class, teaching style, and my condition.

I must say that my students were compassionate, curious, and excellent supporters. They asked questions about my condition and feeding tube. This allowed me an opportunity to increase awareness and teach them about the digestive system which was already part of their science curriculum, so the discussions were more meaningful. They knew that some days I felt better than others, but that I would give all my energy and effort to teach them. If I happened to be absent, they knew it was because my illness was too much to handle that day or there was a medical appointment. I could depend on them to follow directions, work hard, and behave with their substitute.

Having to give up my classroom and teaching career tore my heart to shreds and continues to hurt me. Teaching was my pride, my identity, and an integral part of my life. And yes, I get upset and saddened when I think about how my health and illness took my career away from me.

*

TAMMY DOWNS

Tammy was diagnosed with Crohn's disease, irritable bowel syndrome, spastic colon, gastroesophageal reflux disease, and gastritis in 2006 at age 46, gastroparesis in 2015 at age 56, and motility dysfunction disorder of the rectum and pelvic floor in 2016 at age 58

I did not have gastroparesis when I worked, but will answer the question for when I did work and how it turned out. I was a mortgage processor and it could be very stressful. I had to quit my first job after seven years, and had to make a choice. There were only two of us and I worked long days and sometimes on Saturdays. I looked for a mortgage processing job that had a less stressful environment, and that's when I found out I had Crohn's disease and other illnesses.

I was also injured in a car accident. I started having constant issues that affected my job by keeping me away from the desk and in the bathroom. I had to bring a change of clothes in case of an accident. I ended up in the hospital not once, but five times, because of bacterial infection. Because of neck injuries, I developed migraine headaches and still have them to this day.

Employers want you at work, not out sick or in the hospital, and can come across as uncaring. I thought I was doing the right thing. I had been on the job two months when my boss asked me what was wrong with my health, how long it would take for me to get better, and how many more times I would be hospitalized. I understood they had a business to run. It makes it difficult when we have to make a living and work to pay bills but can't work. I was so thankful for my doctors at that time.

As time went on, I felt I was doing good, but instead another illness flared. I was put on medication for my Crohn's disease. Twelve years later it was discovered that the medication had damaged my bone marrow, caused problems with my blood, suppressed my immune system, and had turned my body upside down. I caught every cold that went under my nose. If someone got the flu, I got the flu. I caught everything. I went online to learn what Crohn's was, how it affected me, why I was in the hospital, and what caused it. But that was the worst thing I could have done; because of that I lost my job. I could do my job with no problem, but physically was unable to be at work. So I understood. That is when my doctors said I had to stop working. That is how it all started.

*

SKYE FALCON

Skye was diagnosed with gastroparesis and other autoimmune diseases in 2006 at age 25

Working in the home, and out in the workforce, I get the best of both worlds. My in-home employees are my family, my children mainly, and they are the most helpful people ever. Unless, of course, there are those pesky teenage mood swings. Whether it is lifting fifty-pound bags of flour for my food business, or carrying my laptop from the couch to my bed when I need to rest, I know I can count on them when I need them. That said, I make it a point to not let my illnesses hinder their childhoods. In the same way that they support me, I give every ounce of myself, the last spoons and bits of energy, to make sure they are kids for as long as they can be.

My coworkers are equally as helpful, and can often tell by looking at me how I am truly doing. When things are rough, they will help me clean my classroom and help prepare for my evening of lectures and presentations. If I need an extra hand at our huge presentations and events, they are there to do the leg work for me. I have worked with this company for over a decade, and in that time, I do not think I have ever felt hostility about my illnesses at work. And for that, I hope my coworkers know how grateful I am, because hostility is something the chronically ill face daily. I am most positive that I push some buttons occasionally, as I know cancelations and changes please no one, but I hope they all know how much I appreciate them, and just how dedicated I am to the company, our mission, and the job.

*

ROBIN MCNAMARA
Robin was diagnosed with
gastroparesis in 2013 at age 55

I have a couple of folks who really support me. Most treat me like business as usual, which helps me feel normal. If there is anyone who harbors resentment toward me for having this disease, that's their problem, not mine. If any hostile situations, biased treatment, or bullying type behavior occur, I deal with the bully head-on and am not bashful going to human resources to protect my own interest.

*

TAMMY PITTMAN
Tammy was diagnosed with gastroparesis and irritable bowel syndrome in 2014 at age 34

When I worked, my coworkers were very supportive and understanding. We were all nurses so they took care of me a lot of times. Some covered my butt at times too.

*

TAYLOR SCHMITZ
Taylor was diagnosed with idiopathic gastroparesis in 2014 at age 22

When I did work, most of my coworkers and superiors were supportive and concerned about me, for the most part. However, there were many who thought I was lying, or being dramatic about my symptoms, or even making it all up.

*

NICOLE STARZYNSKI
Nicole was diagnosed with gastroparesis in 2016 at age 33

I am really tired of using all of my days off for doctor visits, and for when I am too sick to even work from home. It looks like this year they will go to doctor's appointments, tests and another surgery. I would like to take a day off and actually go do something fun besides tests and doctor's appointments. Nobody should have to use that many days off for radioactive eggs, butthole and barium tests.

I am a single mom so I have to work. I am lucky that I have such a supportive workplace. They have accommodated my disease, and done everything they can to aid in my recovery. They have made changes to allow me to work from home more. Not too many places will do that. One thing I am truly grateful for is the support I have from work. Not having that stress to worry about is more valuable than anyone may realize.

For the most part I feel pretty supported at work. I still talk to everyone through chat. When they see me, everyone's always happy to see me and ask how I've been. I was pretty vocal in explaining to everyone what was going on with me. Since it's a small company that eats lunch every day together, it was easy to notice I hadn't been at lunch in almost two years. Other people work from home sometimes and a few actually work remote all the time, so I am not the only person. I still have to request to work from home every single day, which causes me a lot of anxiety; hopefully my fears never come true.

A lot of people have been really helpful, especially when I first started working at home. There were things that needed to be done in the office, and everyone from the owners to human resources, to finance, office manager, and security, I don't think there is a department who didn't lend a hand to help me with something. Everyone I work with has just been amazing in that. I don't think I even realized how lucky I am. See why it's hard to complain about a raise? At the end of the day, what's more important? I deserve the raise, but the fact that I am respected—well, you can't put a price on that.

*

JENNIFER ZUBIK
Jennifer was diagnosed with idiopathic gastroparesis in 2010 at age 27

When I developed gastroparesis and could no longer work, and then once I was able to return to work, my employers and coworkers were very sympathetic toward me and would assist me if able to. They were really understanding if I needed to call off from work for the day, come in late, or leave early. When possible, they would work around my doctor appointments and switch days with me if I could not be there. My current employer has been just as supportive as the others, allowing me flexibility to go to my doctor appointments or letting me work from home if I am not feeling well. The support, care and consideration I have received is remarkable.

*

After all these years, I am still involved
in the process of self-discovery.
SOPHIA LOREN

*

CHAPTER THIRTEEN

Braving Social Advice

> I'll do my best to not judge you after the ignorant comment you just made about a health condition you know nothing about. -ANONYMOUS

As an invisible and seriously misunderstood disease, a common problem is how to explain to others who don't understand. Some well-meaning people suggest remedies in an effort to help. Others make comments that only inflame the conversation. How do you handle questions and comments? What type of advice do you hear most?

*

MELISSA ADAMS VANHOUTEN
Melissa was diagnosed with
gastroparesis in 2014 at age 47

I am generally not too disturbed by well-intentioned advice, even when it comes from those who know little about gastroparesis. Yes, I have heard, "Have you tried yogurt?" about a million times. Yes, I have indeed tried it. It is a minor annoyance, perhaps, to be asked, but it in no way offends me because I understand people wish to find something helpful and useful to suggest. This is their way of showing they care. I try to take such advice in the spirit in which it was intended. What I dislike far more than this is the question which so frequently slips from the lips of most everyone I know: "How are you? Are you feeling any better?" Now, again, I know the people inquiring are usually sincere, and I believe they are genuinely concerned about my welfare, but I have run out of answers for this question.

It is so difficult for people to grasp the difference between a short-term illness and a long-term (perhaps forever) chronic illness such as gastroparesis. No matter how many times I attempt to explain the nature of my illness, people cannot quite get a handle on the concept. It is if they have been conditioned to believe there must be a cure for all ills, and when that cure does not come, they believe I must be doing something wrong. I feel as if I am disappointing them if I answer with anything other than, "Oh, I am doing pretty well." They want me to be healed, and I want to tell them that I am, but that is not the truth. So, I grapple with a good answer to this question.

If, on a good day, I answer that I am doing well, they take that to mean I am healed and will never again have a bad moment. They assume I am eating as normal and will never again experience pain, nausea, bloating, or any of the other unpleasant symptoms which accompany my gastroparesis. They do not realize my condition might change again at the drop of a hat. If I answer that I am doing poorly, they flash that disappointed expression, tell me to hang in there, and walk away believing it will simply take more time for me to improve. It has been three years. I hold out hope that this will change someday, but I know it most likely will not.

Mostly, people do not know how to act or what to say. They are prepared to help and show compassion for brief periods, but over time, they grow weary of devoting themselves to the chronically ill, who never seem to improve, despite their assistance and well-wishes. They grow callous to our situation, not out of malice but because they simply do not know what else to do for us. I do not blame them. My endless needs and frailties are not attractive or uplifting. I am not fun to be around when I am in the midst of my pain and suffering.

The most I can hope for, and what I have generally received, is a sympathetic look or kind word when I tell others I am having a particularly bad day, an offer of assistance when I am unable to complete a task on my own, or an invitation to an event they know I will likely not be able to attend (but extend the request anyway so I will know they thought of me). I am grateful for all small acts of kindness directed toward me and do not expect full understanding or constant support in the manner I see fit. So, I continue my struggle to find the perfect answer to the enigmatic question which haunts me and try to find contentment in, "Oh, I am doing pretty well today."

*

SAMANTHA ANDERSON

Samantha was diagnosed with idiopathic gastroparesis in 2012 at age 26

"You are sick whenever you eat or drink! Whenever!" I used to hear this all the time and it was the one thing that grated on me the most because people would repeat it. I used to think, "Why would I lie to you?" I felt like they thought I was lying. "Even water—just drink water!" Yes, even water, and why would I always want to drink just water? People would often tell me to eat little bits but often and try just liquids, or worse still, "You just need to eat more." Generally, I would let it run over my back. I know that people don't understand it and need to be educated. I only really get offended if people repeat themselves and seem to not believe me.

I had some people looking up and sending me different diets to help me. Before I had my pacemaker, these wouldn't help me; keeping anything down, even liquids was very difficult. But people didn't understand this if I told them. I was, and still am, incredibly happy they took the time to look it up. People thought they could help me with their cooking and looking after me (especially family abroad) and wouldn't understand that they couldn't cure me like this. They would only understand if they saw and spent time with me.

Since having the pacemaker, things are slightly different. I can keep more down. I still vomit most days, but it's much better now. I need to follow these diets more; they might help relieve my symptoms. I can't eat lactose or gluten, and at the moment seem to be better with purees. Again, I value people wanting to give advice as long as it isn't pushed on me and people listen to me. Then I am thankful that they take the time to want to give me advice.

*

JOLI ATKINS
Joli was diagnosed with
gastroparesis in 2015 at age 36

I am lucky that I do not get a lot of advice from people. Most people want to hear more about my condition and what is wrong. They do not try to give me ways to make it better. They ask me what I have tried and if there is anything else that the doctors can do.

*

TRISHA BUNDY

Trisha was diagnosed with gastroparesis in 2013 at age 35

Gastroparesis, as well as other issues, is a hard illness to understand. It doesn't matter if you are trying to explain the illness to medical professionals, family members, friends, or strangers. Well-meaning and unsolicited advice is sure to make its way to your ears. Many times the advice I hear has been spoken and shared by someone with good intentions. I understand that. Advice from my immediate family is often a result of them feeling helpless and desperately wanting to assist me in finding improved health. I can accept that. Having gastroparesis limits the volume and types of liquids and foods that I consume, as well as the energy I have available for living life. Having an ileostomy adds additional limitations to my diet.

I have heard all kinds of advice from a variety of people in my life. The most common suggestions I've heard over and over have been:

"If you eat more, you would have more energy."

"Drink more water so you won't become dehydrated."

"You should eat healthier; more vegetables and beans may help."

"You need to run tube feeds at a higher rate or volume or possibly change to a more calorically dense formula, so you can intake an adequate amount of nourishment."

"Get outside and try to be more active."

"Have you tried_____________?"

"Just think more positively. If you stop thinking about it, things may improve."

"You can eat_________or have you tried___________?"

"If you continue to lose weight, your body may find its desired weight and then feel better."

"Congratulations. You look better since losing so much weight!"

Lack of awareness and education about gastroparesis and digestive motility disorders in the public eye and medical field does not help matters at all. If others could realize the severity of the pain, bloating, nausea, and dry heaving or vomiting, they may have a better chance of understanding our misery. Healthy foods are actually the most problematic for most gastroparesis sufferers, as the fiber slows digestion down even further for us. It is suggested that gastroparesis patients have a low fiber and low-fat diet, staying away from fresh fruits, fresh vegetables, and anything with skin. Add an ileostomy to the picture, and seeds, nuts, and many cooked vegetables have to also be eliminated as well due to increased chances of blockages.

I, personally, am unable to handle much volume or substances orally. I have found a few items that are tolerable at times in small amounts, though I often still have to deal with consequences afterwards. Since I am dependent on tube feeds for my nutrition, I don't take too many risks. Since I am taking a risk each time I drink or taste something, I make sure it's something that I enjoy and feel safe with. Though they may not be the healthiest of choices, my safer comfort foods that I try to occasionally include small amounts of certain brands of ice cream, popsicles, crackers, yogurt, or a hot drink, such as cappuccino with skim milk and no whipped cream.

In regards to my outlook and positivity, I do remain optimistic the majority of the time. If you don't see the positive me, then there's a reason at the moment. Either I had to miss out on a special event or occasion that I was really looking forward to, or I've been experiencing more health challenges than normal recently. The times when someone should worry about me most is when I am overly positive, as those are the times that I'm trying hard to convince myself and others that I'm okay, even though I'm not in that particular moment.

When unsolicited advice comes my way, I usually handle it by ignoring the comment altogether or use it as an opportunity to educate the person advising me. I can't say I've never been hurt or angered by someone's advice, but I try not to let it bring me down. What outsiders and strangers need to know is that I have close family members, online gastroparesis friends, and a fantastic medical team who help make meaningful, and at times, difficult medical decisions. In the online support groups, we share and discuss our conditions, what medicine or therapy is effective or ineffective, and why.

When chronically ill, we have to be mindful and cautious, as normal treatments or medications for an average person facing similar symptoms but without the same illness, may cause additional problems and risk. Over-the-counter medications, herbal supplements, and controversial natural remedies need to be considered very carefully by the patient and their medical team, as each of our bodies are so different. What sounds like a simple solution to try, may cause us to waste valuable money and time, add additional doctor visits to endure, and create complications with our body and other medications, throwing us in a downward spiral.

When people outside of my medical team offer this advice, especially when they are not familiar with my daily health issues, I tell them, "Thank you. I'm in great hands with my current doctor and trust their opinion. I may discuss your suggestion with them to see if they believe that it would be in my personal best interest or not. But for now, I am going to stick with the treatment plan that my doctor and I have in place." It's not that I don't want to hear advice from other people, as they may suggest something that could be very beneficial or that was simply overlooked. However, I do want others to be respectful of my personal needs and choices.

*

LISA COLANDREA
Lisa was diagnosed with
gastroparesis in 2016 at age 42

When people offer me advice, it can be somewhat frustrating. I know others mean well, but at the same time I'm reminded of all the treatment options there are and I've tried them already. Gastroparesis isn't easily understood and affects people in different ways. The types of advice I hear most are people telling me to eat healthy or follow a certain diet. What a lot of people don't understand is that diet doesn't help most people and most people can't eat the foods that they suggest. The hardest is when people say things like, "Think positive," or "It will get better." What they don't understand is it doesn't get better, there is no cure, so it's frustrating. I usually just thank them when they say things like this, and take everything with a grain of salt. It's not what I always want to hear but at least they are saying something so I am thankful for that.

I wish people would pay more attention when I try to educate them on my illness. It does feel disheartening at times because I feel like no one really knows how much I suffer. If you tell someone you have cancer, people can understand the severity of it. But when you say you have gastroparesis, people don't quite understand that it is as serious as cancer. There is no cure and people do pass away from complications of this illness.

*

TAMMY DOWNS

Tammy was diagnosed with Crohn's disease, irritable bowel syndrome, spastic colon, gastroesophageal reflux disease, and gastritis in 2006 at age 46, gastroparesis in 2015 at age 56, and motility dysfunction disorder of the rectum and pelvic floor in 2016 at age 58

I found a gastroparesis support group who has been a big support. They directed me through the support group to files that help with smoothies and other foods to try. My son's girlfriend is a surgical nurse and she has been very helpful when my blood pressure drops and by helping me stay hydrated. When you have people who can give some direction and advice, it's a big help. When I got dehydrated and malnourished, my nurse, Amy, helped me so much. Just little things and support is better and bigger than you know.

I've run into problems with people who just do not understand. I don't think it's because they don't want to understand. I think it's because they do not listen to what you have to say. For example, I may go to a get-together and when I have my smoothie, someone may comment, "Oh, I see you have your dinner," or "I'm sure you can't eat what we have." There have been times when I've been invited to lunch and instead of letting me make the choice of where to eat, they'll say, "Oh, I forgot you can't eat. I guess I could try a smoothie at the smoothie shop. What did you do to cause yourself to be sick all the time?" To me, this is uncalled for. It's how people come across with questions and how they say it to you.

People know how to use a computer. If you truly want to understand, look it up or go to a doctor visit. They don't though. Maybe I am being sensitive. People sometimes just do not know what to say, I guess. I do feel that if someone has not experienced an illness of any kind, it's very difficult for them to relate to how you feel and what you go through. People who haven't experienced illness are the first to make nasty comments.

I have to remind myself that everyone is not like me. I try to understand others by looking up what they have so I can relate to them. I don't want to make them feel bad. People have no compassion for sickness, and do not realize that sometimes all we need is a little understanding. Instead, they would rather be nasty and hateful. I do not wish illness on anyone.

*

SKYE FALCON

Skye was diagnosed with gastroparesis and other autoimmune diseases in 2006 at age 25

"Give it to God."

"Have you prayed about it today?"

"God won't give you what you can't handle."

"Have you changed your diet?"

"Stop being so lazy!"

"Have you tried Atkins?"

"Maybe if you tried exercising more."

"Stop focusing on the negatives!"

"Maybe you should try this Moringa supplement, because it cured my disorder."

"I sell this new essential oil blend that will cure you!"

"You are not praying hard enough!"

"Those medications are just going to make it worse."

"Just call upon Him; He'll take these burdens from you."

"Man! Avoiding candy is as hard as your liquid diet!"

"If you only focus on your sickness, it will take over your life."

"You know what you need? You need a..."

"Sex. Just come over for sex. It will fix everything."

"It can't be that bad."

"Just one bite won't kill you!"

"You should come to my church, because Jesus will save you."

"I thought you were stronger than that..."

"At least it isn't cancer."

The advice I hear the most of is not really advice, but more people telling me their thoughts, to give it to God, and expressing their own uneducated feelings on the matter. This is incredibly awkward for me because I'm not very religious; I'm more spiritual and connected with nature. I do not do the church thing, and have been told I have more of a hippie view on life. That said, I do not discriminate against anyone, any religion, or pay much attention to folks and their religious practices and beliefs. I find it increasingly aggravating that people, some who do not even know me, are so quick to bring religion, God, prayer, and the like into conversations about chronic illness. I often get in very large debates, because I cannot fathom how I am supposed to beg the man above (God, to most) to take away the issues that he gave me in the first place, because I am apparently strong enough to handle it. There is little respect in these types of conversation, especially when my beliefs do not line up with another's. I am expected to listen, agree and understand their views, but they have no patience for mine, which really means they have no patience for my illnesses or gastroparesis, either.

My strategy for handling these types of people and conversations are to attempt to change the subject, ignore, or avoid. I have always had a knack for reading people and situations, so I can often see what is coming before it is happening. This saves me from being trapped in conversations I do not want to be in, or explaining parts of illness to those who could really care less. I also always wear sunglasses to avoid making eye contact with people and starting any of these types of situations. It is very hard to be faced with conversations and people who refuse to listen, or even try to understand. Their advice, their cure-all supplements, and constant need to be right overtake most everything.

These days, I find that most people avoid the topic of my gastroparesis or other illnesses entirely, so I guess that takes the guesswork out of worrying about bad advice! In that slim chance that one slides by and engages in this type of conversation, I politely smile and listen, nodding my head every few seconds to make it seem like I am intently paying attention, and simply wait for it to be over. No harm, no foul. Just a few wasted minutes, and the realization this person is not what I once thought.

All of this can be such an emotional, anger-filled time because the very people who get frustrated when you will not do it their way, are supposed to be your supporters, friends, and sometimes even family. Then, because I will not fill them in further or argue with them about my treatment, they completely withdraw from my life. These circles feel a lot like being punished for being sick, over and over again. And that circle of punishment does not make being constantly sick, throwing up, and dealing with the physical ailments of gastroparesis any less challenging or lonely.

*

ROBIN MCNAMARA
Robin was diagnosed with
gastroparesis in 2013 at age 55

Well, I try to explain that some of their ideas or brainstorms do not work for me and my illness. If they persist, do I get angry? I certainly do. I walk away and never look back. I try to remember the phrase, "Love isn't what you say, it's what you do." If someone is full of words, they no longer belong in my world. Sounds cold, but there are a number of self-centered, selfish people out there who seem to get off by being able to tell others how good they are to the sick one, and expect a round of applause. Yup...they are not part of my world.

*

TAMMY PITTMAN
Tammy was diagnosed with gastroparesis and
irritable bowel syndrome in 2014 at age 34

I get tired of hearing, "Have you tried holistic medicines?" Also, "If you'd get out more often and move around, you'd have more energy." Those make me want to just say something not nice. Usually, I bite my tongue and get away from them.

*

TAYLOR SCHMITZ
Taylor was diagnosed with idiopathic
gastroparesis in 2014 at age 22

In the beginning, hearing advice constantly was very difficult and overwhelming. People always told me I needed to suck it up or to try harder. As I've grown older and more accustomed and in-tune with my body, I've definitely grown more patient. Most people around me know that I'm sort of a pro by now! But there are still people who say I need to try this new diet, or this amazing cure-all wrap or shake. I simply smile and tell them how thankful I am for their advice and concern, and leave it at that. I don't snub them or downplay their advice at all.

*

NICOLE STARZYNSKI
Nicole was diagnosed with
gastroparesis in 2016 at age 33

Sometimes when I tell someone that I have gastroparesis, they know someone with it or they think that it's something that is easily treatable. I have heard numerous times from people:

"Gastroparesis—I know someone with that. They just watch what they eat and sometimes eat smaller meals."

"Have you tried probiotics or drinking vinegar?"

"Have you tried the Fodmap diet?"

"How can you drink a cola? I'm sure that's not helping you."

"Why can you eat this but not that? That doesn't make sense. I read you can just take medicine and your food will digest."

"Are you sure you don't just have irritable bowel syndrome? My grandma had that and she took medicine."

It's frustrating, but at the same time people are trying to be helpful. I can't be angry at them for their ignorance to a disease I didn't even know existed until I had it. I usually take the opportunity to educate them if possible about gastroparesis and all the things I have been through. I know my mom takes it personal when someone makes a comment to her about things I should do. I tell her she shouldn't let it bother her. It doesn't matter what these people think, if they were really important they would see me at my worst and understand that there is no cure in a box.

It can be frustrating if the same person continues to offer the same bad advice. That's when I get to the point when I avoid those people. I'm not going to be put down or questioned by someone continually. So I move on and push it out of my mind. There is so much more to worry about. I guess I have learned, at the end of the day, what these people say or think doesn't help me one way or the other. So why stress about it? The people who matter most in my life, know because they live it. They have all become advocates for this disease, especially my daughter. If my child was smart enough to research the disease and educate herself, there is no reason why an adult can't do the same thing.

*

JENNIFER ZUBIK

Jennifer was diagnosed with idiopathic gastroparesis in 2010 at age 27

Gastroparesis, just like any disease, is not only physically strenuous, but emotionally strenuous as well. Because this disease is uncommon and the awareness is insufficient, people around us can't give adequate advice.

"What do you mean you're nauseous and can't eat? I get nauseous after every meal and eat Tums or Pepto, can't you do the same thing?"

"You know you wouldn't feel so tired if you would eat. Food would give you energy."

"Just do it, suck it up and shove it in your mouth and swallow."

"You know what you need? You need to smoke marijuana. It will help with the nausea and give you the munchies at the same time."

"Are you sure you are not just anorexic or bulimic now?"

"Pray. Go to church and pray."

Some people just don't think before they speak. Others just don't understand, and with good intentions try to help, but sound silly when the words come out of their mouths. Though it was frustrating and maddening to hear some of what people would say, I considered the fact that all they were doing was caring. If they didn't care, they wouldn't think of that comment that came out, even if it was ridiculous or hurtful or may have seemed inconsiderate. I would never argue when given advice I didn't ask for, no matter how upsetting it could be. I tried to not let it bother me and would explain why what they suggested would not work. I would educate them and make them aware of the disease and the difficulties. As they would try to help me battle and get better, I would try to help them in return by giving them knowledge about gastroparesis.

One string of advice that I will never halt from saying and encouraging is, "Don't give up. You need to be strong, not only for yourself, but for others, too. We need and want you to be here with us. Do not give up on hope or ever stop believing." My mother, bless her soul, would remind me of all that every time we spoke. Patience and hope are key factors to survive this dreadful disease.

*

CHAPTER FOURTEEN

Coping with Malnutrition

Courage does not always roar. Sometimes courage is the quiet voice at the end of the day saying, "I will try again tomorrow." -MARY ANNE RADMACHER

Good nutrition is critical to overall health and well-being. But daily nausea, vomiting and early satiety are chronic issues among gastroparesis sufferers. Low appetite results in inadequate food intake which puts us at risk for malnutrition. Have you been at risk of malnutrition?

*

MELISSA ADAMS VANHOUTEN
Melissa was diagnosed with
gastroparesis in 2014 at age 47

To date, though I am frequently weak and fatigued and struggle to maintain good nutrition, my clinical levels have been stable and within normal ranges (though at the low end). I believe most of us, me included, are almost always at risk for malnutrition though. One bad extended flare can send any of us into crisis. But my greater fear is the long-term damage this is doing to my body. While I am not currently in crisis, I know I'm not meeting my caloric or nutrition goals, and I worry this will cause long-term, perhaps irreparable health issues.

I struggle to consume even minimal calories, generally between 500 and 750 per day, and I know this cannot go on forever without consequences. I have noticed changes in addition to the fatigue and weakness as well. My hair is thinner, my nails are brittle, and my teeth and gums are frequently sore. My skin is extremely dry and no longer glows as it once did. At first, I tried to pass this off as simply a normal part of aging, but logically, and in my heart, I know the decline has been too rapid to be explained away by passing years. I often wonder how much worse this will get and what additional effects I will experience. I worry about organ damage, especially to my heart, kidneys, and liver. What unknown, irreversible damage is this cruel disease inflicting right now? I wish I knew.

But the greater matter for me, aside from worries about damage to my body, is the cravings I experience due to lack of variety and healthy options. Before being diagnosed, I ate a reasonably healthy diet rich in fruit, vegetables, whole grains, lean meats, and the like. Now, I am entirely unable to eat meats or grains other than small bites of rice-based products every now and then. The few vegetables and fruits I can consume are either cooked to the point where nutritional value is practically nil or come in the form of baby food, which is not the tastiest option. I can occasionally tolerate fruit smoothies, but not frequently. I miss salads, breads, pasta, cheeses… well, almost every food imaginable, I guess. I miss the variety and I miss not having to worry that the food I am ingesting will turn to poison inside my body.

I try my best to eat the healthiest foods possible from my ever-shrinking list of safe options, which are never truly safe because the list can change at any moment without warning, and can even vary from day to day. I make certain every calorie counts in terms of nutrition. I do not fill my stomach with empty calories if I can avoid this scenario. I also take many supplements: multivitamin, vitamins B, C, D, E, biotin, calcium, magnesium, and a few others. I drink vitamin water and coconut water daily as well. In addition, I consume broths which are meant to calm and line the stomach and which are mineral-rich and nutrient-dense. I drink Kefir and protein shakes to ensure I get the greatest amount of protein possible, and, when I can, I eat Greek yogurt, which provides calcium and is packed with good bacteria.

I also do my best to engage in physical activity. Prior to my diagnosis, perhaps three years or so before, I had taken up running and had begun working out on an elliptical machine. I had been gaining ground and, at the time of diagnosis, I was probably the healthiest and most physically fit I had ever been in my life. This all came to a crashing halt the day I began experiencing the symptoms of gastroparesis. After my hospital stay and several weeks of sheer exhaustion and physical collapse, I began my exercise routine once again, and it was nightmarish! For weeks all I could do was tightly grip the bars of my treadmill and take snail's pace steps for a couple of minutes at a time. I was determined to improve, and week by week, I have gained ground, but it is clear to me I will never be able to return to my pre-diagnosis self where physical activity is concerned.

Still, I work hard to maintain the best exercise routine I can. What once was a speedy forty-five-minute run is now a slow twenty to twenty-five minute run (or sometimes a walk), and I cannot always manage to do this daily. I run when I can for as long as I can. I have also tried to substitute new activities to make up for the loss of the old. I have added extensive stretches to my routine as well as arm weights. On the days when I can walk only on my treadmill, I incline it to add to the burden. My goal these days is not to achieve great speeds or distances. It is simply to be as physically fit and heart-healthy as I can under the circumstances. That is a difficult mental adjustment to make, but it is necessary.

In short, I do my best to provide my body with the essential nutrients it needs to function based upon my very limited options. It disturbs me that I cannot meet normal nutritional and physical fitness goals, but I have had to learn to forgive myself for this failing and recognize I am doing the best I can. It is the only means by which I can survive mentally and physically.

*

SAMANTHA ANDERSON

Samantha was diagnosed with idiopathic gastroparesis in 2012 at age 26

Compared to others with this condition, I have been lucky. I've had several issues with dehydration and had to have intravenous fluids. I have also have had intravenous vitamins on a few occasions to combat malnutrition. Plus, I had a nasojejunal tube fitted for a while (which unlike many amazing others, I couldn't tolerate) to help.

I now have the pacemaker and although struggling, I keep a little more down. My struggles with this have been a lot less, but are not over. Although I'm in the emergency room less, my journey to recovery still continues.

*

JOLI ATKINS
Joli was diagnosed with
gastroparesis in 2015 at age 36

No, thankfully I have not been at risk of malnutrition, although I am on a very limited diet. I currently am on a diet of Ensure and applesauce on most days. There are very few days when I can eat anything else. I do worry that I will end up losing too much weight and will have to have a tube put in or will end up being malnourished. The doctor assures me, however, that I am healthy and will continue to stay that way as long as I keep doing what I am doing.

*

TRISHA BUNDY
Trisha was diagnosed with
gastroparesis in 2013 at age 35

Even though I'm technically a little overweight, I have struggled with my nutritional intake since February 2013. Being unable to handle an adequate amount of fluids, food, or both, keeps me chronically dehydrated, and at times interferes with my lab values. My doctors, family, and I are concerned about malnutrition. Besides dehydration, I have had issues with iron deficiency anemia, low potassium, low magnesium, low blood sugar, orthostatic hypotension, tachycardia, vitamin D deficiency, vitamin B_{12} deficiency, low zinc, possible muscle deterioration, and so on. In order to keep my nutrition stable, we must keep a close eye on the levels.

To improve nutritional intake, I have a gastrostomy-jejunostomy (GJ) feeding tube which feeds my small intestines directly. We've had to change the formula that I'm using on a few occasions because my body was not tolerating them well. Currently, I'm using Peptamen AF (which is semi-elemental). To improve my hydration, I infuse one and a half liters of IV lactated ringers five times a week. At times, I have had to supplement necessary vitamins either orally, through my feeding tube, or at the infusion clinic.

These nutritional issues are a challenge to my physical and emotional health. They impact my fatigue, weakness, mood, pain, mental clarity, and balance. In addition, the lack of nutrition can create other health problems such as organ damage, but thankfully, so far that has not been the case for me.

*

LISA COLANDREA
Lisa was diagnosed with
gastroparesis in 2016 at age 42

In the past year I've been malnourished several times. Since the pyloroplasty surgery didn't work for me, I had to decide whether or not to get a feeding tube placed because of malnourishment. I ultimately decided to get the feeding tube after receiving another gastric emptying study and endoscopy, showing severe gastroparesis. The doctors made it clear that without this feeding tube, I would not be able to thrive and sustain any type of healthy nutritional status, and I would continue to decline. As of right now, it has only been six weeks having a feeding tube, and I'm still trying to accept it and learn how to live with it every day.

*

TAMMY DOWNS

Tammy was diagnosed with Crohn's disease, irritable bowel syndrome, spastic colon, gastroesophageal reflux disease, and gastritis in 2006 at age 46, gastroparesis in 2015 at age 56, and motility dysfunction disorder of the rectum and pelvic floor in 2016 at age 58

Back in March, I had started having problems with my blood pressure dropping, along with lightheadedness and feeling dizzy like I was going to pass out. And I had lost so much weight. I was looking for any doctor who would help me. I went to a doctor in Gainesville, but I had an allergic reaction to everything he put me on, and my insurance covered only five out of the fifteen prescriptions. My bloodwork kept coming back low on some things and high on others. My blood pressure was dropping, and the last blood test they did showed I was dehydrated and starting to become malnourished. They checked to see if by chance my adrenal gland could have malfunctioned. I went through a lot of tests and bloodwork for this.

My nurse was so supportive and gave advice to help me as best she could. When my blood pressure started dropping, she recommended I drink Propel to replace my electrolytes. I also had to get protein in me and my doctor told me to get Boost to try to put a little more weight on. My nurse reached out to a bariatric doctor she worked with who was supposed to be the best in the country. He told me I was a potential candidate for subtotal gastrectomy to resolve my gastroparesis pain syndrome. This would require Roux-en-Y. gastrojejunostomy construction.

However, I am currently being worked up and treated for hypogammaglobulinemia and other blood issues because of the damage to my bone marrow. Until they can get my blood straightened out and treatment started for the hypogammaglobulinemia, and determine whether my adrenal gland is functioning or not, they can't do the surgery. What's even crazier is that the adrenal gland malfunctioning has a lot of the same symptoms. Thank goodness my adrenal gland wasn't to blame for my losing so much weight so fast, but my body has again got off balance and has affected my blood pressure.

*

SKYE FALCON

Skye was diagnosed with gastroparesis and other autoimmune diseases in 2006 at age 25

Until a few years ago, I was able to maintain myself and stay at a plateaued weight. While I was limited on what foods I could eat, I did not gain or lose weight. During this time, my doctors felt that just maintaining and not taking evasive action was the best plan. Any time we would change things or alter my medications, other issues would morph and change into new, often scarier, monsters. These past two years, however, have been a completely different story, in what feels like an ailing, barely-hanging-on at times body. My weight has been in a steady decline recently, every appointment shows another few pounds missing. With each passing week, it seems one of the things I could eat, I can no longer tolerate for whatever reason. My diet is a rollercoaster, and one that frequently derails. I have reached the point of being afraid to eat.

In the beginning of my gastroparesis diagnosis, I was already gluten-free, avoiding red meats, and packing food in whenever I was hungry. There was no set plan from any of the doctors, only to keep doing what I could to keep on the weight and keep calories coming in. About two years ago, my gastrointestinal system completely stopped working. Even the simplest nutritional beverages were causing crazy amounts of pain, blood in my stools, and constant vomiting of foods from days before. Again I was told to just keep on going. I could feel anything that was taken by mouth course through my entire abdomen, and I had the ability to follow the food masses through my system by feel only, for days. Amid all of this happening, I had a failed attempt at tube feedings, a failed Bravo test, and a few growths removed from my esophagus, thanks to all of those proton pump inhibitors I had been taking over the last decade to function.

These days, I try to stick with mostly liquids and very soft, already broken down foods. Lots of creamy soups with protein powders, low fiber fruit purees, and small amounts of fresh juice from my trusty juicer are my crutches. Sometimes I will indulge and attempt four to six ounces of some sort of lean protein, or mushy-vegetable bake. Baby food packages make snacking and traveling to events do-able, although they are still incredibly tricky to plan. For example, I recently had a two-day event, and three hours into that first eight-hour day, my body was screaming for heating pads, rest, medication and calories. Trouble is, having anything by mouth trips the intense abdominal pains, all the stomach trouble and more, pretty much the second it hits my esophagus.

Even with the options of baby food, travel snacks, and being prepared, there is no real way to be ready for the pain that shoots through your entire abdomen when your gastroparesis issues flare. My biggest cravings and what I desperately want when stress is heavy are always tacos, fried chicken, and A1 sauce. I have not had them in so long, that just typing the words now made me drool a little.

I have an incredible fear of not being able to maintain myself or the calories I need, and that by the time anyone figures out how to handle gastroparesis, it will be too late. The clothes I was wearing last month are now tents, and my twelve-year-old has offered to share her clothes. My skin is losing tension, my veins stand out like I am elderly, and the purple bags under my eyes now look like large travel totes, permanently in place. There is a certain feeling your body acclimates to when it has no energy, no calories, and no drive. The sheer energy it takes to parent, be married, to live, and to run businesses is so intense. It is one thing trying to get people to understand what gastroparesis is, let alone trying to get them to understand that you cannot do the things you did last month or year, because now your body is internally eating itself and its muscle content to stay alive.

I worry constantly that I will just drop one day while at home with my home-schooled kiddos, and force them into a situation to have to call emergency medical services or use their own resuscitation skills. That alone makes it harder to get out of bed some days. I worry that without their mom, my guys will be destined for a life of therapy sessions, and worrying about their own issues, which unfortunately mimic my own.

*

ROBIN MCNAMARA
Robin was diagnosed with
gastroparesis in 2013 at age 55

When I was first diagnosed, I wasn't really eating anything that offered much substance, let alone vitamins or minerals. Over time, I was able to introduce soft foods such as plain cooked seafood, rice, spinach and asparagus tips cooked until mushy. I was borderline anemic. Today, I'm maintaining pretty decent nutrition. I still eat a lot of fish. My bloodwork has been good, so I don't have many concerns about malnutrition.

*

TAMMY PITTMAN
Tammy was diagnosed with gastroparesis and
irritable bowel syndrome in 2014 at age 34

Malnutrition is an ongoing issue. I have gone weeks with the inability to eat due to pain and nausea. Ketones and protein were noted in my urine for over a year. My family doctor stated that I was in starvation mode and to follow up with the gastrointestinal motility specialist. Because I'm obese, the specialist didn't think it was necessary to think about alternative nutrition until I'm down to eighteen percent of my body mass index.

I have had many trips to the local emergency room for IV fluids due to dehydration from malnutrition. Many emergency room doctors told me that my specialist needs to figure something out and gain a better plan of care for me. When relaying recommendations to my specialist, I was told there was nothing they could do that the local emergency room couldn't handle. I was told at one emergency room visit that they can't continue to be my source of fluids every time I get dehydrated. It's a lose-lose situation in trying to maintain nutritional needs.

*

TAYLOR SCHMITZ
Taylor was diagnosed with idiopathic gastroparesis in 2014 at age 22

For the past few years, I have desperately struggled with malnutrition. I am five-feet five-inches tall and I got down to eighty-six pounds at one point, a year ago. My naturopathic doctor and my acupuncturist are the ones who put me on the right path toward health, by changing my outlook on the things I actually put into my body. My main concern now is QUANTITY of QUALITY. There is no one over the other.

The common diet that doctors give a person diagnosed with gastroparesis, is one of low fat, low fiber, and highly processed. These are bad foods that do damage to your entire body, and cause major issues down the line, even short-term. The classic gastroparesis diet started to fail me almost immediately, as my weight declined rapidly and my body began to lose all muscle, and all energy.

To this day, I can't go out and get the dog food; I have to wait for my husband to do it. Also, I can't climb the stairs to our bedroom sometimes; I have to crawl up them. My body has been so malnourished, that I wouldn't have my menstrual cycle for over six months at a time, then have a terribly painful one that lasted a couple of weeks. Malnutrition is definitely something I have struggled with, and continue to struggle with, but I have a much better perspective on my health now, and value what I put into my body. God has blessed me so much, and He blesses me at every meal that I attempt to ingest.

*

NICOLE STARZYNSKI
Nicole was diagnosed with
gastroparesis in 2016 at age 33

When you are barely eating or keeping fluids down, the risk of malnutrition is always a concern. I've been told several times, if my weight reaches a certain mark we need to put in a nutrition tube. Every time I have bloodwork and they email the results, there is a moment when my stomach drops and fear sweeps over my body. Fifteen new conditions have been added to your profile! What the? Then you log in and see it's just vitamin deficiencies and other deficiencies all related directly to the fact that even on a good week, you're lucky if you get 1,200 calories in for the entire week.

You have to read food labels to avoid salt, fiber, or too much protein, because you want things high in calories. In my smoothies I might add honey or, if I can get away with it, jelly or a weight booster. Any place you can add calories, you do. Sometimes it's not as easy as taking a vitamin supplement, because your stomach may not absorb it and the filler may make you sick.

I've had kidney stones because of malnutrition a few times, but there are many people not as lucky as me. That's very sad because I shouldn't consider myself lucky simply because I haven't had to have a feeding tube. This disease affects so many in different ways; you can't compare yourself to others who are worse. Everyone's journey is different and that also affects the outcomes of many.

Sometimes you're not eating any food but your weight isn't really moving, so the doctors think you're fine. Meanwhile, every time you put a bite of food in your mouth, you're praying you're not going to pay for it for days. Sometimes if I am feeling somewhat good I will avoid food, but eventually I end up lightheaded and dizzy from not putting anything in me. It's a constant balancing act. No matter what you do, there is a negative outcome, which is incredibly frustrating.

I remember being overweight and going on crazy diets. If I had known then that one day food would be like poison, I would have stuffed my face until I was a whale. It would have only given me more time. Crazy thought when you put it on paper but it's the truth. Most of my life I was overweight. I was never skinny. As a kid, I was teased and called names. I dreamed of being skinny. Today when I look in the mirror, sometimes I don't recognize myself. You can see the bones in my chest. My arms, legs, stomach and face are significantly slimmer. And can't forget my boobs that used to be there, those left too. It's sad that for so long all I wanted was to be thin and healthy. Now that I'm thin, I am so far from healthy and I'd rather be overweight and able to eat anything I want. This is different than saying, "I have curly hair and want straight hair." I've lived that want as well, ha ha. I can't make anyone possibly understand how it feels to look at pictures of yourself, or the vision you still believe you are, and the reality of what you have become.

Since my first surgery I have gained some weight, but I am not healthy and am severely deficient in fifteen things at the moment. At this point, I do not have any tubes, but accept that the reality of that happening is possible. You learn that things you could never have imagined having to do, you end up accepting so that you have a chance to fight for the life you deserve. Nobody deserves to be at war with their stomach every day; food should never be your enemy. One of the most important things I have learned is that when I was overweight, I was still me. But I was living a healthy life with no fear that a disease would eventually claim its victory. I wish I was still that me all the time.

*

JENNIFER ZUBIK
Jennifer was diagnosed with idiopathic
gastroparesis in 2010 at age 27

Every aspect of gastroparesis is scary. Not being able to get adequate amounts of nutrition leads to so many other problems. I was losing weight and energy so fast, it was terrifying. Hair loss, bruising, weakness, fatigue, skin problems, being able to see my bones. I feared if I fell, I would break in half. I had emergency room visits for IVs and nourishment. My levels were always so low or out of whack. My doctors told me to try taking gummy vitamins and supplements, which surprisingly worked for me. I didn't exactly feel better, but my levels were closer to normal. My white blood cell count has always been high since I got sick, without any explanation about what we need to do to correct it, it's still a mystery.

I literally thought I was dying, and if not soon then this disease would kill me eventually. Within three months of getting sick, I prepared my living will, general power of attorney, medical power of attorney, and last will and testament. I was terrified but wanted to at least make sure I had all bases covered if anything would, god forbid, happen. I needed to make sure my daughter would be taken care of if I was not around to do it myself. Fortunately, as time passed, with doctor's orders, supplements I could tolerate and gummies, I managed my levels sufficiently. Unfortunately, everyone is different, and may have to go to other extremes. We do what we must do to survive, and help and support those in need along the way.

*

CHAPTER FIFTEEN

Mental Aspects of Pain

It's not just pain. It's a complete physical, mental, and emotional assault on your body. -JAMIE WINGO

The pain-brain connection is an established and widely accepted theory that receiving nonstop pain signals can result in rewiring, making those with chronic pain more susceptible to mood disorders. Further, the brain may not be able to attend to other tasks efficiently because it's preoccupied with pain signals. How does the pain from living with gastroparesis affect your mental health?

*

MELISSA ADAMS VANHOUTEN
Melissa was diagnosed with
gastroparesis in 2014 at age 47

One of the topics that comes up frequently in my gastroparesis support groups is the refusal of some physicians to believe that there is pain associated with gastroparesis. It is a common occurrence for members to post that their doctors have told them, "There is no pain with gastroparesis." Gastroparesis-associated pain has been fairly well recognized and documented by motility experts. It is noted as one of the concerns in the Guidelines for the Management of Gastroparesis, established by some of the top experts and researchers in the field and shared on the American College of Gastroenterology website (see below). It is also discussed by the National Institutes of Health and various clinics known for their innovation and excellence in the treatment of gastroparesis. In addition, there are thousands upon thousands of members in our support groups who have been diagnosed with no conditions other than gastroparesis who regularly post about their daily battle with pain.

gi.org/guideline/management-of-gastroparesis/

www.niddk.nih.gov/health-information/digestive-diseases/gastroparesis

www.mayoclinic.org/diseases-conditions/gastroparesis/basics/symptoms/CON-20023971

consultqd.clevelandclinic.org/2016/03/new-program-offers-multidisciplinary-treatment-hope-patients-gastroparesis/

Despite the facts, many physicians, family members, and loved ones still refuse to believe pain is a typical part of gastroparesis, and so countless of us are reproached for faking this pain. Although I have never faced this accusation personally, I see the toll it takes on those who have. It is devastating to try to cope with ongoing, debilitating pain only to be told it is all an invention of the mind. Some doubt themselves and others grow angry. They feel unsupported and rejected by the very people who should be of greatest help. They bear the burden alone.

And while I am blessed to have supportive loved ones and physicians, this unfortunately does not diminish the effects of the pain associated with my gastroparesis. Indeed, it is both the most significant physical symptom and the most difficult mental and emotional burden I shoulder. I am not certain I can adequately describe what it is like to wake up every day knowing that if and when I eat, I will experience pain. I must decide every day whether eating will be worth the excruciating pain I know without doubt will ensue. Many days, I go as long as possible without eating to try to put off the inevitable. But I do not wish to die, so eventually, I must eat, and though I consume only gastroparesis-friendly foods and liquids, the pain still comes.

The most agonizing moments are those just before I fall asleep. Most nights, I go to bed in pain, and as I lie there in the silence, with nothing to do but review and contemplate the day, I am saddened at all I have endured. But worse yet, I know I must wake up tomorrow and face the same torturous dilemma, to eat or not to eat, day after day after day. Every single day, without fail, I must find a way to get through the pain, knowing there is no foreseeable end. It is agony, pure and utter agony.

I do what I can to lessen the physical and emotional pain, but it is never enough. I face it the only way I can: day by day and sometimes moment by moment. I frequently write about my attempts to overcome the mental torment resulting from the physical pain, and I share a sampling of these writings as follows.

PIECES OF THE WHOLE

By Melissa Adams VanHouten

Something less than human,
Pieces of the whole,
Cracked and broken open,
Have mercy on her daunted soul.

A puzzle missing pieces,
Never quite complete,
A riddle, an enigma,
An unfinished music sheet.

There is something she is lacking,
Once held but now is lost,
The key to all her questions,
But the chasm she cannot cross.

The labyrinth engulfs her,
Cannot see above the walls,
The answer, it eludes her,
As she roams lost within the halls.

What happened to the person
Who once was unimpaired?
She has been found wanting,
Frail and weak and scared.

Must rearrange the pieces,
Put them back in place,
Decipher the information,
Before it is too late.

The woman who now queries,
Once knew where she belonged,
Planned a different future,
One that has gone so wrong.

Caught up in this dilemma,
She cannot see the light,
Feels her way through the darkness,
Seeks an end to this black night.

Who can help this poor blind soul,
Guide her back to where it's safe?
Who can gather the parts,
Assemble them in their place?

Those masters of comprehension,
Vast knowledge to impart,
Should perhaps review the problem,
And respond instead with their hearts.

For this being who is divided,
Split and incomplete,
Requires compassion and healing,
Not scolding and conceit.

Her solitary hope in this life,
Lies in the One above,
Who can mend her tattered soul,
Offer grace and comfort and love.

He holds all the answers,
Carries her through the maze,
He erects the bridge
From despair to brighter days.

He is her Saving Grace,
The One who keeps her sane,
Who never fails to remind her
That her searching is not in vain.

He is patient, though she falters,
Failing to understand,
Holds the fragile fragments together,
Dries her tears and takes her hand.

He silences her doubts and fears,
Calms her shattered mind,
Fills in the missing pieces,
Pens a symphony warm and sublime.

He alone can restore her,
Shape the parts into a whole,
He is indeed the Great Healer,
The one who completes her soul.

* * *

FACE IN THE MIRROR

By Melissa Adams VanHouten

This face in the mirror,
Sullen and gaunt,
Like a stranger in the daylight,
And my dreams it does haunt.

Eyes peering back at me,
Sunken and dull,
Light that once danced there,
Dimmer than before.

Lips that once sang
And laughed without care,
Now silent and thin—bitter?
Sweet music no longer there.

This body is ravaged,
Battered, drained, and thin.
How do I reclaim the light
That once shined from within?

What I once was is gone,
Cruelly wrenched from my hands.
Of all the existences I imagined,
This was not in my plans.

I long for an answer,
To this bewildering twist of fate,
Search my troubled mind,
For a means of escape.

As I finish the day
And turn in for the night,
Try to find the courage
To make it to light.

Arise in the morning
And begin it all again,
Face the face in the mirror,
Days without end.

I question my purpose,
Do not like what I see,
And wonder what happened
To the person I used to be.

But there remains a flicker,
A glimmer of hope, far below,
In those strange sunken eyes,
Buried deep in my soul.

I cannot see a path out,
But I know there must be,
For I am Your creation,
And You watch over me.

You know the stranger,
And You guide her path,
You know her purpose,
Help her find her way back.

The face in the mirror,
Sad and forlorn,
Still has a connection
To the one she was before.

This new path is foreign,
And not one I wish to take,
But with the stranger before me,
Amends I must make.

For we have a purpose,
And You have a plan.
Though I cannot always grasp it,
I know my life is in Your hands.

So the face in the mirror
And the face I once knew,
Must find a means together
To begin each day anew.

We must pull ourselves up,
Blink back the tears,
Find a way to go on,
And face all our fears.

We are frail and uncertain,
This stranger and I,
But despite our misgivings,
We will fight to survive.

Please forgive me my failings,
My worries and doubts,
And help me find comfort,
Seek solace throughout.

For with Your great mercy,
With Your kind loving grace,
Though it may not be easy,
This life we embrace.

I have heard it said that pain changes people, and I believe this. Although I would never willingly choose this fate, this agony is my constant companion and has, in a peculiar way, restored my soul and fashioned me into a stronger, yet ever more delicate, creature. It has taught me I can bear far more than I once imagined, with dignity and grace. It has brought true meaning to the words perseverance, determination, and resilience. It has driven me beyond barriers and obstacles I once set for myself and believed I could not breach. It has placed me on a course vastly superior to the path I once believed I should walk.

It has turned my blind eyes and deaf ears toward the suffering that surrounds, that has always encircled me, but that I once chose to discount. These cries now tug at my heart and allow me no peace, no rest—and that is proper, for there is great need, and someone must answer this cry for justice, mercy, and relief. It has created in me a passion for altering the fate and suffering of others and has developed in me a level of compassion and understanding I never knew could exist. It has grown in me a love and appreciation for the smallest of things, the mundane moments, and the humblest of beings.

Yes, pain has changed me. And I thank God for that. It now molds me, defines me, and guides my footsteps to the hidden pathways I would never have encountered nor willingly traveled, but so desperately need to walk.

*

SAMANTHA ANDERSON
Samantha was diagnosed with idiopathic
gastroparesis in 2012 at age 26

How gastroparesis has affected my mental health is a hard one to talk about, simply because how much do I admit to myself? Let's be honest, I think it is fair to say everyone has their issues. I have struggled with my confidence and being very critical of myself for almost as long as I can remember. Did I ever feel stupidly low to the point of depression? Heck yes! However, since getting gastroparesis I have had all-time lows and definitely had depression for long periods of time. I have wanted it all to end too many times. Although I have always struggled with my confidence, it's so much lower than before. I didn't think it was possible to feel this low in esteem and confidence. Don't get me wrong, I will act like I'm okay and fine, and will get on with everything without most people knowing any different. But how I'm actually feeling is totally different.

When I first got ill, they made me feel like I was doing it to myself and it was my fault. This made me question everything I was doing, to the point where I wasn't sure if my symptoms were all down to me. I felt like I was losing it! And yet in a way, I still often feel like it is my fault and that somehow I deserve it. I often don't feel worthy of people's help with my illness and needs surrounding it. I feel this so much so, that when I couldn't get funded by the National Health Service for the gastric pacemaker, I wasn't surprised or shocked, just hurt. I expected it, as I felt like I was less deserving than others to treatment.

As gastroparesis is quite unknown, people are less sympathetic and say, "Well, at least you don't have this." So I think this didn't help and hasn't helped to how I feel about it now. Although I feel like this about me, I feel the total opposite toward others who have gastroparesis—they deserve all the help they can get.

I now suffer much more from panic attacks and anxiety. The thought of being sick or fainting around people, being in crowds and going out is awful. When around friends and people I may know, the worry about being boring because of my illness is significant. Yet I still want to be social and around people. I have a constant battle of wanting to be around people, but not wanting to be around people and trying to be positive even though I feel completely negative. This is without throwing in actual tiredness, fatigue, and exhaustion like I have never known it before!

Having gastroparesis is an absolute rollercoaster. There are the bad moods, feeling completely alone, feeling like no one really gets me, and then having to mentally prepare myself for the day and for getting through the pain. After six years of having gastroparesis and things slightly improving with it, I still don't know if I can ever get to half the place I want to be and be as good as I want to be. But then we could go back to age long issues.

*

JOLI ATKINS
Joli was diagnosed with
gastroparesis in 2015 at age 36

I suffer from depression as a result of this disease. Not just because of the pain, but also from the loss of my normal life. I do use the term normal in a relative way. Everyone's life has a different normal but I miss the life that I had before this disease. I was an active person. I was able to work four jobs and go to school and still have a life, but I cannot do that now. I am limited in my activity, and depression makes me want to stay in bed most days. I have to fight that demon every single day and it is hard. I have never thought about ending my life though, because I know that it could always be worse.

*

TRISHA BUNDY
Trisha was diagnosed with
gastroparesis in 2013 at age 35

Living with gastroparesis, other chronic illness related issues, and medical therapies can be extremely challenging. I am trying to learn how to focus my attention and worries over what I can control and not dwell on things outside of my control. I write in my blog often about the challenges that my illness has on all areas of my health. I've found that writing helps me understand and deal with the experiences and my emotions with more clarity. In my situation, I have been faced with figuring out how to accept and cope with life's uncertainties.

How do I discuss the unknown with my children? I want to be honest with them, yet still protect them from worrying too much. I don't have control over the unknown, but do have control over what I share and how I share it. Which is not always an easy decision.

Will I ever be able to return to fun and active experiences with my children? If so, will it be soon enough, or will it come too late to enjoy great times with them before they're grown? Once again I have some control of keeping a positive and hopeful mindset as well as trying to find and choose new meaningful experiences that fit within my realm of possibilities. However, I do not have total control over what I'd like to do due to my health situation.

I'm uncertain over how much to push myself to take risks and test boundaries or how much to give in and accept. My level of control varies in these respects on day-to-day perspectives, attitudes, and situations. It is still a balancing act that I sometimes succeed at, and yet too many other times struggle with.

I'm uncertain about how to respond to family members expressing their concern over my health and limitations, as well as their fears of if I'll die as a result of my illness. I have no control over other's opinions, emotions, or fears, at least not directly. I do have control over how I choose to respond, but just don't know how sometimes. I don't necessarily agree with their observations, but can't deny that I've wondered the same things, especially during the very difficult and painful times when better days ahead are hard to believe. Of course I can't share those feelings with them as it would only increase unnecessary worrying on their part.

I am uncertain how to respond when my medical team is bluntly and genuinely concerned, yet don't know what else to really do. I appreciate their honesty and compassion, as well as their communication and empathy, and while it softens the blow, it's still a hard pill to swallow. It's definitely a reality check when the ones you trust actually recognize the struggles on the body and see some of what you are experiencing before you even speak or share what's going on at the moment.

I'm uncertain if I will ever regain the strength and energy to return to the teaching I loved so much. Once again, I do not have direct control over this. It's very dependent on my health and who knows when, how, or if I'll ever improve enough. The only control that I have in this situation is to have an open mind, take it day by day to see what happens, and follow the medical advice I am given—even if it's all trial and error at this point in time.

Another area of uncertainty is how much advocating I'm comfortable doing on my personal Facebook timeline. This is in my control, yet I'm just not sure. While I know it's important, and I have a desire to help others, sometimes it is tiresome and grueling. We need people to hear and visualize the truth so family, medical professionals, and friends are aware of the conditions that plague our lives. Yet, at what cost? While some see it as being brave or inspiring, my family and I are forced to face the painful memories and scary realities.

I have currently chosen to be less vocal around my kids and careful about what I decide to share and with who, taking into consideration how my children will see and respond. I believe that they need to be aware, however, I don't want them seeing all the negative stories and lose sight of positivity or hope. They see enough from their own experiences with me, the sickness and pain (physical and emotional at times) that they've actually witnessed and visualized, to the individual research that I've recently learned they independently have done, and are doing. Which in fact may be spiking some of the questions I'm being faced with recently.

My daughter asked me again the other day whether I will I be like the other people who haven't made it? Will I die like them? How do I know? My son has been wondering and questioning if I will ever improve, would transplants be worthwhile and worth the risks, what else can we try? My stepdaughter has been expressing her concerns as she learns more about nutrition and related health risks. She's applying her new collegiate knowledge to my condition, basing it on her perception of how I look and feel as well as what she's heard us talking about after doctor visits. Her goal is to double major in health promotions and nursing with a concentration in nutrition. I honestly don't even know where or how to begin explaining, comforting, or reassuring my children or other family members when there are so many unknowns and uncertainties.

I'm uncertain why I became ill in the first place, even if the why doesn't really matter. It is what it is, and I have to find a way to simply deal with it. Unfortunately, that doesn't make it any easier.

I am uncertain about how to remove the emotions I feel building up inside me at times. How can I allow myself to cry tears or vent personal frustrations, fear, and even anger without losing control, falling to pieces, or allowing others to see me as fragile, torn, and weak? Writing helps my mind relax and allows my thoughts to flow, but even then I sometimes build barriers to protect myself from falling to shambles. Sometimes I just wish I could find a secret soundproof safehaven to scream, cry, or act out without anyone ever knowing. But even if such a spot existed, I'm not so sure that I'd be able to allow myself to freely express my emotions, in fear of not regaining control afterwards.

I still have uncertainty and doubts over when to contact my medical team, when to ignore symptoms, when to try to tough it out, and sometimes how much to actually tell them, especially when I fear their responses or answers. I'm aware that these choices are completely in my hands and under my control. I'm trying to trust myself and medical team enough to handle these individually as they arise. I know that honestly communicating my concerns and needs is essential if I'm going to depend on them to help determine if it's important enough to adjust my treatment, begin or end a treatment, investigate further, or if it's safe enough to ignore and just monitor.

I'm uncertain how to react when someone I respect tries to help me think positive by offering messages of hope, even if at this point it sounds like they are building false hope. I would love to believe them, as I know that we never know what tomorrow holds and things could possibly one day change. I usually agree, smile, and even catch myself repeating some of their very words to sound positive or hopeful myself, even if I don't truly feel that way. Why? Possibly because I know that I should feel that way or maybe because I believe that others expect me to feel so optimistic and hopeful, or sometimes because it's the only thing I can grab onto and say to help them feel better when things look and feel so bleak. When in all honesty, as much as I would like to think things could turn around, I don't truly expect it anymore.

I feel as if we don't have the answers available and may never have the answers to find lasting improvements. Instead we have to just figure out a way to help manage symptoms and try to prevent other issues that seem to happen all too often in our online community. I'm uncertain where I fall on the scale of things. I am aware, however, that my issues are more progressed or severe than many, yet thankfully not complexed with additional chronic illnesses that some have along with their digestive struggles. Learning that I'm able to offer possible treatment options that others haven't yet tried and may want to discuss with their doctors, is meaningful. But realizing that the majority of options I hear about, I have already tried with unsuccessful results or they are not recommended in my situation, sucks and just leads to more uncertainties about the best route of action for myself.

I admit that I have occasional negative uncertainties, and emotional pain that I try to avoid but still occurs at times, such as, why am I even here? Am I being unfair and a burden to my family? Rehashing how I am disappointing them by constantly failing at getting better. Yes, I know that it's not my fault and in some degree out of my control, but am I adding additional pain or troubles in their lives that I could minimize in some way? Is my health negatively impacting their health? I know I shouldn't, but I do occasionally consider if they could be happier and better off without me, maybe not immediately but after they have time to cope and grieve.

I'm uncertain about what comes next and what I should do. I'm uncertain about how to keep functioning like this, because living with my health conditions and all that goes with them is tough. However, seeing my loved ones concerned, worried, scared, and sad as a result of me, my health, and my actions (or lack thereof) is even tougher. I'm uncertain of how to remain strong enough and positive enough for them so that so much of their lives are not always worried about mine.

Sometimes I just want to say, "To heck with all of it," and just pretend that everything is better in the presence of everyone else (family, doctors, everyone) and just suffer in my own little hidden world all by myself until I just completely collapse or deteriorate. I know that this is not the answer and not even remotely possible. I may be uncertain about many things, but I am certain that my family loves me enough, and many times my medical team understands me enough, to realize when I'm being secretive or stubborn about sharing how I'm truly feeling. Even if I did decide to return to the "I'm okay," or "I'm feeling better" cop-outs.

It's discouraging for my family to continually witness my bad days and moments. And it must be discouraging for my medical team to continue hearing that I'm still struggling with the same symptoms, just at various degrees or levels. I can promise that it's equally, if not more so, discouraging for me to report that I'm once again not feeling better simply because for one, I'm certain that it's not what anyone wants to hear, and second, I'm certain that I'm sick and tired of repeating and hearing those exact same words myself. I know that I would likely not be successful with the "I'm okay, I'm better" scenario though, as the people closest to me can read me all too well now.

The truth of the matter is that life is full of uncertainties for each and every one of us. I am not supposed to have all of the answers. The journey of life is just too complex for me to ever comprehend. Instead, I should be certain that my heart is in the right place and that I hold on to faith and love to get me through whatever obstacles or battles come my way. My health may be uncertain, but there is one thing I know for sure, and that's how blessed I am to have a God so loving and gracious that he has surrounded me with some truly remarkable people to help me navigate this journey.

I may be uncertain about the path that I'm enduring and embarking upon or uncertain about how to best respond or react, but I do believe that one day (even if it's not until I'm in heaven), all of this will make perfect sense. I am certain that even though I may feel awful most days and that I may be confused about living with constant illness, I am still blessed beyond measure in so many other ways!

*

LISA COLANDREA
Lisa was diagnosed with
gastroparesis in 2016 at age 42

The pain I feel from gastroparesis affects my mental health on a daily basis. I find myself constantly thinking about what will become of me and when. The panic I feel has an effect on everything I do. I haven't felt suicidal. However, I do feel helpless and hopeless living with this illness every day. Because of that, I do have days when I feel like I want to give up.

*

TAMMY DOWNS

Tammy was diagnosed with Crohn's disease, irritable bowel syndrome, spastic colon, gastroesophageal reflux disease, and gastritis in 2006 at age 46, gastroparesis in 2015 at age 56, and motility dysfunction disorder of the rectum and pelvic floor in 2016 at age 58

Just having the disease and everything that comes along with it can get very depressing. The pain and nausea is just the tip of the iceberg. If those went away, it would be okay. If the rock in my stomach would disappear after eating, that would be even better.

There are times when just having a smoothie, soup, or eating just a piece of baked chicken or sweet potatoe causes everything to pile up in the stomach and lead to vomiting. It's a constant circle. When I eat solid food, I get bathroom issues which can be pretty bad. It plays with my mind and causes depression and anxiety. I just want to feel better.

When I was diagnosed with Crohn's disease, I had a lot of support from the doctors at both the office and hospital. Once I got the idea of what I had to do, and eat and not eat, I was able to control it, and was able to accept and understand more. I am not quite there yet with gastroparesis, and I was diagnosed a year ago this past April.

Gastroparesis is a stomach problem that needs a lot of help. I feel like we turn into guinea pigs. "Let's try this to see if it works." Or, "Try this medication. By the way, side effects are symptoms of Parkinson's disease, and when you stop the medication the symptoms won't go away." We take major chances of getting added problems.

I have found I can eat or drink something once with no issues, but the next time I try it, it will make me sick. I can cook it the same way I did before, but it doesn't matter. There is no rhyme or reason. The only thing I know for sure that work for me are liquids, smoothies, chicken noodle soup, and cooking with almond milk. No green vegetables. I have to cook my food very soft. I can eat baked chicken, shrimp, scallops, rice, a little bit of mashed potatoes, sweet potatoes, and yellow squash cooked real soft in the oven. I can eat baby food with fruit, stage two and some stage three baby food. But even these solid foods I don't eat every day. I try adding them two to three times a week, depending on how I feel and how my stomach is doing.

I really hope one day gastroparesis has a cure or a medication that can help, or a clinical trial that can give people hope that something could help. Too many wonderful people are dying. Why? Because there is no information and doctors don't know what to do to help these people. Why?

*

SKYE FALCON
Skye was diagnosed with gastroparesis and
other autoimmune diseases in 2006 at age 25

My pain levels have been quite high for years. Due to my overly reactive body, I cannot and do not take prescription pain medications, opioids, or the like. Instead of helping me through the pain, those types of medications often throw me straight into a flare, trigger every side effect listed on the label, and do not nix the pain. As my abdomen has become more and more taken over by scar tissue, furthering my adhesions to organs, intestines and the rest, the pain increases almost with every breath, and movement. It is a challenge to keep from acting the way I feel, which is often exhausted, lousy, and over it.

Because of how people react to my bad days, I tend to hide them and become a recluse, as most everyone with chronically awesome issues do. Somedays it is easier to slather on a fake smile and push through the pain rather than admitting what I am really feeling or experiencing. The mental anguish that comes from knowing that at any time my body could just quit, and I could be alone in trying to bring myself back again is hard. Day trips have to be planned, bathrooms scouted out ahead of time, and even more planning if there is any sort of food involved.

Facing every day with constant pain makes focusing on life that much more difficult. Sleep no longer happens regularly, only in spurts of an hour here, or twenty minutes there. There is little comfort, even when lying down, as no position is comfortable for longer than ten minutes. My bony protrusions require frequent movement so bruising and blood pooling does not occur, causing even more pain. Recently, I managed to pinch a vein on my shin, causing a small blood clot. Dealing with those pains, on top of my normal pain, was extreme.

These severe pains often create an unstable temperature in my body, and I fluctuate between overheating and turning blue from cold. The overheating is mixed with my defunct hormone levels and early onset, surgically induced menopause which means I go from six hundred degrees to negative six degrees every other minute. Once the Raynaud's phenomenon is tripped in a pain flare, it can take me hours to re-regulate enough to return to a normal body temperature, stop shaking, and be able to use my hands, arms, and legs again. Because of this, I am almost always connected to heating pads or electric blankets, even in the dead of an Indian summer, and allow them to provide the heat I cannot make for myself.

Dealing with the pain in the past led to cutting, although, not for the purpose of suicide. The release of a controlled pain, in whatever area I chose, was just the burn needed to remind me I was, I am, still alive. However, this coping mechanism is just no good, hard to explain, and something few truly understand. As time went on, I turned to the art of tattooing, and now sport a few dozen tattoos all over my body. Every tattoo tells a story of a specific incident, medical turn, new diagnosis, or life tragedy. I take my daily pains and mental anguish and turn it into the most positive energy and productiveness that I can muster. In my life, I have known many people who have chosen suicide in their path, and that is not something I could, or would ever do to those who mean the most to me.

Keeping the mental aspects of chronic illnesses in check is complex. There are so many levels to first establish, and then regularly deal with, both within the illness itself, and within our own human need. Just when I adjust to how things are, I wake up the next day and something totally new, unexpected and often challenging has presented itself. And those things that I just adjusted to? They are gone. And if I wasn't already sure that I am not certifiably crazy, I would think that I was, and had imagined it all. Being able to deal with sudden shifts, worsening and constantly morphing issues is a huge mental challenge. It is wearing, exhausting, and gets old so fast. But I feel that I only have two options. I can let the pain, depression, anxiety, and every other horrible thing that comes with gastroparesis living engulf me and just fall victim to this disease. Or, I can take a stand and make my life about learning, loving, and living, about giving back, and being as open and honest as I can about the things I face, so that I might be able to help another through their own issues someday.

*

ROBIN MCNAMARA
Robin was diagnosed with
gastroparesis in 2013 at age 55

I am one of the lucky ones. In the beginning, my entire abdomen hurt and was beyond uncomfortable. I will get stomach pain here and there, but it doesn't leave me doubled over in pain; it's more of a nuisance. In the beginning, I thought I would die because I was so miserable and had been mishandled by my former gastroenterologist. I can honestly say the thought of self-harm has never crossed my mind.

*

TAMMY PITTMAN

Tammy was diagnosed with gastroparesis and irritable bowel syndrome in 2014 at age 34

Pain itself doesn't affect my mental health as much as the bloating and nausea. I suffer from depression, and gastroparesis as a whole makes it worse. When I'm in severe pain and have to go to the emergency room, only to be told they can't find anything wrong, it depresses me because I know how I feel and I can't change it. At times, there are thoughts of giving up and letting it control me until the end. I feel like I'm a burden to those around me. I'm surrounded by very unsupportive family, and at times I just want to disappear.

*

TAYLOR SCHMITZ

Taylor was diagnosed with idiopathic gastroparesis in 2014 at age 22

The first few years were the hardest. As previously mentioned, I served in the military, and after my deployment, I was diagnosed with post-traumatic stress disorder. My biggest threat was the depression, and the extreme anxiety coupled with panic attacks. Unfortunately, gastroparesis thrives on mental illness. Even the slightest bit of stress triggers a flare, and after a while, I would give myself panic attacks because I desperately wanted to avoid eating at any cost. I was terrified of food and the pain it caused, and the panic attacks would not stop coming. My husband was so desperate to help, but he was frustrated, not knowing what to do. This fed my depression.

When I was kicked out of the military because of my disease, and they told me it had nothing to do with them and they wouldn't help me with it, I spiraled. Thoughts of not belonging in this world, thoughts of everyone I loved being so much better without me, being a worthless person, and being crazy, were too overwhelming. The PTSD gave me nightmares and unwanted thoughts all the time, but the gastroparesis made them seem real, until I found God again. I decided to follow Him, read His words, and not be afraid of what I couldn't control. My family needs me in ways I probably won't understand, but they need me. God put me here for a reason, and He is with me in my battle. No matter how hard it gets, I know I can overcome as long as I have my faith.

*

NICOLE STARZYNSKI
Nicole was diagnosed with
gastroparesis in 2016 at age 33

Mentally, gastroparesis takes a huge toll. I have never wanted to commit suicide, because I am fighting to live for my daughter. I do feel hopeless sometimes though. How can I live the rest of my life this way? I have called my mom crying so many times, and cried to Josh. I'm tired of being sick. I just want to wake up every day and feel good. I have a lot of panic attacks because I'm sick. Sometimes being sick triggers a panic attack. Fear of losing my job creates anxiety, and fear of not being able to leave my house. It's scary. What if I eat this, what's going to happen? I do have some extremely low times but even sick, life is much too precious to throw in the towel and give up. Sometimes it might feel like you are dying, you are so sick.

Many times the pain and puking were unbearable, and I just laid on my bathroom floor. I wanted to die but eventually got up, and each day I will continue to get up. It may not be a good day, but I'm alive. I can still talk and see my beautiful baby every day and that's all I need to remind me there is so much more in life to live for.

I do take Xanax for anxiety. I am on a very low dose but it has helped me from having complete meltdowns. With any chronic illness comes so much emotion and fear. When I am well enough, I make time for things that help my mental well-being, things to help my mind relax. Obviously how I feel dictates what I am capable of doing, but I've found things that relax me all over the spectrum, from coloring, find it puzzles, making bracelets, knitting, taking a walk, and—if I am really having a good day and feeling ambitious— a long bike ride or hike.

I've learned to try to take each day as its own day and not focus on the future or the past. I'm not Susie Sunshine, but being negative by choice, and being negative because of fear and a sense of hopelessness are entirely different. Normally those lows are followed by either self inspiration of pushing myself out of it and being positive, or my mom, Josh or my daughter saying, "Snap out of it. You have come this far and you can't give up now." Fear is always something hovering over me but no matter what happens, I am never going to surrender. I am not sure I would feel so strong about living if it wasn't for my amazing support system: my daughter, Josh, and my mom.

Every story I have read about another warrior taking their own life breaks my heart and sends chills through my body, and is always on my mind. They weren't a coward; they had decided the fight wasn't there any longer. People don't realize how many people with gastroparesis take their own life. Their stories deserve to be heard. Most of the stories include doctors ignoring them and families and friends not believing in them. It's heartbreaking to believe that anyone could treat a loved one like that, but it happens and it's because there isn't enough out there about gastroparesis. It's not on the news, and there isn't fundraising for it everywhere, so people have a tendency to think people with gastroparesis are overreacting or extremely dramatic. They don't realize that negativity is the difference sometimes between fighting and surrendering. Sometimes I do feel like I can't do this another day, but I'm quickly reminded that no matter how bad I feel, I'm alive and I am not giving up.

*

JENNIFER ZUBIK

Jennifer was diagnosed with idiopathic gastroparesis in 2010 at age 27

Fear is an understatement when describing my emotions and mental state during the worst time of my battle. I never once thought about harming myself, but at my lowest point I did not want to live under these circumstances forever. With the excruciating pain and overwhelming nausea, plus all the other effects, I felt that I did not have it in me to endure this for the next fifty to sixty years. With one breath, I wanted to grow old with Lou, watch my daughter become a successful woman with a family of her own, and have fun with grandchildren. With another breath though, I didn't want to live that long with this disease and symptoms and suffer. How would I be able to help my daughter plan her wedding and be a fun-loving grandma if I could barely leave my house or take care of myself? Who is going to take care of Lou if he ever needs assistance and I can't?

I felt as if I was hindering Lou and my daughter from so many experiences in life. Lou and I wanted to have a child together, but this disease prevented me from being able to give him that gift. My daughter is from a previous relationship. Lou has known her since the day she was born and began taking care of her when she was three years old. He loves her as his own, but would have loved to experience the news of us being pregnant, seeing a sonogram, listening to the heartbeat, the birth and instant love of a baby, and watching his child grow from the beginning. That choice has been taken away from us, and it breaks my heart we couldn't experience that together.

I feared we would never get to travel like we had dreamed about in the past, or even just go on fun family vacations to give our daughter some amazing memories. I cried all the time, every day. The guilt of ruining Lou and my daughter lives was unbearable. My daughter was so young and deserved so much more. She deserved to be a happy child with a happy childhood. I became severely depressed with high anxiety. Because of the anxiety, I developed an extreme case of obsessive compulsive disorder as well. Since I didn't seem to have control over the major aspects of my life, the other smaller things I would obsess about gave me a sense of control in a way.

Again, the effects of gastroparesis were overtaking our lives and I began seeing a therapist and psychiatrist for help and stability. Unfortunately, every anti-depressant my psychiatrist prescribed me made me sick, except for Ativan. With a combination of therapy several times per month and medicine, I could cope with all my fears and disappointments in life. I learned to accept what was out of my control and make the best of what I had left. Acceptance, another key factor you need with this disease. You can accept the fact of having the disease and the unfortunate consequences that come along with it, and still make the best of what and who is around you. For each day I get to see my daughter's smile and kiss Lou and hold his hand, that is a good day that I am thankful for waking up to.

*

The moment you accept yourself,
you become beautiful.
OSHO

*

CHAPTER SIXTEEN

Facing Our Fears

> Your illness does not define you. Your strength and courage does. -ANONYMOUS

Gastroparesis is a riddle wrapped in a mystery inside an enigma. It is a complex and misunderstood disease, resulting in confusion, myths, taboos, and sometimes permanent damage. At the root of it is a person in pain. What do you fear most about living with gastroparesis?

*

MELISSA ADAMS VANHOUTEN
Melissa was diagnosed with
gastroparesis in 2014 at age 47

I no longer fear anything regarding my own fate, really. I do not fear death, although I used to, especially in the early months just after diagnosis. This fear intensified for quite some time as I watched helplessly while others in my support groups, my friends, passed time and time again. I watched as they fought with everything they had to escape this fate, yet succumbed to it because it was beyond their control. Sometimes no action we take, no matter how valiant, can change the course of our lives.

Due to my role as group administrator, I have the unenviable task of posting the deaths in our community, and this wears on me. I see the strain these passings cause loved ones and the members of my gastroparesis community. I see the fear they incite. It breaks my heart. I miss those who have passed and I ache for those who share this sentiment. But mostly, I am angry. I am angry with family and loved ones who do not understand the struggles my community members endure. I am angry with the doctors who lack empathy, knowledge, and the will to treat us properly. I am angry with the researchers who cannot find a cure and the insurance companies which deny us basic, necessary treatments which could relieve a bit of our suffering. And I am angry with the media and the general public who turn a blind eye and a deaf ear to our plight. I am angry with all those who are blessed with good health and who choose to ignore the green candles I must post time and time again, the burning flames which represent the passing of each beautiful soul in our community. These are human beings—mothers, fathers, daughters, sons, sisters, brothers, friends. They are not statistics, numbers on a page. They matter. Their lives matter. These are needless, senseless deaths.

It is these deaths which led me to begin advocating for the gastroparesis community. I well remember the day I made this decision. It was a few days after a twenty-five-year-old young woman in our group, a good friend, died from the complications of gastroparesis. I posted the following on my social media sites:

"Okay, here is what I am going to do. I hope some of you will join me, but even if you do not, I am going to do it. I am going to do it because I am tired of watching my friends suffer and die. I am tired of watching them get pushed around and bullied—of being accused of lying, making up symptoms, and wanting attention. I am tired of them not receiving good treatments and medications—or even being treated like human beings by the medical profession. And I am not going to sit around and be told that I can't make a difference any longer. I am not going to wait for bills, or lobbyists, or patient associations to come and rescue us either. I am not going to request funds or request that funds be sent to any of the existing groups that claim to represent us. I am going to write a letter, and I am going to send it out to every congressional representative, every senator, the president, the SSA, and maybe even a couple of committees and subcommittees. I am going to write every drug company and nutritional supplement company I can find, write and call all media sources I am aware of, and send my letter to every hospital I can.

Furthermore, I am going to put a copy of this letter up here for you. Use it as is, plagiarize parts of it, pretend it is your own, alter it, whatever you want to do. Or simply write your own. Use my story, or tell about your own experiences. Send it to any or all the places I have mentioned. If you need additional help, please do not hesitate to send me a PM. I will gladly help."

Shortly afterward, I created an online Facebook group, Gastroparesis: Fighting for Change, and have not looked back. I have posted many deaths since, and I make no apologies to those who grow weary of this. I am angry and sad—and too determined to bring about the changes we seek to allow the opinions of others to influence me.

Our cause is just and right, and we need awareness. So, much to the chagrin of many of my non-gastroparesis friends, I make many posts like the following:

"Over the last two years, since my diagnosis with gastroparesis, I have gradually become more comfortable with publicly sharing information about gastroparesis as well as stories regarding both my personal struggles and the types of hardships I see every day in our support groups. I am not certain how my non-gastroparesis friends feel about this. I am guessing they sometimes find it boring or even annoying. In any case, it is not something for which I will apologize, nor is it something I will cease. You see, the message is too important for that. We need awareness, and not just within the gastroparesis community. We need the non-gastroparesis world to know our plight.

But as important as it is to extend our message to the world around us, the one thing I have refused to do from the beginning (and will continue to reject) is to publicly name those in the gastroparesis community who have passed away. I am sure you have noticed the far too many green candles that have appeared on my page over the last couple of years, and perhaps even wondered about the lives these candles represent. We have chosen, as a community, to largely keep this information confined to our private groups out of respect for the people who have passed and their loved ones.

What I can tell you though, in general, is that gastroparesis itself is not considered a terminal illness. Good news, right? Only it is not quite as rosy as it first appears. While gastroparesis itself may not directly cause death, the conditions resulting from it and the effects of our illness on our bodies over time most certainly can and do lead to death. Many times, there is an underlying cause of gastroparesis (such as diabetes or an autoimmune disorder) that contributes to this. It is also somewhat common for people with gastroparesis to have a cluster of other conditions such as IBS, mitochondrial disease, lupus, Lyme, etc. that can contribute to decline in condition. Further, those with tubes, ports, and PICC lines must constantly be alert for infections and other complications that can lead to crisis. But there is also another contributing factor, one that is sometimes not pleasant to discuss but must be confronted nevertheless, and that is death due to outright malnourishment and starvation.

Malnutrition and the gradual decline and starvation resulting from it is what we all fear, and yet many in the outside world (and some within the gastroparesis community) wish to pretend that the threat is not real. Well, let me tell you, it is, sadly, quite real. On a very good day, I am able to consume about 750 calories or so, but many days, I do not achieve 500. Five-hundred calories per day. Did that register? Can you imagine the toll that this must be taking on my organs, my appearance, my cognitive abilities, my very being? I read stories every day from group members who are losing their hair, their teeth, their energy, their organ function, and their ability to function mentally. It is overwhelmingly difficult to function with so few calories and such poor nutrition.

We try to prepare ourselves (as if that is possible) for the loss of those around us the best we can. But how do we as a community and as individuals process all of this? We rise every day knowing that we may hear of yet another death in our community. Will it be someone we know? A close friend? How long before it is us? Death surrounds us, and the unspoken fear that this will be our all-too-soon fate as well is ever-present in our lives. We push it to the backburner so that we can get through the day, but when someone we know, someone we love, someone we spoke with just yesterday passes, it becomes a little more difficult to confine the idea to the corners of our minds. And we wonder, am I next?

So, when you see my articles, blogs, stories, awareness and advocacy efforts, petitions, and the like, and when you see the green candles that I have come to detest, please try to understand that this is an attempt to garner attention and to win the support and assistance of those in the outside world who might intervene and perhaps alter our fates. It is, indeed, an endeavor to honor those community members who have earned my respect, admiration, and love by virtue of their existence and by virtue of their struggle to survive. It is an effort to keep their deaths from being in vain.

And though I may not be able to share the names, rest assured that these are real with families, friends, hopes, dreams, goals, and wishes. These are people who have fought hard to survive, who never gave up but through no fault of their own have been forced to pass from this world far too soon. These are not stories or statistics to me—they are my friends. They are people who mattered, who touched my life and the lives of so many others. They are people who needed help and deserved far better than this fate."

These deaths and the deep emotions they stir in me have spurred me into action. But while these passings make me angry and sad, they no longer provoke fear in me. Indeed, now, I am almost certain there are worse things to fear than death—constant pain is but one example. I recognize death remains the biggest terror for many in my community, and it is an overwhelming fear for my own family. But some days, truthfully, if it were not for my loved ones, I think I might welcome death, at least that is my fleeting feeling. It seems, at moments, it would be a release from this cell. These are my dark flashes, of course, the times I allow myself to forget my family, my loved ones, and all those in my support groups who mean everything to me. These are the times I walk a tightrope between loathing and welcoming death. I have written about death's seductive, yet dishonest, appeal on numerous occasions.

DEATH DANCES

By Melissa Adams VanHouten

Death dances, swirls, surrounds me,
He presents his bittersweet ballet,
Haunts me, taunts me, longs to seduce me,
Lures me closer with his sad serenade.

He burns the candles and dims the lights,
Promises nothing short of the divine,
Romances, entices, whispers sweet nothings,
Ensures me the pleasure is all mine.

His icy-cold fingers brush softly against me,
Almost feel his numbing embrace,

He's had countless lovers and courted far more,
With his kiss a multitude have been graced.

Entwined together in a Danse Macabre,
I nearly accept the deception,
His words drip softly, but his lips tell lies,
Become aware of my misguided misconceptions.

Our passionate tango begins to unwind,
His embrace is a death grip, heart-stopping,
The room spins around me—deceived, no escape,
Let me go! To my knees I am falling.

Past lovers do mock me, scoff and deride me,
"Did you believe you were favored or special?"
My paramour delights in my confusion and terror,
My horror brings him laughter and pleasure.

At last the fog clears, break free from his grasp,
Not my lover, but a tempter, a beast,
He distracts me, cajoles me, ensnares me,
But this courtship leads only to grief.

Past partners not cherished nor valued,
Though mesmerized by his slow, sad tune,
Mourn the losses, count the costs, and awaken,
They were betrayed—mere victims of the tomb.

But there's another, my first love, my true love,
Though scorned, He reaches out His gentle hands,
He offers comfort, solace, and tranquility,
Forgives my failings; He sincerely understands.
His romance is tender and eternal,

Light His burdens and few His demands,
When I allow, He guides and directs me,
And I know that perfect are His plans.

I blow out the candles, but I am not in the dark,
Indeed, in His true radiance I am bathed,
Can still hear the music, but fainter it calls,
Leave the dancefloor, though not completely unscathed.

Death dances, swirls, surrounds me,
He presents his bittersweet ballet,
Haunts me, taunts me, longs to seduce me,
But I take no notice of his sad serenade.

As with death, I also used to, but no longer, fear decline. I once worried my symptoms would worsen and I would one day be entirely unable to function. But that is almost my expectation now, and I have determined I will simply deal with it when it comes. I do still fear the pain. Or, rather, I fear I might not be strong enough to overcome it. But I try very hard not to allow myself to be consumed by such matters. I cannot control my illness nor prevent any deterioration which may follow. Many of the scenarios I imagine might never occur. It seems pointless to dwell on the what ifs.

No, my biggest fear, the one I am still unable to tame, rather than death or decline, is the thought of what might happen to my family should I die. I want to watch my daughter grow up. I want to see her graduate, get married, and have children. I want to see what career she chooses. I want to see what sort of woman she becomes. But mostly, I do not want her father and her to suffer because of my absence. I do not want her scarred by such a traumatic experience, and I do not want her to struggle as a result of it. I do not want it to change her, and I do not want it to hinder her from becoming all I know she can be. Quite simply, I do not want her to have to grow up without a mother. I also worry about what my husband will endure. I fear he will be unable to function and will neglect his work, our child, and his own life out of grief. We planned to grow old together. He should not have to alter those plans, and I know he will struggle insanely with having to do so.

So, in the end, I choose to live for as long as I am permitted and battle the fears which still remain. I fight for my daughter, my husband, my caring friends, and all those in my groups who are so dear to me. I endure and push the fears aside because I wish to correct the injustices daily inflicted upon my community, the wrongs which drive me to action and inspire my advocacy efforts. And, ultimately, I confront the fear and battle to survive because I serve a loving God who directs my path and who has determined this is my purpose. Who am I to argue with such a God? He knows my limits and my destiny, and so, I try my utmost to fulfill His will.

*

JOLI ATKINS
Joli was diagnosed with
gastroparesis in 2015 at age 36

Every day when I see another person in my support group has passed from this disease, it makes me worry that it will someday be me. This disease needs a cure and it needs to be soon. Too many people are losing their life because they cannot eat. I worry that I will have to be tube fed one day because I will not be able to eat. I worry that I will be bedridden one day because of the depression and lack of energy. I worry that my boyfriend will say he's had enough and leave. I turn my fears over to God and let him handle them. I cannot always be worrying or I will never have a life. I turn to my friends and my family and my support groups for support when I am down. That is what they are there for, in our times of need.

*

TRISHA BUNDY
Trisha was diagnosed with
gastroparesis in 2013 at age 35

I experience emotional sadness every time I see the green candle on Facebook announcing another death in our online gastroparesis community. We've lost so many in our groups lately, many of whom I've been familiar with, many that I corresponded with often in the groups, and others who I've formed wonderful friendships with. Most of them are close to me in age, were true life-fighters, helping others even when they were having their own challenges, helping spread awareness in their own personal ways, and willing to share their life joys, fears, and personal struggles. Each death causes me sadness and hurt. I don't know if it's because my circle of connections has grown larger or if more members are actually dying. I do know that the deaths seem to be closer and closer to me, not just people I've heard of, but friends! Facing the grief of so many young people dying, increases the worry that I have for my other close friends who are currently struggling right now.

I honestly don't know how to handle these heartaches anymore. I know that people die every day. People lose friends and loved ones, it's only natural. But somehow, being aware of so much death makes me contemplate how I can protect my heart, if that's even possible. Due to my own health recently, I have tried to continue advocating. I honestly feel like advocating is one of the best ways that I can have an opportunity to help others while also fighting for myself.

Yes, my heart is broken! It breaks for so many wonderful people! There are so many people struggling, pleading for better medical care, searching for needed physical and emotional support. It breaks because I want to help, but I don't feel like I'm succeeding at making enough of a difference. I know it's a tall order; I know it's an unreachable goal to help everyone. I know that I don't have control over when life begins, improves, or ultimately ends. I know I can't make someone's body accept the nutrition it needs. Geez, I can't even figure that out for my own body. But if a fellow group member or friend needs to vent with someone, if I can help ease a few of their worries, or answer some of their questions, then I want to be able to help them.

Yes, I get hurt, concerned, and frightened at times. I become scared when I consider how many more friends I will lose to this illness! Scared of who will be next! Scared of distancing myself and secluding myself from friends who understand my struggles and are able to help during the difficult times, friends whom I can return the same empathy and support to. Scared of isolating myself in hopes of protecting my heart from losing them later, even if we need each other now in the present moment. Scared because I see myself in some of these deaths, similar battles with similar results, prior to their passing. Scared because I don't want my medical team to give up on me. I hear about that happening to fellow gastroparesis sufferers all the time. Scared because I don't want to give up on myself. Scared because I don't want me or my friends to have to face our problems alone.

These emotions are real and can't be denied. Fortunately, I am able to navigate and continue forward with emotional support from God, my family, my closest friends (most of which I've met along my medical journey), and my current health team. Whether it's praying, venting to a loved one, opening up to my best friend online, writing, reaching out to an online support group, listening to my favorite music, talking with my psychologist, or spending a few minutes exercising mindfulness, I know that I have someone to turn to when times are most difficult.

*

LISA COLANDREA
Lisa was diagnosed with
gastroparesis in 2016 at age 42

The thing I fear most with gastroparesis is death. Most doctors say you can't die from gastroparesis. However, you can die from complications. People die from malnutrition alone. It's really hard for me to work through this fear with the not knowing. For me, this illness has progressed since being diagnosed just one year ago. I fear what will happen to me. I'm scared of not living my life the way I want to, or not being here for my family. I've been fortunate to gain support from strangers through online support groups, especially since most friends and family haven't been as supportive as I thought they would be. I haven't known anyone personally that has passed from gastroparesis. However, several people within an online support group that I am part of have passed away from complications of this illness. When I hear about someone passing, I start to get more scared. I think about my own life, and all I can think about is someone finding more treatments or a cure.

*

TAMMY DOWNS

Tammy was diagnosed with Crohn's disease, irritable bowel syndrome, spastic colon, gastroesophageal reflux disease, and gastritis in 2006 at age 46, gastroparesis in 2015 at age 56, and motility dysfunction disorder of the rectum and pelvic floor in 2016 at age 58

I do not like always referring back to my Crohn's disease or other issues. It's just that it has all had such a big effect on my life. I do not like the dehydration and malnutrition. I had that with Crohn's at the beginning and my weight dropped from 140 pounds down to 89 pounds. The only thing I did not experience was vomiting. Instead I had diarrhea, and everything I ate went right through me.

With gastroparesis, I went from 135 pounds down to 99 pounds. Everything I ate, I vomited up. I had very bad nausea, and pain like I had a rock in my stomach. I do not have vomiting as bad as others. I do have migraines, which I've had for a long time, and being unable to eat doesn't help. With a disease like this, I worry I will die before my time. I feel I have so much to live and see yet. Sometimes it is difficult to do that though, because of feeling so sick. I do not want to do anything but stay in bed or on the couch. When I force myself to get up to clean the house or do laundry and move my body around, sometimes it helps and sometimes it makes it worse.

It would be great if there were cures. I have grandchildren who I want to see grow up and get married. I have my family, so I have to keep going. I love my family and just want to feel better. I love to laugh and have fun, but it doesn't always work that way. I wonder sometimes if all my health issues come from having a lot of fun when I was younger and enjoying life too much.

All I can do is just keep going and hope that I can always keep myself above water. When my times comes, that is when I will go. I have twenty years or more to live, I hope.

My wish is for this book to help others. It is a difficult disease, and when you have multiple diseases that butt heads, it's hard to figure it all out. I hope everyone with gastroparesis is able to help one person somehow, some way. Just getting the word out is a very big accomplishment toward helping others.

*

SKYE FALCON

Skye was diagnosed with gastroparesis and other autoimmune diseases in 2006 at age 25

Next to death, my biggest fears are being alone, forced into a gastrostomy (G-tube), a jejunostomy (J-tube), or an ostomy. Not because of the tubes themselves, or what they do. More because of the side effects, limits, and general life changes I am just not ready to give up at this point. I also fear being unable to function and bedridden. After the failed nasogastric tubing and the horrendous eighteen-hour liquid feeds that made me sicker, plus the horror stories from my tubie friends, it is something I am wholeheartedly against at this point in time. I have always maintained that if malnutrition takes a drastic turn, I would of course do what I needed to stay alive, regardless. But tubes… tubes are a huge step and I am just not there yet.

I have been threatened with them multiple times in the past year, told that the inevitable is on its way, and that I just need to bite the bullet. I have a few close friends who have the same issues I do. While it is so wonderful to have people who truly do understand your worst days with little explanation, it is torture when something happens to them, their tubes, or their person. It's also hard when their illness takes a new turn, or when they leave this world all too soon because no one knows what to do about gastroparesis.

I find the most support in my local support groups, online support groups, and people who have like illnesses, chronic or terminal diagnoses. I believe that while many have the best intentions, and do not hold ill will toward me about my illnesses, they still do not have the time or patience. Nor do they really want to fully understand. In my experience, when people do not know much about the reality of these illnesses, especially the gastroparesis, they tend to say ridiculous things, offer poor advice, or make generally stupid comments. Those who deal with these types of illnesses often have more compassion and empathy; they just know how to treat another struggling human.

When a friend dies who has the same issues that you struggle with every day, you automatically take stock of the entire situation, even if there are blatant differences from your own. You compare their treatments, their extra methods, and note everything that was not working for them. If you are close to the person, you feel like a piece of your heart is missing, and your mind is inconsolable because this could be your truth too. Just last week I lost two friends, one to suicide and one due to the malnutrition of the disease, within hours of each other. Losing both hurt in completely different ways. I could understand her need to end things, but knowing that he had no choice in the matter and would give anything to still be here with his kids and wife, gave me the perspective to see things from all sides.

I fear being alone because I have watched how this, and other illnesses, have pushed so many people completely out of my life. I see the impacts of my illnesses, the trials, setbacks, successes and failures in the eyes and actions of my marriage, and it hurts on so many levels. I find myself offering my husband the easy way out when things are too much, too stressful, and too complex, because he didn't sign up for this sort of nonsense twenty years ago. I fear that I will become incapacitated and require more help from people who will build more resentment toward me personally, or my illnesses. I fear the disgusting outcomes that gastroparesis causes will eventually become too much for my husband, or others. I fear that the burden of taking care of me as my conditions continue to deteriorate will further the gaps between us, and cause us to divorce. I fear the troubles and things my children are witnessing now will make them resent me and what I could not do for them in the future. My fears with gastroparesis and chronic illness living are endless, and the list gets longer every day.

*

ROBIN MCNAMARA
Robin was diagnosed with
gastroparesis in 2013 at age 55

My biggest fears with gastroparesis are that I will go backward to when I was first diagnosed, and that I won't be lucky enough to skip a feeding tube. There are some wonderful women and men on Facebook who live with this horrible disease and are in very bad physical shape. I read their stories and I thank God I'm not struggling to stay alive like some folks are. The groups on Facebook are wonderful because we all get each other, and during times of struggle the entire community rallies around those who are having a rough time.

I have a couple of really wonderful friends who listen to me when I complain, and will say something simple that puts everything into perspective. I also have a sister who has been wonderful to me from start to finish. If I start going off the deep end, she slaps me back into shape (she doesn't really hit me, although sometimes she may want to!). My gastroenterologist has also been a wonderful resource for support. He offers me hope.

*

TAMMY PITTMAN

Tammy was diagnosed with gastroparesis and irritable bowel syndrome in 2014 at age 34

Fear is part of my life with gastroparesis. Fear of starving, fear of rejection everywhere I go. Fear of not being able to take care of my children, fear of my children suffering from the distress this disease can do, fear of watching my fifteen-year-old son going through this. Fear of losing my fellow gastroparesis brothers and sisters, fear of taking a chance at anything. Fear of the unknown and what's next with this debilitating disease. There is very little support at home from my parents. My son helps me during difficult times. I have a huge support system in groups on Facebook. The groups keep me going ninety percent of the time. We exchange happy mail during difficult times.

*

TAYLOR SCHMITZ

Taylor was diagnosed with idiopathic gastroparesis in 2014 at age 22

My biggest fears are simple: I'm terrified of driving my family crazy by being such a burden, and I'm terrified of not living my life because of how scared I can be of food and my limitations. One day, I know I'll be strong enough to live my life, and maybe one day I will be healthy enough as well. Who knows?

*

NICOLE STARZYNSKI

Nicole was diagnosed with gastroparesis in 2016 at age 33

Gastroparesis feels like the devil in disguise. Have you ever seen the movie *Ghost*? The black invisible demons that come from the ground to take lives? The way gastroparesis kills reminds me of that. When I was first diagnosed, I joined a bunch of support groups and read online stories like "The Mighty," both of which served a positive and negative impact. It made me feel comforted that others had stories similar to mine. From Google+ to Facebook, there are definitely numerous places to find people living a similar nightmare.

There was one girl whose story I was following because I really felt that she was living my life. Her battle was my battle. Her health began to decline and one day when I went online, someone had posted that she passed away. She was in her early twenties, just a baby. She was not skin and bones, she didn't have nutrition tubes. I never met or spoke to this woman directly, but her death really impacted me. I felt a connection to her. Within a few weeks her health had plummeted and she lost her battle. After that I stayed off the support groups for a while. I didn't want to think that her future could be my future. Then one day I realized that I also received positive support from people who understood me in a way that my family couldn't. So I still visit support groups. Sometimes it is a very harsh reality, but sadly, having this disease, you need to accept that there are some harsh realities we would all like to ignore. They're there and they aren't going away. You just have to learn how to use that fear as fuel to never give up and keep fighting to beat the demons of this invisible illness. That's something I have learned, and just like anyone else who tries to be positive, the negativity does take over. That's normal, and it's normal to be scared and have fears. Don't keep them in. Sometimes it helps to just talk to someone, or read how someone surpassed all odds. That little bit of hope beats all the unknowns and fear.

In just a few short years they have made tremendous strides in treatment for gastroparesis. It doesn't seem like that until you consider that prior to 2000, they didn't have a SmartPill test, gastric stimulator, or gastric peroral endoscopic pyloromyotomy (G-Poem/POP). Most of these have just come in the past ten years. The medical field is researching so many different things to aid in the battle of gastroparesis. I continue to research clinical studies across the world, and talk to people who have this disease about procedures they have had. Educating myself is one of the most invaluable tools that I have control over. The more I know about nutrition, digestion, and treatments available, the better advocate I am for myself. I wouldn't be where I am today if I hadn't done all my own research and took a chance reaching out to doctors who specialize in treating gastroparesis. I may not be cured but I know what is causing my symptoms and I've already started the war to win.

*

JENNIFER ZUBIK

Jennifer was diagnosed with idiopathic gastroparesis in 2010 at age 27

What I fear most about living with gastroparesis is probably the same as many others: losing my battle. This disease can cause so much damage and lead to so many additional problems. I fear the uncertainty of what could happen to each one of us because of this disease. I admit that I am not on social media and do not follow any gastroparesis groups. When I was diagnosed, I knew nothing about the disease and researched a lot online. I entered one group one day and read a few stories with death outcomes. I was horrified about what my destiny could be and could not bear to read anymore. Excuse my ignorance, and maybe even selfishness, but I did not want to believe the reality of how dreadful and bad this disease truly was. I took it upon myself to travel this road on my own, with the only knowledge given to me by the doctors who knew about gastroparesis. The doctors at the Cleveland Clinic became my only source of information, which was enough for me since that is what they specialized in.

My husband, daughter, mothers, fathers, sister, brothers and niece were my support group. Their love and encouragement gave me the will to not give up. I recently reconnected with my old best friend from high school who I had lost touch with. Coincidentally, she was experiencing stomach problems that seemed similar to mine, so I tried to help lead her in the right direction. She too was diagnosed with gastroparesis shortly after our reunion, unfortunately. She has been very active with the gastroparesis groups and community and has kept me informed and up-to-date with the news.

It's odd; gastroparesis has come so far since my diagnosis and experience. When I think back to how doctors did things compared to how they do it now, it amazes me how much has changed. It saddens me to hear there are so many who experience the awful symptoms and effects, and then about those who lost their lives due to this disease. I would never wish gastroparesis upon anyone. Perhaps I should reconsider, and become more involved and partake in encouraging and assisting fellows in need—yes, I should, and yes, I will.

CHAPTER SEVENTEEN

Confessing our Struggles

Walking with a friend in the dark is better than walking alone in the light. -HELEN KELLER

Gastroparesis and other motility disorders can do permanent damage, both emotionally and physically. What is the hardest aspect of living with gastroparesis?

*

MELISSA ADAMS VANHOUTEN
Melissa was diagnosed with gastroparesis in 2014 at age 47

By far, the most difficult aspect of living with gastroparesis, for me, is letting go of the past, holding on to the positives that still exist, and finding a way to make a new, beautiful life despite the horrors of this illness. My life has been completely altered by my gastroparesis in both positive and negative ways. I have been forced to make drastic and nearly constant adjustments, physically and mentally, to survive and thrive in this new reality. I wrote the following on my one-year anniversary and much of it still rings true today.

ONE YEAR ANNIVERSARY

Please forgive me if I am a little "off" today. I don't usually remember dates; I am actually really bad about that. So, I didn't think I would remember this "anniversary." That is pretty foolish of me. Try as I might, I cannot forget that it was one year ago today that I was diagnosed with gastroparesis—and my life instantly changed forever. Seems like ten years ago. I won't bother retelling my story. Most of you have heard it before. It is funny; this year has been both harrowing and uplifting at the same time.

I know there might be some right now who are thinking, "Oh, no, she's talking about her illness again. That's all she ever does." But how can I not? It is my constant companion. The physical and mental aspects of this disease are unimaginably bad, and I don't believe anyone who has not experienced it first-hand can truly understand. Physically, I battle with much pain, exhaustion, and weakness. Mentally, there is isolation, anxiety, stress, and depression to fight. And it never goes away.

There is not one single day when I wake up and do not have to face this. There is never a break, not even for a moment. Every morning I wake up and know that though I am hungry, if I eat, agony will follow. Every day I try to balance my hunger and nutritional needs against that pain. We live in a world centered around food, so that is tough. It is everywhere. It is on my television and on my radio; it is on billboards and in magazines; it is at every social gathering that exists. It is in my own house. Normal people eat. They eat three entire meals a day, but those of us with gastroparesis cannot. And every time I take a bite, I feel like a complete failure.

I sometimes fall into the trap of believing that because I occasionally give in to my food cravings, and take a mere bite of something, I am weak. How can something that is a basic need for every human being cause me such agony? Why do I feel like I have somehow failed because I want what every person on the planet wants? It is not a case of eating too much and then regretting it. It is taking a bite, a single bite, and then wishing I could take it back. Food is a basic need, and yet I am denied it by this cruel disease. I likewise fall into the trap of believing that because I cannot always keep up with daily chores, or work a full-time job, I am lazy. But I know people who are too weak physically to even make it through their daily hygiene routine. Many truly expend every ounce of energy they have just trying to fight the pain and nausea. Are we weak? Do we lack willpower? In what world? Why should any of us ever have to feel that way? In reality, we are stronger than most. Do you know how much effort it takes to resist food when you are literally starving? Do you know how physically exhausting it is to try to tackle even the most basic chores when you have been fighting nausea and pain all day? You likely do not. That takes a special kind of willpower and strength that (I hope) most will never experience. We are truly warriors.

Beyond the physical aspects, there is much mental anguish associated with a chronic illness such as this. I am mostly confined to my home and can hardly ever leave. I joke that the only time I go out is to a medical appointment—and yet, that is the truth. I do not travel or vacation. I miss my child's events, and I endure much guilt because I cannot attend even the most important family functions. But I have it better than most. Many people I know no longer have any family support, and their friends have deserted them because they cannot participate in the social activities they once did. Yet, when we mention this, when we talk about feeling alone and isolated, we are labeled whiners and complainers who are simply seeking pity. Again, I ask: In what world? We are among the strongest people alive to be able to endure this day upon day and still have the guts to wake up and do it all over again the next day.

This disease is merciless, and it has made for a rough year. But as difficult as it has been and still is, it has not been entirely darkness and gloom for me this past year. When I was first sent home from the hospital with no clue as to how difficult things would be, I was forced to accept assistance from family and friends. I had no choice; I simply could not manage daily life without them. This was a new experience for me. I do not like being helped. I like to think of myself as self-sufficient. But this acceptance of help had a strange effect on me. It softened me. It forced me to experience humility and dependence on a level previously unknown to me. It made me view my life and the people in it quite differently, and it marked the first step down a very different path for me, the beginning of many changes.

I have never told anyone this, but a short while after being diagnosed, I actually wrote letters to many of my family members and close friends, basically telling them goodbye. For the first few awful weeks after being diagnosed, I was unable to imagine I would still be alive at the end of a year's time. Truly, I did not think I would last a few months. Seemingly overnight, I was thrust into facing just how fragile life is. This realization, coupled with the kindness shown to me by my family and friends, made it possible for me to put down in writing my deepest feelings for many of the most important people in my life. For the first time, I understood that they needed to know that their part in my life was not meaningless. I needed them to know, before I left this world, that they had made a difference to me, that they had meant something to me, that their kindness and love had mattered in my life.

Writing the letters was a very difficult thing to do. Believe it or not, I am not a person who wishes to talk about my personal feelings. To this day, I have been unable to write those letters to my husband and my child, the two people who matter most to me in this world. Maybe in time, I will grow brave enough to do that, but today, I still cannot face the thought of leaving them.

In any case, the letters were another step in my journey down this difficult path. But something even more eventful happened after I wrote those letters, something even more eye-opening. Somehow (through God's grace, I believe), it occurred to me that I should try to find others who might be experiencing the same thing as me. I was unable to leave the house, and so I was limited, but I thought maybe I could find others online. Well, we all know that I did. And oh, my, what a world these support groups have opened up to me. These groups have truly saved my life.

I have gained much knowledge about my illness from these groups, of course, but I have gained far more than that. To begin with, they have given me the courage to share my personal story in a very public way. That has helped me immensely. It has shown me that I do not need to hide my vulnerability. I can open up to others about how I truly feel, and the world will not end. I have received support, caring, and kindness on a level I never knew existed. In a matter of a few months, I have made friendships that will last a lifetime. I can honestly say that if I were miraculously cured tomorrow, I would not desert these people. I would still be here every day, all day long, talking to them and fighting for them. I would just be able to do a far better job of it. The people I have met in this online world have shown me more commitment, more dedication, and more acceptance than I could have imagined. Because of this otherwise wretched disease, I have met beautiful people, and I have opened up to them and others in my life in ways I previously thought impossible. That is a very good thing.

And that is not the only thing I have gained this past year. Over the course of this journey, I have developed a passion and purpose in life that I never even knew I had been missing. I have seen unimaginable suffering and need. My eyes have been opened to it, and I have discovered that I want to help people—these people. I know now that I can. What I am doing matters to me. I believe it matters to God as well. I have made no secret of the fact that I am a Christian. I do not force that upon people, but my faith is what gets me, personally, through the toughest days. And over the last year, I have seen that though I feel worse physically than I ever have, I grow spiritually stronger every day. I am often overwhelmed with compassion and concern for the people I have met. They have touched me deeply, and I am far more aware of the blessings I have been granted.

This is a tough anniversary for me. I have mixed emotions about it. I am sick. I am not getting better. I know I must face this devastating disease every day for the rest of my life, however long that may be. But it is a good life—one worth living, one worth fighting for. And there are people in it who matter, who count on me, and who love me. This gives me hope and strength to go on. It gets me through each day. Thank you all for what you do for me and for what you mean to me. I truly love you all.

* * *

I have written about my struggle many times since that first anniversary, but the theme remains the same: take the good with the bad and find a way to move forward, live a meaningful life, full of grace, compassion, and joy. It is not simple, and I have hit many bumps along the way, but I refuse to allow this illness to take my faith or to force me to lose my passion for life and my drive to be a better person. Those goals and dreams remain and are perhaps stronger than ever. Hardships have a way of defining, molding, and refining a person. That is what my gastroparesis has done for me.

TURN THE PAGE

By Melissa Adams VanHouten

She pens her poetic story,
Marks the callus pages of time,
Bittersweet winding journey,
Inscribed upon her restless mind.

Chronicles her ever-changing existence,
Notes the infirmities and grievous pain,
But her tale runs far deeper than this,
For of this saga much more remains.

Turn the page on what you are thinking,
This novel does not end that way,
Life is seldom what we envisioned,
And the best-laid plans can go astray.

Turn the page.

It began as most all accounts begin,
A child with high hopes and dreams,
Plans for a long and bright future,
Life wide-open and joyful, it seemed.

No time to stop and ponder,
Whether the story was compelling,
Adding chapters at whim, at liberty,
On unhappiness, there was no dwelling.

No concern about the lesser beings,
Mere minor characters to she,
Bad reviews and strong critiques,
Not considered, not noticed, not seen.

Turn the page.

But swiftly fly the pages,
And a new chapter soon began,
No foreshadowing this turn of the tables,
Takes place in a dark, foreboding land.

Turn the page on the life that she once knew,
Gone the carefree, the light, and the green,
Trapped in a desolate desert,
New chapter, new verse, new scene.

Turn the page.

The tone and the mood have been altered,
Cheerful setting now shadowy and bleak,
A land full of agony and misery,
One from which there is little relief.

This chapter, indeed, feels the longest,
Though the page count is relatively brief,
Not a grand proportion of the story,
But yet the focus, she somehow believes.

It is suspenseful and intriguing,
Though quite gloomy and melancholy,
It speaks of opportunities missed,
Highlights shallowness and foolish folly.

It encompasses the tear-stained pages,
Which recount the troubles and deep despair,
Of a heartbroken soul who does flounder,
Searching for meaning, in profound disrepair.

Turn the page.

The pages seem ragged and tattered now,
The cover is faded and worn,
The binding is barely holding on,
The edges are frayed and torn.

But the narrative has taken a thoughtful turn,
Greater definition and sensitivity than before,
The protagonist is growing—and learning,
That in a meaningful life there is so much more.

Turn the pages and keep reading onward,
Though the setting is still exacting and cruel,
The plot is growing ever thicker,
The epic novel ever richer and truer.

Turn the page.

Our heroine is gaining wisdom,
Acquiring compassion and full perspective,
She no longer wears heart blinders, protectors,
Becoming sincere, empathetic, reflective.

Turn the page on all the grief and anger,
She longs for a shiny brand new edition,
Delete the harshness and omit the anguish,
Insert new hope, with the author's permission.

Turn the page.

Turn the page on past chapters and sections,
Too difficult to remember anyway,
All new content and improved format,
Are the goals for this castoff castaway.

Turn the pages and write the future,
Not just for herself but for those who surround,
Change the setting and the well-worn theme,
For the whole community she has now found.

Edit out the pain and suffering,
Introduce a world fresh and anew,
One with hope and gentle tenderness,
With understanding and mercy through and through.

Turn the page.

Our heroine is now weak and shaken,
For she thought that everything she knew,
But she was most sadly mistaken,
Her grand plans and lofty values all askew.

She believed herself to be the novelist,
Though deep down she should have known,
She was nothing more than inconsequential,
The True Author holds the author's throne.

And He is an accomplished playwright,
A true poet, a genuine Nobel Laureate,
A superior author and skilled illustrator,
Whose stories are nothing short of glorious.

Turn the page.

The story is of yet unfinished,
But the foreshadowing is rather clear,
The heroine's one true mission,
Begins from the new beginning point—here.

All before was but an introduction,
Setting the stage for our protagonist's role,
She does not belong among the others,
She does not need to be physically whole.

Moves the plot along very nicely,
When the heroine recognizes the theme,
To support, serve, and guide the devalued,
Though minor characters they once seemed.

Turn the page.

She is made whole through the mission she is given,
And only then is her tale at last complete,
Only through her attendance and dedication,
Does the bittersweet once again become sweet.

Turn the page on the life that she once knew,
Filled with suffering, questioning, misery,
One with all manner of horror and pain,
New chapter, new verse, new scene.

Turn the page.

The pages have now all been published,
For all who have eyes and care to see,
Our heroine is no magnificent author,
But a master storyteller is He.

* * *

CHAINED TO THE BEAST

By Melissa Adams VanHouten

Chained to the beast,
Who would rob me of my soul,
Haunted by this nightmare,
Who can make me whole?

Sentenced to this fate,
But I have done no wrong,
My captor, my companion,
He appears to be so strong.

Trapped in this dungeon,
While the monster rages on,
He will surely slay me,
When his taunting's finally done.

How can I defeat him?
Release my daunted soul?
Who is there to rescue me,
To unbolt the prison door?

I fear my days are numbered,
His looks have grown so cold,
I'd like to ask his reasons,
But I am not this bold.

I know not why he chose me,
Why this burden I must bear,
But there is little question,
I must soon escape his lair.

My body falls to ruin,
But that's of little concern,
The greater battle blazes,
Reaches the point of no return.

The beast inflicts great sorrow,
His misdeeds do take their toll,
But though he ravages the body,
He must not reach my soul.

For he may hold the power,
To bedevil, inflict great pain,
But he must not persuade me,
That my life is lived in vain.

Shackled to my tormenter,
But inadequate is his reign,
My soul is mine alone,
And my choice it does remain.

Confined by the walls which surround me,
But my spirit can surely sing,
No cell can tether my soul,
Nor the hope to which I cling.

Chained to the wretched demon,
Who seeks only to devour,
But he knows not the day,
Nor the minute, nor the hour.

His power is but an illusion,
My fate transcends his command,
The key is beyond his reach,
But within the grasp of my hand.

My oppressor, my constant companion,
Unleashes his bitter fury,
He rails and rages against me,
But my fear, at last, is buried.

Though bound to the beast within me,
My spirit's, unrestrained, free to soar,
This body is enslaved in his Hell,
But my fearless soul has been made whole.

*

SAMANTHA ANDERSON

Samantha was diagnosed with idiopathic gastroparesis in 2012 at age 26

So much is hard when living with gastroparesis. The lines of one thing being more difficult than another are so blurred. On different days, weeks, months and maybe even years, it changes as you change, as the illness progresses (gets worse), stays the same or gets better.

The feeling of never really feeling well is a strange one. I feel like I am complaining when I say I don't feel well, or feel worse than usual, simply because I never feel particularly well. I generally feel poorly, dazed and not properly with it; it has almost become the norm. I have had to accept that this is generally how I feel now and to get on with it, but allowing myself to believe that is another thing. Acknowledging and living with the fact that I can't do as much as I used to, or would like to do, or as much as others, is a constant battle. It's definitely something that plays on my mind a lot. I often feel stupidly lazy now, even when it's pointed out to me how much I do, considering what is going on. I want to do so much more. I want to live so much more, but not in a mist. Feeling a bit more human would be amazing. I understand people often feel like this without having gastroparesis or other illnesses. I know that everyone's problem is hard for them to deal with, otherwise it wouldn't be a problem. And I know there are people out there who have symptoms of gastroparesis a lot worse than me. I do consider myself a lucky one of the sufferers in many ways.

Even though I often don't feel strong, I feel like I always have to be. It makes life easier to push as much negative feeling away as possible. I believe in positivity even when it is the hardest thing to do.

Just living with pain all the time is a struggle. The condition and the pain, especially, affects my sleep. My sleep is now constantly disturbed. I equate it to just napping on and off throughout the night. On the other hand, I've always said since getting ill, if I could get rid of all the other symptoms, I would live with the pain happily. In all honesty, it wouldn't be happily, but maybe more contently and freely. However, I know this is a very personal thing.

Then there is feeling like I have to rely on those closest to me for all kinds of support, and feeling like I do it too much and am maybe burdening them. Seeing the effect that me being ill has on them, particularly emotionally, is horrible, heart-rending and makes me feel guilty. Yet I also have the feeling that I am alone and that there is no one who really understands how I am feeling physically and mentally. I know now there are people who do understand, however gastroparesis symptoms and the severity of symptoms are very vast. The spectrum is large and thus not everyone in the gastroparesis community truly understand how we each feel. We can, without a doubt, empathize more with one another though.

Do I need to even broach the subject of being a foodie? Of loving food and knowing that so much of life is surrounded by it? It is hard to get away from, yet the effects I get from food (and drink, in many circumstances) is disgusting and awful. I am actually lost for words to effectively describe it. The nausea, the vomiting, the bloating, the belching, the extra pain, the acid and, at times, the heartburn. The list is long. I am lucky enough to not get very hungry. I suppose I'm hungry a little more often since getting the pacemaker, though. But it is the missing food, the social aspect of it particularly, that is hard. Yes I can still be social, I'm learning more and more as I go along, but then I'm dealing with educating others and trying to ensure they don't feel guilty. I know many of my family and friends often do feel guilty, and that's the last thing I want. When I actually carry sick bags around with me, and feel very uncomfortable when I'm out and don't have one, it can make something fun seem a little bit of a chore.

I often feel like my life changed dramatically for the worse when I got ill. Although things have got better, life has remained a little bit static. I have watched people move on with their lives, get new relationships, get married, have children, get new jobs and promotions and go traveling, and I am so happy for them. It makes me smile. But my life has stayed the same, and not in a particularly enjoyable way. I'm not saying I haven't had fun or good times, because in life you get both and need to enjoy the simple things. I just want my good times to be a little more like others have. What you see isn't always what is going on, but I hope you get the gist of how I'm feeling.

*

JOLI ATKINS
Joli was diagnosed with
gastroparesis in 2015 at age 36

The hardest part of this disease is losing my life. I have a different life now and it is hard to understand. I have good days and bad days but I never know what my day will be like until I wake up. I want to be the active person I was two years ago, before this all started. I want those days back but I know that it will never happen that way again. I want my boyfriend to look at me the same way he used to before we had to worry about what my day was going to be like, and before we had to worry if I could make it through the day without getting sick.

*

TRISHA BUNDY

Trisha was diagnosed with gastroparesis in 2013 at age 35

The hardest aspects of living with gastroparesis for me are accepting the physical and emotional changes that have occurred in my life, without becoming helpless or giving up, and witnessing the impact it has on my loved ones, especially my children. This illness has changed my life in ways I could never have imagined, literally overnight.

One day, I was able to eat anything I desired, and the next day, I was unable to tolerate any foods or liquids. Instead, I had to depend on a feeding tube for nutrition. I was an active parent, wife, daughter, and teacher before my illness. I was obese, but otherwise healthy and felt great prior to getting sick in February 2013. I have lost two hundred pounds due to the inability to receive adequate nutrition, and on most days feel too awful to be active in any form or fashion.

At first, I told myself that this stupid disease would not own me, control me, or affect my daily life. I felt strong and brave, thinking I could handle this disease and live my life the same as always. I would just have a different way of receiving my nutrition. Instead of eating, I would tube feed. In the beginning, I tried feeding at night so that I could feel and look normal during the day. But as time passed, I began to see how foolish that was. It didn't matter how much I tried to appear normal, my normal had changed. I was struggling to get through my day at work, just to come home and literally crash on the couch or bed during time I should have had with my family.

I gave up trying to hide my illness and decided to begin wearing my backpack during the day to run my feeds, in hopes that my energy would improve. I wear my backpack the majority of my day, regardless of where I go. When my family and friends eat, whether it's at home or in restaurants, I just sit there and watch, unable to eat myself. I look in the mirror and see the backpack and tube that feeds me instead. Occasionally, when my nausea is at its lowest, I do attempt to taste a couple of bites of food, but usually regret it soon after when I am forced to cope with the agonizing pain and nausea it created. Thankfully, I rarely have an appetite or desire to eat. Some days I am weak and fatigued to levels I did not think were possible. I can barely concentrate and function enough to do everyday tasks. I had to resign from my career as an elementary schoolteacher, a career that I loved, because my body could not keep up with the physical demands.

Since 2013, my gastrointestinal issues have led me down a path of numerous surgeries. Since diagnosis, I've seen multiple doctors and nurses in a variety of settings including but not limited to immediate care visits, emergency room visits, hospitalizations, diagnostic testing, outpatient clinics with my routine doctors and consultations with various specialists. In many of these situations, the medical providers (aside from my gastroenterologist) were either clueless from never having heard of the condition or having heard of it, but unfamiliar with how to best treat my symptoms. I have had many return visits to the emergency room for dehydration, uncontrollable pain and nausea, feeding tube issues, surgeries, infections, and so on. Every three months I have to return to interventional radiology and have my feeding tube replaced, sometimes sooner if it clogs or falls out. I have had my colon removed (colectomy) and now have an ileostomy due to colonic inertia, my gallbladder was removed due to stones and inflammation, and I use my central line port for IV fluids at home five days a week due to chronic dehydration.

When I look at myself in the mirror, my personal self-image can change drastically depending on how I view my body and medical appliances at that particular moment. Most days, I can credit the feeding tube, accessed port, ileostomy bag, and scars as battle wounds that keep me alive and with my kids, welcome additions to help improve my overall health. But there are also times when I feel disgust at what I've become and how my unclothed body now appears to my eyes. As a wife, I do sometimes worry about what my husband must think. How could he not be bothered by all of these unsightly changes?

Anger, lack of patience, and increased irritability all find their way to me at times. I'm sick of feeling so sick! I try to psych myself up, pretend to be okay, try to be strong, and try to remain positive. I smile when I feel like screaming or crying. I try to motivate, encourage, and distract myself by listening to music, blogging, using social media, watching movies with the family, and sometimes playing board or card games with my kids. I do become discouraged and frustrated with my body for how easily it becomes drained and fatigued. I often wonder why it is so necessary for me to exhaust all my energy and ruin my tolerable moments to attempt forcing nutrition or activities, just to end up sick, miserable, and defeated time and time again. Each time I fall, it becomes more and more difficult to recover, more difficult to rise to the person and character that I envision for myself. I just don't get it anymore! I'm worn and weary. I accept that my life isn't normal, may never be normal, but I do not want to accept that this is all that's left! My mind, spirit, and body desperately need a break. A break long enough to enjoy life with my family with little or no symptoms, have a chance to completely recharge, and create exciting memories together without the dreaded consequences afterwards.

I have received help and support from family members, friends, acquaintances, and some medical providers, which I am most grateful for. I have had some amazing doctors along my medical journey that have taken my condition seriously, discussed the treatment plans thoroughly, and always made sure that I was comfortable with the choices before moving forward. I wish I could say that about all of the doctors who have been responsible for my health care. Knowing that I have to keep optimistic and continue fighting for improvements with everything I have, but accepting the fact that it may never get better, is extremely difficult at times, especially when my body and mind are already so tired. Having an awesome support team is a valuable asset that I will never take for granted. My heart is full of appreciation and love for everyone who has been by my side, or still is by my side, to comfort, care, and assist me along my path through life.

*

LISA COLANDREA
Lisa was diagnosed with
gastroparesis in 2016 at age 42

The hardest aspect for me personally is both physical and emotional. They go together. It's knowing that when I wake up the next day, nothing really changes and my illness is still there and it's never going away. It's physically difficult because of the pain and suffering I feel, and sometimes the medicine doesn't work. I'm also a really emotional person. It's emotional knowing I wake up every day feeling horrible, and knowing what it's doing to my family as well. I am not waking up and living the life I had hoped and planned for. It puts a strain on my finances, my family, and not knowing what my future holds. The emotional part of it is just as much a struggle as the physical part.

*

TAMMY DOWNS

Tammy was diagnosed with Crohn's disease, irritable bowel syndrome, spastic colon, gastroesophageal reflux disease, and gastritis in 2006 at age 46, gastroparesis in 2015 at age 56, and motility dysfunction disorder of the rectum and pelvic floor in 2016 at age 58

My family, grandchildren, and others support me, and try to understand what I'm going through. A lot of times, I just keep going. Sometimes I just act like I'm fine, and I do not bring it up. If I am asked how I am doing, then I will discuss it.

People have a hard time when their family or friends have some kind of illness that they do not understand and there is no cure. I just have to stuff my emotions in further like I have done a lot of through my years of dealing with health issues and life. Having gastroparesis, blood problems, and then finding out I had the motility disorder along with it, makes it even worse.

*

SKYE FALCON

Skye was diagnosed with gastroparesis and other autoimmune diseases in 2006 at age 25

The hardest aspect of living with gastroparesis is just trying to get through everyday life. Starving constantly, being burdensome, having little understanding from the social world, and knowing you are a living, breathing guinea pig who is being used for their doctors and medical staff to learn from is hard to deal with. For me, being unable to keep up with my old self is disheartening, and seems to worsen by the year. The physical aspects bother me the most, because I have no control over the abilities I am losing. Watching my once muscular, fit body become frail, thin, and weak shows how never-ending these illnesses are. Being that my issues began to seriously flare when my stint with motherhood began, I have never really gotten to experience being a mom and having energy, or being able to push through the day without wondering when I will fall over or need some extra medical intervention to make it through.

Being faced with uncertain terms in life and difficult, painful illnesses makes everything emotionally charged, especially when the pain is great. So much of my focus every day is spent on taking a breath, counting calories in hopes I can retain what I need, calming myself and my racing blood pressure back down, controlling the vomiting, and not freaking out that there is again blood in the toilet, from one end or the other. Having chronic illnesses and gastroparesis, and a load of unfortunate violent crimes and family events over the years, have really helped put the meaning of life into perspective for me. Sure, I fight every day to just get through, and my pain is off the charts most every week. But I have seen worse, dealt with those who are more unfortunate and in worse situations, and seen the worst parts of life that can sneak out of even the darkest closet unexpectedly. I know that if I put one foot in front of the other, I will make progress regardless of how slow or imperfect. What I can give to another truly does matter, and that is where I focus my emotional energy, rather than solely on my illnesses.

The challenges I face with my gastroparesis are always on the move and always changing, both physically and mentally. For example, I am an avid green-thumbed gardener but my abilities have changed drastically in just the past five years. Five years ago, you would find me in my garden, hand-tilling to perfection, followed by mowing, raking, and more planting all in the same day. Three years ago, I began spacing out days in between planting for my gardening, and what once took me two days, then took fourteen. Mowing is now something that my teenagers do, and I miss. Two years ago, I could no longer bend over to easily plant, or reach my gardens, so new, taller raised beds with seats were made so I could still do what I loved.

Now in 2017, I am lucky to spend two solid hours outside, and I need to go in and rest for an hour. If I push myself more than that, my heart races, I begin to vomit for hours on end, and my gastrointestinal system shuts down for days, triggering a myriad of other issues, ailments, and side effects, and that good ole circle cycle begins again. My hands that were once strong and covered in calluses are now boney, veiny, and fragile. The hardening tissues inside are making it difficult to make fists, and bend my fingers. I am not ready to give up anything that I love, so I alter my methods, plans and how I do things to ensure that I can still physically make it. I tend to do this with all my extra activities, businesses, and family activities. Everything is planned. Everything has its own method, plan of action, and prepacked travel bag.

*

ROBIN MCNAMARA
Robin was diagnosed with
gastroparesis in 2013 at age 55

The hardest thing for me is not being able to drop what I am doing and go out or away. I'm always concerned, wondering what will I be able to eat? Will I get somewhere and have nausea strike out of the blue? Physically, I've held up pretty good, and do not expect that to change. Emotionally, at holidays and special life events, my emotions are either in check or food just makes me angry. I'm angry that I cannot eat the same food and enjoy it. Instead, I just sit there, listening to people say, "Aren't you going to eat anything?"

*

TAMMY PITTMAN
Tammy was diagnosed with gastroparesis and
irritable bowel syndrome in 2014 at age 34

I would say the hardest aspect of living with gastroparesis is the poor education on what the disease is and its potential. Many of us are verbally abused by strangers, friends, doctors, family, and the legal system. This disease is called the silent killer because that's exactly what it does. People who are uneducated on this disease can't comprehend that just because we don't look sick, doesn't mean we aren't struggling from day to day to achieve the smallest tasks, such as getting out of bed.

People look at me and almost always see a smile or laugh. That's who I'm portraying to be, my old self. Behind that smile are tears that can't fall because I'm cried out, teeth with decaying holes in them from the malnutrition, and bald spots from hair loss due to malnutrition. There is pain that has consumed my life, depression from the inability to perform tasks like cooking, fear of the unknown, and anger at everyone who doesn't understand. There is also the hurt from knowing my fifteen-year-old son is just starting this battle, hopelessness because I've tried and failed as a nurse, a wife, a mother, a daughter, as a person.

*

NICOLE STARZYNSKI
Nicole was diagnosed with
gastroparesis in 2016 at age 33

The hardest part of living with gastroparesis is the unknown. Will the disease continue to kill the working nerves in my stomach? What will happen to me over time? Will I eventually be dependent on tubes for nutrition? Will I have to accept what the doctors say, that having my stomach removed is inevitable? That the chances of me living a normal life are slim? They have no way to know what's killing the nerves so they can't stop it. They have absolutely no way to find out the answers to questions that I think of every day. What if the stimulator does over time stimulate the nerves to work? What if newer treatments come out? I don't want to have my stomach removed, and then any new treatments aren't even an option.

What my life might be ten to fifteen years from now is very scary. I try to stay positive, and I won't stop fighting. But what is my life going to be? Sometimes I totally lose it in the shower. I cry so hard, just frustrated with all the failed treatments and never-ending tests. I have doctor appointments that make me feel like I should lose all hope. It's hard to stay positive all the time, when there are so many unknowns. I could do everything there is available and be the biggest advocate for my health and still end up losing to a mysterious disease that nobody seems to really understand.

I go through lots of ups and downs. Depending on my symptoms, I may feel like no matter what, I am going to beat this. Then after a bunch of bad days, I start to wonder, or some doctor wants to force their stomach removal on me. I'm thirty-four. I am not having my stomach removed until I have exhausted all other treatments available. I might be making the wrong decision but it's the decision I feel the most comfortable with. That, I have learned, is so important to living with an incurable disease. You have to be in control. Do your research, and think about your choices. No doctor can force you into doing something while you are of sound mind.

Since being diagnosed, I have had to make sure I have advance directives, a will, and so many other things that sent me into a mini depression. It's hard to imagine that I could become so ill that I can't make my own decisions. When I was going through completing all the papers, I cried a few times, and even weeks after I was still upset about going through that entire situation. Then the fear left and I felt protected. Protected that the people I put in charge know what I want and understand the choices that would need to be made. That's hard when you're thirty-four and a single mom.

I worry about my baby growing up without her mom around. That's when the fight comes back and I tell myself no matter what, I am going to do what it takes to kick butt. I'm not letting any disease take me from my daughter. She deserves to have me here. I want to watch her grow, go to college, have a career, and eventually I want to be a grandma one day. No disease is going to take that away from us. Sometimes it's just hard to stay positive when the only news you hear is negative.

I have never been more relieved to have a stomach flu (Norovirus) in my entire life! One Sunday, I started to get nauseous and it kind of came and went. Then came stomach pain and all those other fun things that the stomach flu brings. However, this is how I have felt for the past fourteen months and immediately in my mind I thought, "Oh no, the surgery didn't work." I honestly almost had a breakdown. It took a few days to shake it away, but I was so happy it was just a stomach bug.

As my health continues to decline, some days seem like there is no hope of ever beating this, and that eventually I am going to look like the crypt keeper. The fear of this disease winning sometimes plays havoc in my thoughts. Support groups are supposed to be helpful but if someone is dying or has died every day since you joined, you start to wonder. Am I fighting hard enough? Is that going to be me? What if the surgery doesn't help or what if my nerves continue to die? I'm scared at the thought of having some electrical device control my stomach. Freaks me out! But it's my only option at this point and if I want to kick this disease's butt, that's what I have to do.

No matter what challenges I may be presented with, I always try to keep a positive attitude and stand firm in strength.

*

JENNIFER ZUBIK
Jennifer was diagnosed with idiopathic gastroparesis in 2010 at age 27

This disease was damaging both physically and emotionally. I feel the hardest part of living with gastroparesis is facing the unknown and living with the what ifs. We all know and have that fear of this disease taking our lives, but when? How long can I survive with the complications I am currently experiencing? What other complications am I going to experience because of this? At the beginning, I knew there was a possibility of organ failure and my heart stopping due to malnutrition and starvation. It was just a matter of time and when. I was afraid that I would not survive emotionally with this disease, even if I could survive physically.

I am very fortunate to be able to say that my challenges have changed. Since getting the gastric neurostimulator implanted, I have miraculously improved and have been given back the quality of life I had before this disease took over. I have gained all my weight back, plus a few pounds more, and I am not upset one bit because that extra weight was gained by enjoying the foods I missed so much. I am living my life without any limitations once again. Although, let me rephrase, I do have limitations with the stimulator as far as going through metal detectors, or if having any surgeries, I need to go to Cleveland to have the stimulator turned off, or not being able to have certain tests because of the stimulator. Otherwise, I can eat and drink anything I choose to. I no longer have any medications to take at this time. I understand that this too could all change one day.

Unfortunately, this stimulator that was placed inside me has a glitch and the doctors are unable to tell when the battery is going to die. Due to insurance not covering a random replacement now before the stimulator dies, I must wait. I was told I will wake up one day and be sick again, and will be sick for however long it takes to get another surgery scheduled to have it replaced. And even when that happens, will the outcome be just as successful? Knowing that is terrifying. Knowing that I will one day have to experience this all over again is unexplainably scary.

However, the time I have had being well now, is more than I could have ever asked for, especially because I didn't ever think that day would come. The stimulator was truly a blessing for me. The doctors cannot believe I recovered so well and had so much success with it. Even with all the uncertainty and risks involved with implanting the stimulator, I was not ready to give up and took a chance. I literally gambled with my life. I took the hand I was dealt and risked it all. I was fortunate to have the opportunity even though there was a lot of time and hassle involved to get it. After my insurance denied the surgery and my doctors appealed it three times, I was granted the lease for another chance at living a wonderful life. As my mother would say, "Honey, don't give up. You need to be strong, not only for yourself, but for others too. We need and want you to be here with us. Do not give up on hope or ever stop believing."

God bless her soul.

*

CHAPTER EIGHTEEN

Importance of Hope

Be like the birds, sing after every storm.
-BETH MENDE CONNY

Hope is the fuel that propels us forward, urges us to get out of bed each morning. It is the promise that tomorrow will be better than today. But chronic pain has a way of redefining what hope means to each person. What does hope mean to you today?

*

MELISSA ADAMS VANHOUTEN
Melissa was diagnosed with
gastroparesis in 2014 at age 47

I read a quote a while back: "Have defiant hope because reasonable hope is not really hope at all." I agree with this wholeheartedly and have adopted it as a motto of sorts. I used to hope for a good career, a nice home, lavish vacations, good health, and financial stability. I never imagined my life would take the turn it has. The meaning of hope and the things I hope for have changed dramatically over these past three years, and are far more basic than ever before. Hope is a real, tangible, nearly material item to me now. It is something which keeps me going on my darkest days. It is, indeed, not ordinary hope... but defiant hope.

What is defiant hope? Well, to me, it is akin to hoping against hope, believing in something most people would say defies all odds. It is finding a way to face a future that is, perhaps, mere survival at best. For those of us who live with serious invisible illnesses, such as the gastroparesis which seeks to destroy my own body, it is a way of life.

Beyond aspiring to survive the day, those in my community seek defiantly, rebelliously, to live a full and meaningful life in spite of this cruel disease. We hope for strength and stamina to face the pain, nausea, and fatigue that we daily confront. We hope to be able to push our symptoms to the back of our minds and deep inside our bodies and somehow be able to complete the tasks of the day, or, on a particularly successful day, attend some sort of outing or event. We hope to have the courage and will to interact with our families and friends in meaningful ways, show up for our jobs, attend church, and join in the other many activities we participated in before our diagnosis. We hope to enjoy a bit of life instead of simply enduring it.

But rather than further define defiant hope, I offer the following illustrations. Defiant hope, for those of us with invisible illnesses such as gastroparesis, is:

- the woman who enrolls herself in college courses, though she knows she will struggle greatly to attend classes and complete the work, because she wants to fulfill her dream of creating a nonprofit that will benefit others in the community.

- the mother who rises every morning and seeks medical answers for her two children who, like her, have been afflicted with this devastating illness, despite being told time and time again that nothing more can be done.
- the husband who, because his wife cannot bear to lose him, fights back tears and musters up the courage to drive himself to the local emergency room where he knows (almost) beyond a doubt they will mock, accuse, and offer little assistance.
- the mother who undergoes surgery after surgery, sacrificing more of her body and soul each time, so that she can survive a little longer to take her children to their baseball games and Nascar races for a few more seasons.
- the father who drags his tired, beaten body to work every day and faces the less-than-understanding glares of his coworkers and superiors because he is the sole income-earner and has small children at home, and who dreams he can get through this day, this month, this year, for their sake.
- the woman who sends cards to others in her community, despite barely being able to hold her head up, because she wishes to add cheer to their otherwise dreary and lonely days and believes beyond reason that this simple act of kindness will give others cause to go on hoping.
- the daughter who pulls herself away from her mother's hospital bed and forces her own tired and failing body to post awareness articles, memes, and encouraging words on our social media sites because she believes this sharing will enlighten others and spur them into action that will one day save us.

- the husband who spends his life savings and sacrifices his comfortable retirement plan to take his wife to the newest, best treatment facility in the blind faith that the doctors there will know of a new or more effective treatment that the other facilities somehow overlooked.
- the child who begs her sick and down-hearted mother to please try a bite of the food that has failed her a thousand times before because, "Mommy, this time might be different."
- the wife who books a flight for her family's next vacation in a faraway paradise, though she cannot for the life of her figure out how she will make it to the airport, let alone survive the entire two weeks of adventures, and who knows, she might have to cancel before all is said and done.
- the cousin who begs, pleads, and ultimately nearly forces his loved one to take her medicine, regardless of the fact that it is obvious to both of them it is no longer effective, and who picks her up and carries her to the hospital rather than giving up when it does indeed fail.
- the advocate who wills her frail, weak soul to pick herself up, seat herself at her computer all day long, every single day (as she has done for the last nearly three years), writing, emailing, tweeting, and calling every medical professional, politician, government agency, and media source she can find about her illness, despite rejection after rejection, because she defiantly believes that someday, someone will help her make the invisible visible.

Yes, my community and I defiantly cling to hope. Beyond logic, we hope to someday make our invisible illness visible to those around us who do not yet see. If they are not willing to open their eyes to us, to our illness, perhaps they will open their ears and hear us. If we are loud enough, persistent enough, and refuse to go unnoticed, maybe we can one day make ourselves known to them. So, we continue our rebellion.

We defiantly hope for a cure and anticipate that medical professionals will gain understanding of our illness, that we will no longer be viewed as hypochondriacs or drug-seekers, that we will be given the medications and treatments we know to be helpful for our condition, that our pain will be adequately addressed, and that we will be guided toward options that can provide us with better quality of life. Further, we defiantly expect that the Food and Drug Administration will not deny us those options, that our insurance companies will cover them, and that pharmaceutical companies will search diligently for safe, effective treatments and refuse to charge outrageous prices for our lifesaving drugs.

We defiantly hope to be financially secure despite the costs associated with our illness. We hope we will not lose our jobs, homes, and possessions due to the effects of this disease. We hope, one day, gastroparesis will be treated as the devastating disability we know it to be, that our government officials will recognize the seriousness of our situation, and that we will be granted necessary research dollars and policies beneficial to us.

But above all, we defiantly dream of a day when we will be understood, appreciated, and cared for by all those who surround us and impact our lives. We long to see our children grow up, grow old with our spouses, realize our dreams and goals, and once again enjoy life without pain, nausea, and fatigue. We defiantly hope for a full life, a bright future, and an end to our seemingly ceaseless struggle to merely survive. I defy you to take that defiant hope from us.

HOPE

By Melissa Adams VanHouten

I taunt myself sometimes,
With the hope that I could have a normal life.
Dress up, go out, converse, fake a smile,
Shatters, crumbles around me, no longer meant to be.

In the deepest recesses of my haunted mind,
There's a dream, a longing, that is still alive.
But it is much fainter, much paler, than in days before,
Will it continue to dim, till it is no more?

Surely something better waits for me,
The object of my yearning, that's alive in my dream.
At times, I reach to grasp it, often timidly,
Beyond my boundaries, but perhaps soon won't be.

*

SAMANTHA ANDERSON

Samantha was diagnosed with idiopathic gastroparesis in 2012 at age 26

Hope is something I have found myself clinging to for the past six years and will continue to, so much so that I have a Hope and Love tattoo with a gastroparesis ribbon under my left collarbone. I do hope for a cure, but like with many other illnesses, know this is going to be hard to come by. Often, once one thing is cured, something equally as horrible or even worse comes along and takes its place. However, I hope that less people get gastroparesis and that it becomes much easier to treat, so people living with it can do exactly that—live a more fulfilling life.

For me, personally, I would like it to just disappear. At the very least, I want to be able to cope with it all better, which will enable me to live more of a life that I would like to be living. I won't say a life like before I got ill, because although there was so much of it that was good, I have learned, grown and become a different person. I know that I am stronger than what I was back then, that I still need to be less hard on myself, and that there is so much to life. Some days, I may not say or feel like that at all, if I am being honest. To wake up and to go to bed not feeling yucky would be amazing. I suppose hope is wanting things to be a little bit easier, a little bit nicer; not a miracle, although that would be nice too. It is that sparkle, that thing that keeps you going; it gives you something to live for.

*

JOLI ATKINS
Joli was diagnosed with
gastroparesis in 2015 at age 36

Hope is waking up each day and seeing my boyfriend next to me. Hope is feeling my son hug me tight. Hope is having a good day and not regretting it. Hope is watching the chickens in the yard and being able to enjoy it because I've made it out of bed that day. Hope is feeling the sun on my face. Hope is just all of the good things in life that I get to enjoy and not thinking about the bad.

*

TRISHA BUNDY
Trisha was diagnosed with
gastroparesis in 2013 at age 35

Hope can have a few different meanings. To me, when I think of hope, I think of events that I anticipate or want to happen. In regards to my health journey, my definition and thoughts about hope are constantly evolving. When I first became ill, my hope was that my doctors would be able to quickly diagnose and treat my condition. I knew that something was wrong and that I felt extremely sick, but felt confident that my doctors would know how to fix me, how to take away the pain, nausea, dry heaves, vomiting, and inability to eat. Little did I know that many doctors would be as confused and perplexed as me, without an effective treatment plan or solution.

When I first received my feeding tube, I was full of hope. I felt as if I could finally receive the much needed nutrition and hydration that my body needed, and would be able to return to teaching. I thought a feeding tube would get me by until my body could reset itself and begin functioning correctly on its own again. It wasn't easy; it was definitely a life-changing event, but I was still hopeful that my life would soon return to normal. In the midst of learning how to effectively use my feeding tube, I patiently tried numerous medications. Prior to chronic illness, I was used to medications solving illnesses and infections, ending symptoms, and healing me. It was a wake-up call when medicine after medicine continued to fail and doctors began having no answers or explanations as to why this was happening to me or how to correct it. Weeks turned into months,

months followed by years, and I'm still plagued by this relentless and frustrating illness.

As time progressed, as my symptoms and ailments continued day after day, as trial and error symptom based treatments steadily persisted, my hope for lasting improvement dwindled away. I began worrying that I would never completely feel better again. In time, my hope of returning to my normal life, a life of feeling healthy and being actively involved was diminished. My hope for a cure, my hope for continuous relief, disappeared. I lost hope for fully recovering and no longer believe that I will ever be able to return to eating like a normal person. I no longer expect to return to my old normal self.

However, I do attempt to hold on to some sort of hope that my new self can become healthier and my symptoms can become more manageable and tolerable. Each change or treatment that is offered or tried adds additional challenges, hopes, and unfortunately, sometimes disappointments. While striving to remain optimistic, I also have to remain realistic. New medications, treatments, adjustments, side effects, changes within my medical team, surgeries, physical therapy, psychological therapy, family's opinions, my personal perception, and even deaths occurring in the gastroparesis online community ALL impact how hopeful I am at any given moment in time.

When considering my hope for today, as nice as it would be, I no longer expect or ask specifically for healing. I hope that new information and treatments will become available. I hope that my medical team stays invested in searching for what's in my best interests medically. I hope for knowledgeable, compassionate, and empathetic doctors and nurses in hospitals across the globe, including but not limited to ones that will treat me. I may not believe a different treatment will create a drastic improvement for me, but I am willing to keep trying in the off chance that one day I may be pleasantly surprised. I've learned the hard way that placing too much hope in upcoming treatments often crushes and chips away more and more of my spirit, leaving me feeling defeated or even like a failure. Instead, I have to prepare by constantly reminding myself that it may possibly help in some ways, but that there is no cure currently available. Trust me, this is more difficult to experience than it is to say. In time and through practice, I am having to learn how to alter my perceptions.

I may no longer hope or expect a concrete and lasting cure to be discovered for me personally, but I do have faith and believe that I am surrounded by an amazing support team. With God, family, friends, and key doctors by my side, I can stay open to all possibilities, and consider which actions may move me closer to my goal of improved health. I am motivated to push past the pain and obstacles that get in my way, and trust that my struggles will eventually pass as better days are possible. We may never know what tomorrow holds, but I honestly hope and pray that God, my loved ones, and the medical world will never give up on me, even when I feel like giving up on myself. I also hope that sharing my health journey will somehow help others better understand what it is like to live with invisible illnesses such as gastroparesis and even aid in the push for new research, more awareness, better treatments, and hopefully one day in the future, an actual cure.

*

LISA COLANDREA
Lisa was diagnosed with gastroparesis in 2016 at age 42

Hope for me is waking up another day and getting through it. I have the hope every day that someone is going to help me feel better. Someone is going to come out with some other treatment option or even a cure. I hope something will change, and I won't have to wake up feeling the way I do anymore.

*

TAMMY DOWNS
Tammy was diagnosed with Crohn's disease, irritable bowel syndrome, spastic colon, gastroesophageal reflux disease, and gastritis in 2006 at age 46, gastroparesis in 2015 at age 56, and motility dysfunction disorder of the rectum and pelvic floor in 2016 at age 58

Hope is a cure. Hope is doctors having answers with medication, and finding ways to get gastroparesis in remission. I hope that the public becomes more aware of what gastroparesis is, what our bodies go through and how it can cause other illnesses. I hope doctors can find a way to help us, and have better explanations and better support. They need to be able to help us with what we can do to keep from being malnourished, and to keep us from losing so much weight. We could lose our lives because of how it affects the organs and causes other illnesses to get worse; and then there is no hope. I also hope that the insurance companies get straightened out by learning what gastroparesis is, and then having a better understanding of the medications so patients are not having to fight to get them. Hope is that insurance gets better, for everyone to be able to afford it and be covered. Hope is not having to worry about pre-existing conditions.

*

SKYE FALCON

Skye was diagnosed with gastroparesis and other autoimmune diseases in 2006 at age 25

Hope is the future.

Hope is in my children, their beautiful souls, hearts, and heads.

Hope is volunteering and delivering meals to homebound seniors.

Hope is beginning a charity in my grandmother's name to continue her giving, loving legacy after her brutal home invasion and life-stealing attack.

Hope is planting a garden.

Hope is making plans, even if your next year looks grim and unknown.

Hope is finding a new natural treatment that gives relief, even if only temporarily. Hope is stronger than fear.

Hope is the warm sun rays on your cheeks, and the gentle spring winds blowing through your hair.

Hope is knowing that nothing is promised, and being grateful for every step of the way even if there are very large pot holes strewn about your path.

Hope is carrying out someone's wishes as they wanted, even if it goes against what you feel or believe.

Hope is tomorrow's sunrise. Love is tonight's sunset.

Hope is believing in yourself and your passions.

Hope is being deflated, hurt, alone, and crushed, and extending your hand to another with no expectation.

Hope is knowledge.

Hope is uplifting.

Hope is not judgmental, or self-seeking.

Hope is life.

Hope is everywhere, if you just open your eyes, focus your mind and heart, and live life to the fullest.

Did I always have this outlook? Of course not. As most humans do, I ended up focusing on myself and my children until 2006 when I became my grandmother's power of attorney. This put me in control of her assets, plans, bills, medications, and life. That turned into its own disaster, but because she wanted me in that role, I complied. She was frail and went through a series of rehabilitation centers, senior communities, apartments, and finally nursing homes. It was not until I witnessed her own wishes being completely disregarded by medical professionals that my eyes were opened to things on a new level.

I welcomed this enlightenment, and sought a new journey to educate myself more on senior and elderly living, and into my own medical disasters. Knowledge truly is power, and the more you know and educate yourself about medical issues, and life issues for that matter, the easier of a time you will have navigating through the maps of the illness or issue. I choose to find hope in everything, because I cannot imagine how life would be with none.

That said, finding hope in the darkness and grim times during a chronic illness is difficult, to say the least. I find myself struggling every day to find the good, and now take the time to really focus on multiple great things, small accomplishments, and my children's smiles. During the instances when I cannot get out of bed, I remind myself that bad days do not last. During the times of judgment and when things seem impossible, I remind myself of my track record. During the moments in time I wonder if my marriage will make it, I cling to the good memories, and the reasons why we started in the first place. Many periods in my life, I have been labeled dark and morbid. Even in those times, wallowing for too long in any pile of self-pity or horrible situation is not my style. I am just a realist, taking what life has thrown at me in the most honest, open way possible. There is always hope; sometimes you just have to search in places you never thought you would be looking to find it.

*

ROBIN MCNAMARA
Robin was diagnosed with
gastroparesis in 2013 at age 55

Hope is something that I expect or want to happen. Before an event, it is, "I hope the weather is good." Today, my hope is that someone will find a magic pill to make gastroparesis go away. Today, I hope I can have a good day and eat the foods I can without nausea. Today, I hope for a cure and hope that people with this disease can hang on for that cure. Today, I hope that I do not become a statistic.

*

TAMMY PITTMAN
Tammy was diagnosed with gastroparesis and irritable bowel syndrome in 2014 at age 34

Hope to me is based off my faith in God. I can hope for a cure all day, every day, but having faith in God's power to heal, gives me hope. Hope is probably one of the most used words in the world. We hope to be accepted by friends and family. We hope to make the team. We hope for a raise in salary. We hope we can live long enough to watch our kids grow up. So to me, I have faith that God will guide me in the path he has intended me to take.

Hope is just a thought that leaves a person to ride the fence between expecting a positive outcome or a negative. Having faith lets me, you and everyone push the negative outcome out of our minds and focus on the positive. In turn, this decreases stress and anxiety on the situation. I have faith that if the negative outcome is what we're handed, there's a reason. We don't have to understand it, but have faith in God's plan for our lives.

*

NICOLE STARZYNSKI
Nicole was diagnosed with gastroparesis in 2016 at age 33

When I think of hope, this quote always sticks in my mind: "She is clothed in strength and dignity and she laughs without fear of the future." Being told countless times that my pain can't be controlled, or that we are going to play Russian roulette with medical tests and postponing treatments, can be very frustrating at times. I always tell myself the tougher the battle, the more rewarding the victory will be. I have an invisible chronic illness that has permitted me to discover not only my purpose in life, but also how much internal growth I have encountered during my journey. I love the person I've become because I have surpassed all odds to become her.

The truth about chronic illness is that it's always a part of your life regardless of how you are feeling. Even on your best day, it's lurking, ready to strike. I've come to the conclusion that I was given this life because I am strong enough to live it. I may have gastroparesis, but it doesn't define who I am. Only I can define me!

The thought of being thirty-four and having a device control my stomach is scary. What happens five years from now? If I have already reached grade three, gastric failure, what does my future look like? How do I beat a disease I see someone dying from every day? Well, I know I am stubborn and I don't like losing. I am hoping that is what pushes me through this, that and my daughter. Long term, I fear the removal of my stomach, and worse. That is something I battle mentally every day. It may not be the main thing on my mind but the fear is there every day. Which makes me incredibly thankful for the littlest thing in life that others don't appreciate.

There are a lot of unknowns in my life because of gastroparesis but I have a lot to be thankful for. Having this disease isn't easy but I choose to live life and enjoy the moments I'm given. I'm surrounded by love and happiness, and those people who matter the most to me. At the end of the day, I might be sick but I will never let this disease consume me.

*

JENNIFER ZUBIK

Jennifer was diagnosed with idiopathic gastroparesis in 2010 at age 27

Hope is a feeling of expectation and desire for a certain thing to happen. It is exactly what it is defined as. Hope is also courage, strength and strong will. Keep believing and dreaming for the best to come. The path you are walking on may not be what you had desired, but trying to make the best out of the wall you are facing is all you can do. Attempt to enjoy each day, yet hope for a better one to come tomorrow.

I would try not to dwell on how dreadful it was. I took every day I was given and ran with it the utmost way I could, yet always hoped for better. Today, hope gets me through each day of my life, as I run with one hand in my husband's and the other in my daughter's.

*

All of life is peaks and valleys. Don't let the
peaks get too high or the valleys too low.
JOHN WOODEN

*

CHAPTER NINETEEN

Walking the Journey

> I don't want my pain and struggle to make me a victim. I want my battle to make me someone else's hero. -ANONYMOUS

Every journey is as unique as one's fingerprint, and yet we are never truly alone, for more walk behind, beside, and in front of us. In this chapter lies the answers to the final question posed to the writers: What would you like the world to know about how it feels to live with gastroparesis?

*

MELISSA ADAMS VANHOUTEN
Melissa was diagnosed with
gastroparesis in 2014 at age 47

What would I like the world to know about how it feels to live with gastroparesis? There is so much, and I hope I have conveyed a portion of this through my writings. If I must sum it up in a few words though, it feels misunderstood and overlooked. Most people have never heard of gastroparesis, and those who have do not comprehend it, or see its true effects. They believe it to be a stomachache, a passing phase, something that while perhaps not always pleasant, is not any big deal in the grand scheme of things. Only… it is.

I want the world to know how my community struggles, and what a huge impact this cruel disease has on our lives. I want them to know how inadequate friends and family, the medical community, the insurance and pharmaceutical companies, the media, the public, and the legislators and policy makers are at meeting our needs and understanding our plight. I wrote the following a little while back in an attempt to describe our situation to those who are blind to our misery, and I share it here so that you might know.

STARVING FOR HELP

I had a good week, a very good week. I probably managed to consume between 500 and 600 calories per day this past week, every single day. I thought I was doing so well. I was feeling pretty good this evening, so I decided to take a couple bites of a cookie—merely a couple of bites, not the whole cookie. I am doubled over in pain now, and I am in tears. It is agonizing. Who would believe this kind of pain could stem from tasting a couple of bites of food? I only wanted to taste a cookie. I miss food. I want to eat… I just want to eat! I want to have a normal day again, just once—one normal day, the way it used to be. It has been more than a year now since I have been able to consume a meal, and I don't think I will ever be able to eat one again.

I have a pretty good attitude toward my life and my circumstances, but the fact remains that like so many of my friends, I am not getting any better. I am dying, and it is a slow death, attributable to starvation. I am dying, and there is no help, no cure, few treatment options, and little concern about it from the media, the public, the policy makers, the doctors, and the researchers. I am dying, and no one wants to hear it, or face it, or stop it from happening.

Does this matter at all to the people who make the decisions that largely determine my fate? Does it matter to the medical world, the lawmakers, the insurance companies, or the news people? Not enough. Most of them have never heard of gastroparesis, and the ones who have, don't fully understand it or decide to ignore it, and dismiss it as if it is a stomachache. Well let me tell you, it is not just a little tummy trouble. I am not certain that anyone who has not experienced this disease personally can ever really grasp the true horrors of this disease, but if these decision-makers and life-shapers could spend a week in my support groups, perhaps they would begin to comprehend the never-ceasing torture we endure day in and day out. Perhaps then they would see what I see: tremendous physical suffering due to pain, nausea, and the inability to eat, seemingly endless doctor visits, emergency room trips, surgeries and procedures, isolation, loneliness, depression, resignation, financial distress and ruin.

Perhaps the medical world would understand the lack of compassion and concern we face on a daily basis. Many in my groups are in and out of emergency rooms, must tolerate lengthy hospital stays away from their family, and are forced to endure surgery upon surgery in an attempt to simply survive. Many of us have no effective medications or treatments and are denied insurance coverage for the few necessary drugs, treatments, and supplies we do have. Maybe after a week in my groups these doctors would see that we are frequently mistreated and even downright abused by a medical community that lacks knowledge, understanding, or the will to help us. Maybe these same medical professionals would feel guilty for their lack of desire to help, and for treating us as nuisances to be swatted away like flies. This without so much as an ounce of concern or guilt over making us feel humiliated, treating us like hypochondriacs and drug abusers, and for pushing us out their doors without providing any aid or any guidance as to where we might go for assistance. Perhaps they would think twice before leaving us to cry out in anguish while lying in a hospital bed being denied pain medication. Maybe they would reconsider their use of phrases such as, "There is no pain with gastroparesis," and "There is nothing more we can do."

If the media could spend a week in my groups, would they begin to understand our need to be heard? They have no space for our stories, yet they seem to find slots for such pressing matters as the perils of purchasing fake Final Four tickets and the opening of the latest local dog bakery. They can sometimes tolerate the chronically ill when we have sexy, prettied-up stories or when we have overcome incredible odds to survive. They can tolerate us when we are upbeat and hopeful, but they want no part of our messy stomach and bathroom issues, our tubes and scars, and our despair at facing starvation and ultimate death.

Perchance if we could learn to be a little cheerier about our circumstances, and pretend we are not bothered by our skeletal frames and hunger pains, we would gain acceptance. Perhaps if we could hide our tubes and ports and PICC lines, we would be more camera-friendly. Maybe if we could find a way to tie our stories into both local and national events, or manage to summarize our dying pleas in 140 characters or less and get enough people to tweet a certain hashtag, or manage to generate some sort of low-level controversy, we would get a moment of coverage from them. Would a week in my groups change their attitude and make them more amenable to assisting us? Would our pleas for help then cease to fall upon deaf ears?

If the policy makers, insurance companies, and researchers spent a week in my groups, would they put less emphasis on monetary concerns and more on humanitarian issues? Would they be more willing to fund our cause if they saw how ineffective our current treatments and medications are? Would they open their eyes to our suffering and make us a priority? Possibly the lawmakers don't understand that when they refuse to grant us anything beyond a tiny portion of their research dollars, no one is willing to seek treatments and cures for us. Maybe they believe researchers work for free. Or maybe they believe digestive disorders are not cause for genuine concern. After all, what's a little heartburn, gas, and bloating, right?

Perhaps, after witnessing our pain and the tough choices we must make when we cannot afford the potentially lifesaving drugs and treatments they refuse to cover, insurance companies would begin to appreciate our dilemma. Would they then understand what it is like to look forward to a surgery for pacer implantation as your last hope for survival, only to be told it is experimental or not medically necessary and therefore will not be covered by the insurance company to which you have paid premiums your entire adult life? Perhaps after spending some time in my groups and witnessing the tics, cramps, pain, nausea, and heart problems caused by our currently available medications, the Food and Drug Administration would consider streamlining and fast-tracking drug approval or loosening restrictions on risky and potentially addictive medications.

In the early hours of every day, I rise and head for my computer to work as long, and as hard, and as fast as I can to reach the people who might be willing and able to help us with our plight. I sacrifice time with the family I love in the slim hope that I might be able to persuade just one influential person to notice, to care, to help us. I panic if I must fritter away a day due to other obligations (which mostly consist of doctor's appointments) because I recognize that this is time I will not be spending on advocacy. I do not know how much longer my friends and I have left, so I cannot afford to squander my time. Does anyone appreciate that we are people—human beings with the same wants, needs, goals, and desires as others? We are struggling. We are dying. We are STARVING FOR HELP. It's not just a slogan. Does anyone hear us? Does anyone care?

* * *

Sometimes I wonder if anyone is listening, if anyone even tries to comprehend our circumstances. I know there must be a few. But even those few who do care, those who take the time to learn a bit about our illness and do not simply brush us off, cannot truly understand what we endure. There is a difference between knowledge and understanding. Knowledge is a mere accumulation of facts and data, while understanding requires a bit more. It demands insight, sensitivity, and intimacy with any given situation. Sometimes, it necessitates you have borne a particular burden. I am convinced there is a basic lack of understanding regarding the effects chronic illnesses such as gastroparesis have on the lives of those afflicted. But though I recognize this deficiency, I do not believe it must necessarily lead to our abandonment. Please allow me to explain.

You may have knowledge of my illness. Perhaps you can even define it, explain it, and list its symptoms. But you have not lived with gastroparesis nor felt its effects on your own life. As one who is unafflicted, you cannot fully appreciate the agony, the mental and physical torment of this punishing disease. You have not met the horror of being surrounded by a virtual cornucopia of foods, of savoring their tempting aromas, of longing to take just a bite, and of ultimately having to reject them. You have not faced the fear of perhaps never again being able to delight in these tantalizing treats, nor have you desperately clung to the slowly fading memory of what it was once like to partake of them.

You haven't experienced the overwhelming nausea which comes out of the blue and, at times, tethers you to your couch or the bathroom floor. You have not endured the never-ending daily pain which cannot be tamed and drives you to tears, confines you to your home, chains you to your heating pad, prevents you from sleeping, and haunts you as you lie in bed contemplating how you might face it again tomorrow. You have not watched your body wither away, felt the energy drain from you with the slightest exertion, nor endured the bone-deep fatigue and weakness which weigh on both body and soul.

You may have knowledge of the available treatment options associated with my condition and be able to recommend the top physicians in the field, but you cannot comprehend the depths of the disillusionment and rejection which accompany failed medications and contemptuous, cold-hearted physicians. You have not felt the condescending glare of the doctor who has accused you of imagining or inventing your symptoms in hopes of gaining sympathy, attention, or mind-altering medications, who has blamed you for the very existence of your illness, or who has admonished you for not trying hard enough to overcome its effects. You have not spent your life savings, traveled cross-country, and held out hope that a certain new doctor will take your case and finally see your agony and alleviate your misery, only to experience the utter devastation of having your hopes dashed when this tops-in-the-field doctor turns you away with a simple, "I'm sorry, but your case is too complex." You have not anticipated healing and relief only to discover your miracle medicine comes with serious risks and harmful side effects or that, in reality, it simply has no effect on your symptoms at all.

You may know what is best, endlessly reprimand me for my lack of positivity, and direct me to fight through the pain, but you are not the one who must look your child in the eyes and tell her yet again you will miss her latest performance, school activity, or birthday party. You are not forced to deny your spouse a celebratory evening on the town or miss the family Christmas gathering because your body refuses to cooperate with the demands of such an outing. You do not bear the burden of being unable to work or provide financially for your family, help with basic household chores and errands, or contribute in any productive way. You do not ceaselessly relive the memories of earlier times when such tasks were easily performed and such activities were readily attended, nor do you live with the anguish surrounding all you have lost and all you can no longer accomplish. You do not suffer the guilt of constantly disappointing others.

No, you may know of my illness, but you lack understanding on any meaningful level. Nevertheless, you need not wholly comprehend the full effects of my illness to offer your kindness, to co-exist with me in peace and harmony, or to genuinely help. I will settle for your knowledge alone if that knowledge is unaccompanied by judgment and reproach. It is not necessary for you to intimately understand my deepest longings, aches, and needs, my fears and regrets, so long as you will simply offer support in the ways I desire and not in the ways you deem best. You must merely recognize I am truly ill and doing the best I can to survive, to thrive, despite this cruel disease. You need only sit by my side, present a listening ear, believe my struggles are genuine, offer comfort, respect my choices, acknowledge my efforts, forgive me my failings, and refrain from criticizing that which you do not—cannot—comprehend.

I leave you with a couple of poems because they express my feelings best. No one is immune to illness. It can hit anyone, at any time, and leave you unprepared. Put yourselves in our shoes as best you can and see things from our perspective. Show us mercy and offer your assistance. Be kind and gentle with us. We matter.

THE OTHERS

By Melissa Adams VanHouten

We walk among the shadows
And live behind the veil,
Locked in another world,
One dull and dark and pale.

Just a few shades shy of whole,
Peering now through the looking glass,
Mired in this desolate land,
Remembering fonder times past.

We once knew light and laughter,
Lived among the living,
Once strolled among the Others,
No apprehension or misgiving.

We cannot now embrace them,
Just beyond our reach,
They turn as if to stare,
Feel their gaze, but they do not see.

Invisible? No—but shrouded,
Enveloped in a mist,
The others mill about us,
As if we do not exist.

They go about their carefree days,
Oblivious to our plight,
Ignore the gaunt apparitions,
Though we plead with all our might.

Our words, they must be muted,
Our appearance obscured by the haze,
Our struggle to cross back to their realm,
Unnoticed, unaware of our pain.

We yearn to feel the sunlight,
Co-exist in their brilliant world,
We cry out to be resurrected,
They hear, but we are not heard.

Dear Others who have such blessings,
Such contentment and such peace,
"Won't you help us?" we beseech you,
We beg for our release.

Healthy and whole on the outside,
Free from the invisible cage,
You who are dead on the inside
Do you notice our cruel fate?

You who have been granted wellness,
Who know no pain or despair,
Pull back this shroud, this curtain,
That prevents us from joining you there.

Open your hearts to our calling,
Let your ears hear our distant cries,
Shine a light into our blackness,
Shed the scales that cloud your eyes.

For the veil between the worlds
Is your choosing, your will, your design,
And the unseen partition that divides us
Must be removed by the enlightened side.

Your eyes are blurred by callousness,
Instead of heartfelt tears,
But you can remove the blinders,
Your vision, at last, can be clear.

From behind the window, we entreat you:
Break the panes and remove the shards;
Crack open your shielded hearts,
And topple this house of cards.

The ghostly world that entraps us,
Imperceptible but to the chosen few,
Can surely be made apparent,
Can again appear in plain view.

We ache to walk among you,
Leave this world so ethereal and frail,
Endeavor to rejoin you Others,
Are our petitions to no avail?

Who among you holds the mercy,
The tenderness and grace,
The perception and the wisdom,
To save us from our dark fate?

Please hear our unsung malady,
Find the compassion for which we long,
Once again embrace our presence,
Usher in for us a new dawn.

* * *

COMES THE NIGHT

By Melissa Adams VanHouten

In the glistening warmth of the sun,
In the glorious light of the day,
No worries, no concerns, no cares,
All my trials and troubles far away.

No sorrow, no qualms, no regrets,
No frailties or infirmities to be seen,
Hopeful, blissful, and optimistic –
What on earth could happen to me?

Far below me, all creation cries its tears,
But I am blinded by the magnificent light,
Oblivious to the broken and downtrodden,
Turn my eyes from their miserable plight.

Artfully avert my downward glance,
Perhaps all the misfortune will go away,
Walking the enlightened path,
From my righteousness, I will not stray.

The sunshine is simply splendid,
The future burns quite bright,
No need to dwell on hardships –
But all at once, down comes the night.

Comes the night and all the darkness,
Bitter, harsh, and cold,
Frightened, stunned, and shaken,
Chilled to the brittle bone.

What once was mine is lost,
As pleasure turns swiftly to pain,
Lose the day, lose the warmth, lose my footing,
Sunlight transforms into rain.

Hellish beasts and demons,
Appear the creatures of the dark,
Cruelly haunted by my long-dead past,
Become wounds of my once hardened heart.

The tomb that is hollow and empty,
Beckons, calls to me,
The grave, profound and hidden,
Now forever can be seen.

The depths of despair and anguish,
In the ones who are less than whole,
The fate of all the abandoned ones,
Now pierces my once lost soul.

Some will declare their disbelief,
But I know the story far too well,
It lies buried deep inside of me,
And it is mine alone to tell.

The pages turn before me,
Swiftly, fleetingly, they fly,
So far from the glorious beginning,
When I believed I had more time.

I had no great love, no tenderness,
During my days in the blessed light,
No concern or solace for the lesser ones;
They barely entered my mind.

I have found that fate's a cruel teacher,
But an effective one nonetheless.
I have become a scholar in hardship,
A dazzling master of hopelessness.

So I offer up a warning
To you whose hearts and souls are black –
The shades have been thrown open,
Find the mercy you seem to lack.

The sunrise can once again return,
Not only for me but for you,
But you must be willing, be open
Must help those around you begin anew.

Those unfortunates who have passed over,
From bright daylight into dark night,
Need kindness, understanding, and mercy.
Will you take up our burdensome fight?

You soulless souls find it arduous
To pause and peer into the dark,
But you must, for the sake of your own sakes,
Spark the fire in your cold, dead hearts.

Illumination comes from the inside,
And not, as you believed, from without,
Have compassion on the untouchables,
Radiate your brilliance throughout.

For it is only your benevolence,
We anchor our fragile hopes upon,
Only your kindness and gentleness,
That reawakens the dawn.

*

SAMANTHA ANDERSON
Samantha was diagnosed with idiopathic gastroparesis in 2012 at age 26

Living with gastroparesis is like living with a stomach bug or stomach flu constantly, almost round-the-clock. It doesn't just go away, and finding an effective long-term treatment for it is very, very difficult. Some days are slightly easier than others, but even those aren't easy. The simple mundane tasks that most people take for granted and do on autopilot are a struggle, like getting up, dressed, daily chores and eating. There are times people with gastroparesis don't look sick and even do things that seem to be easy, but it doesn't mean they are. Often, to get through the fatigue, you have to swap things around and cut things out of your day. For instance, some days taking a shower and going to work are too much, so using wipes to feel fresh and going to work is your absolute limit. Utter tiredness and being continually drained is a real thing. Drinking more, eating more, eating someone's specific cooking isn't going to cure it, even if it is something all sufferers would love! We don't want to be feeling the way we do. Basic and simple answers to many questions are:

"Yes, a bite of food can be very damaging!"

"Yes, even little bits of food can have a terrible effect on us for hours and hours, but feeling rough is a standard thing!"

And finally, "Yes, most of us are in pain (most of the time)!"

It's a condition that has an effect not just physically, but mentally and emotionally. It's often socially disabling but not through want of trying.

*

JOLI ATKINS
Joli was diagnosed with
gastroparesis in 2015 at age 36

I would like people to know that this condition is not a choice. We do not want to lose weight, lose our hair, and our normal life. We do not want to not be able to eat. We do not wish to spend our time in the doctor's office having test after test done. We do not wish to lose friendships and family because of it, but all of this happens. It happens from the day we are diagnosed, and even more will happen. A cure needs to be found and it needs to be found quickly. Too many people are dying because of this disease and there is no excuse for it. This disease will prove to you just how strong you really are. It will make a strong person out of a weak one and if you are already strong, it will make you stronger. As I close this, I want to leave you with my favorite quote: *I can do all things through Christ who strengthens me* (Philippians 4:13).

*

TRISHA BUNDY
Trisha was diagnosed with
gastroparesis in 2013 at age 35

I am puzzled by the fact that there are more than five million people living life with gastroparesis, yet this illness is not known by the general public. Even more surprisingly, gastroparesis is under recognized and misunderstood by so many medical providers. It isn't uncommon to have doctors or nurses who are cold, turn their backs, or even dismiss our pain and health struggles. Luckily, for the most part (yes, I've had a few bad experiences), the medical providers I've depended on have been empathetic and concerned. Unfortunately, even they don't always have the answers and sometimes don't know enough about the condition to know how to best treat it. This is not always their fault, instead it's evidence of why more research is needed.

It's difficult to communicate to others, especially to my family and self, that there is no fix or cure for this awful disease, at least not yet! It is all symptom treatment and management. Medicine that treats some symptoms, in return creates horrible side effects. Then there is medicine to treat the side effects that were created by the medicines trying to alleviate symptoms. Finally, there are the surgery interventions that make you face a risk of making the illness worse, in the off chance that it may possibly help you improve.

I do get upset with myself at times because I am doing everything that I am supposed to do and I am still sick! One of the most discouraging things to hear from a medical provider is, "I don't know how to help you. We are running out of options." Or, "As much as I want to help you, I don't think there is anything else I can do." However, those words are commonly heard by so many in the gastroparesis community.

It's imperative that one creates a medical team that is knowledgeable, trustworthy, willing to listen to your concerns and cares about your quality of life. You may not always agree or see eye to eye, but you should be able to openly communicate and discuss treatment options together, and at times with other health providers as well. I have many friends who I've met online that are literally starving to death from gastroparesis or similar conditions. They have been turned away or denied appropriate health care because they were too complicated or complex. Gastroparesis may be considered an invisible illness, but the patients that live with it are not. There needs to be more research and awareness in order for new treatment options to become available. You, the reader, can help make a difference in the lives of yourself and others simply by sharing your own experiences with those near you.

Living with gastroparesis negatively impacts multiple areas of my life and the life of my loved ones. All this being said, having an illness, whether it's invisible like mine or not, will have some silver linings. You just have to open your eyes and heart to recognize all of the blessings that surround you. I have discovered new strength that I did not know existed within me, become friends with some of the most courageous spoonies across the world, gained valuable and interesting information about my own health, and have learned how to better advocate for myself and loved ones in a medical setting. Most importantly, I became even more appreciative for everything I love in life and take little for granted! I have also realized how to openly express gratitude to my loved ones and everyone else that helps me along my journey. My health may cause me distress but God has ensured that I am immensely blessed!

*

LISA COLANDREA
Lisa was diagnosed with gastroparesis in 2016 at age 42

Living with gastroparesis feels like a living hell. It's draining. It's a feeling of fear because you never know what the progression will be. Doctors can't give you a timeline or what will happen a week, month or year from now. There is nothing that can tell you what will happen or how much time you have left. In a week's time or even day to day, you can go from one extreme to another. It's something you don't want to control you, but still makes you sick every single day.

I want people to know that living with this illness is just as bad as living with other major, incurable illnesses. People with gastroparesis suffer so much with friendships and families because it's an illness you can't see; people don't believe you. It's a complete burden in life and changes the way you feel about your future. It shatters you and your life. It's hard on you, your spouse, your children, or any other family member that is a caretaker. It feels like there is never that light at the end of the tunnel and that things are just not going to get any better.

*

TAMMY DOWNS
Tammy was diagnosed with Crohn's disease, irritable bowel syndrome, spastic colon, gastroesophageal reflux disease, and gastritis in 2006 at age 46, gastroparesis in 2015 at age 56, and motility dysfunction disorder of the rectum and pelvic floor in 2016 at age 58

It can be emotionally and physically draining. I have no energy, I cannot sleep, I'm in pain, nauseous, and it feels like a rock in my stomach after eating. The gastritis causes burning like I have a match in my stomach. And then there's the acid reflux, Crohn's disease and irritable bowel syndrome. Finally, add in dyssynergic defecation, which is a condition in which there is a problem with the way certain nerves and muscles function in the pelvic floor. The pelvic floor muscles are located at the lower part of the abdomen, between the hip bones, and support pelvic organs such as the rectum, uterus, and urinary bladder.

I have had to learn over the years to do my best to accept what I have, and hope that I can learn how to manage it and live with it. I have learned to pay more attention to the medication that I am given, because all medication has side effects; some of them are horrible, and some you can deal with. I learned the hard way that there are medications that may help in the long-term, but in the meantime they cause even more damage. I have also found you have to be comfortable with your doctor and trust him. You also have to learn your body. Ask for help if you need it. It's a revolving door.

*

SKYE FALCON

Skye was diagnosed with gastroparesis and other autoimmune diseases in 2006 at age 25

Living with gastroparesis and my slew of other autoimmune and medical issues makes living so hard. I do not just wake up in the morning, jump out of bed, and start the day. My days begin hours before I can even move to use the bathroom, swallowing handfuls of pills to keep my systems going and control the vomiting and nausea that plagues my every hour. After medications settle, and the nausea subsides, I begin stretching my joints. First my ankles, then knees, hips, spine, back, shoulders and arms. After I am up, I then have to decide what I am going to work on for the day, and when I could squeeze calories in.

If I have laundry and housework to do, I cannot eat until after I am finished. If I do, I will be down for an hour or two while my body works insanely hard to push the foreign objects (otherwise known as food) through my gastrointestinal tract. Normally I eat twice a day and it consists of an applesauce cup or baby food packet. In the evening, because by this time I am weak, slow, exhausted, and my mind is all foggy from lack of calories, I aim to eat four to six ounces of soft foods. That might be a small bowl of soup, broth, or extremely cooked lean meat or vegetables. Some days, all I can do is liquid feeds. Those days are hardest of all.

After I get it down, hoping not to choke and vomit it all back out before I even have a chance, I have to recline with a heating pad on my abdomen and my back to keep my muscles relaxed and accepting of the food I am trying to get nutrients from. The speed and reaction of my gastrointestinal tract every morning tells me which medications I will need to help digest at night, which determines if I will spend extra time on the commode due to diarrhea and explosive intestines. My insides have usually relaxed by about eleven at night, but then my mind races about everything that I did not get to, need to do, what the kids need from me, what the husband needs, and what I have promised of myself to others. Mr. Sandman and I no longer have regular dates, and I am often lucky to meet with him for more than an hour straight, before the next day begins at five in the morning. Repeat that every morning, and every day.

Not even having fun is easy. Birthday parties, holiday gatherings, parties in the midsummer sun, even swimming in the summer heat; they are all difficult, emotional times. While everyone is sharing cake, pizza, and turkey dinner, they are all repeatedly asking why I cannot eat, why I am starving myself. When I cannot stand in the sun at your backyard party, or swim with the kids in the pool, I am accused of being standoffish, and no fun. Truth is, I cannot and do not want to eat your cake, your pizza, or your turkey dinners, or I might end up in the hospital. Although, you should definitely watch your gravy boats... soupy condiments are my thing. I cannot stand outside in the sun, or my skin blisters, peels, and rubs off, not to mention the stroke-like symptoms that the heat brings on. Now, if something were to be off in my daily routines, say I have a cold, one of the kids are sick, or I have to make an emergency trip to the doctor, everything is thrown off and nothing is as it should be. In these cases it is like I do not even know the body I am living in.

Vacations? If it is farther than three hours away, count me out. Looking back to my childhood, I was a bad traveler then, as well. I was constantly car sick, had to have vomit buckets and be able to see through the front windshield to ease the nausea or I could not manage. I tried traveling a few years back and learned pretty quickly that it was a disaster. Sitting still in a car for twelve hours was not at all what my joints, back, or body had in mind. The pain that coursed through my sore body with each bump and pothole that the tire hit was more than I had bargained for. Every low-dip into the potholes pulled my intestinal scar tissues and ignited a burning fire. The farther away from home I got, the farther away from my comforts, and my bedside medicinal arsenal I was. The farther from my heating pads, my known toilet, and routine was. The farther away I get from home, the more the heaviness of knowing that I am a broken, broken human weighs down. These things, the anxiety that it all brings, the gross issues that keep slowing me down, all inhibit my ability and desire to have fun and be in the moment with my people. And while they never say it, I know that it brings them down, and essentially ruins the intended vacation or fun. This, in turn, crushes my spirit even more.

Relationships and friendships are similar. I do not have the extra time I once had to sit and listen to people gossip and ramble on about nothing. Have you ever really taken the time to understand how much energy it takes just to have a legitimate conversation? To focus and listen to another? It is exhausting, especially if you are riddled with energy-sucking illnesses. And because I do not drink alcohol and cannot eat, going out to dinner or meeting my friends at the bar seems redundant. And being suckered into getting to be the designated driver stinks. I am then kept out too late, overdoing it for drunken idiots who could care less about my issues. Those sorts of things just are no longer worth my energy.

Another often forgotten group of people who are forced to deal with these issues are the children of those adults who are struggling. For these children—my children—they often fear medical institutions, and have an extremely close relationship with their ill parent. They become protective, know the things that cause the illnesses to flare, and often become advocates for whatever the issues their person deals with are. In some ways, I am grateful for my illness in that, my children have gotten the opportunity to slow down with me, and really take in their childhood and everything that is happening in it.

If there was one thing I could implore upon the world, it would be to slow down, be patient, and realize we are all human. We all bleed, we all struggle. We all have challenges, problems, catastrophes and illnesses to deal with. We all have someone with mental issues or disorders. We all lose loved ones. While our DNA is all different, we all exist the same. We all breathe the same air, have the same senses, and feel the same emotions. Just like you would not push an alcoholic to try a new vodka, you should not push food on someone who cannot eat it. Just as you should not make fun of people for issues that you do not understand, agree with, or believe, you should never judge someone because of their issues or the way they choose to live. Chronic, lifelong illnesses are scary, and no one should have to face them alone. Gastroparesis is indeed a life-changer, but just how it changes your life is completely up to you.

*

ROBIN MCNAMARA

Robin was diagnosed with
gastroparesis in 2013 at age 55

At times it feels as though I am not living with gastroparesis. I'm just going through the motions. I want everyone in the world to know that my life is less than; that I cannot eat anything I want, that nausea is not something that anyone should have to deal with. I want the world to know that their twenty-four or forty-eight-hour virus that beats them down physically with nausea, and makes them drop-dead tired, is how I feel every single day. I want the world to know that this disease is so unpredictable; you just don't know what's going to happen as the day goes on. I want them to know that I'll have days when I wake up feeling amazing, and then as the hours pass by, I slip into the black hole and do my best not to be sick. Why would anyone in the world want to feel like they have the stomach flu round-the-clock every day of the year?

I'd also like for people to realize that I have limitations, that their intentions of "Just try to eat this," will only cause me to feel miserable. I want people to know I am thin, skinny, whatever you wish to call it, but I can't eat a lot of food to catch up on calories or I will just be sick.

Most of all, I would just like people to try to understand, and to ask how I'm feeling when they may not hear from me for a day or two. I don't want to hear how difficult their time is on trivial items—sorry, I've lost patience for that. I want people to just be human and care.

*

TAMMY PITTMAN

Tammy was diagnosed with gastroparesis and irritable bowel syndrome in 2014 at age 34

Imagine having food poisoning every hour of every day. No energy from no nutritional intake for days or weeks. Hunger rattles through your stomach but the smell of food causes the worse pain and, often, vomiting. It's like morning sickness, all day. Everything we take for granted each day like brushing our hair or teeth, getting dressed, getting out of bed, tying your shoes, or taking medication, those abilities are stripped from you in a very short, painful period. Losing your hair and teeth that you worked for years to be perfect. Waking up and not being able to fit in the same clothes you wore the day before. Losing control of your bowels or bladder, or vomiting without warning in public.

People look at you and think you have an eating disorder. They tell you what you should do to get better. They tell you it's all in your head or you're faking or exaggerating it, call you lazy or worthless. Never having an answer to anything. Doctors not knowing what to do next. Becoming a burden to friends and family. Losing your career because you can't physically do the job. Being asked how far along you are in the pregnancy because you're bloated and look eight months pregnant. Hurting too much to stand or sit, but not being able to get comfortable lying down. Having gastroparesis has taken almost everything from me, but it will not win.

*

NICOLE STARZYNSKI
Nicole was diagnosed with
gastroparesis in 2016 at age 33

It's hard to understand what someone else is going through until you go through it yourself. I find new struggles all the time. Most of them are just dealing with a chronic illness, when I am told things that I don't want to hear from doctors. Unfortunately, I have learned nobody can explain what dealing with this is like, in words that do the physical and emotional struggle justice. I wouldn't wish that knowledge on anyone. With that knowledge comes an endless struggle to live.

So what is gastroparesis? Imagine having the worst stomach flu in your life every day for the rest of your life. The food that you ate yesterday, last week or even last month is still sitting in your stomach because something happened to the nerve that controls stomach contraction for digestion. You may be able to only eat one or two bites of food and then feel full, bloated and full of pain. Think of food as a missile attack on the inside of your stomach. Some people experience issues when they eat greasy food, dairy, gluten, red meat and numerous other common food allergens. Some people might experience diarrhea, constipation, bloating, stomach pain, and in some cases nausea and vomiting. Now imagine that it wasn't just one type of food; it's every type of food and drink, sometimes even water.

Moments after taking a bite of food, my stomach declares war. It swells and makes angry noises. Sometimes I experience spasms. Once the war begins, the pain starts. It's like being stabbed from the inside out. If you're a woman, childbirth pains are a very good example. For men, kidney stones are comparable. But neither do the pain that gastroparesis causes any justice. No pain medicine helps. Twenty-plus hours after eating something, I can throw it up completely whole and undigested. Sometimes it's not just being nauseous and throwing up. Sometimes it's dry heaving until every blood vessel on my face is exposed and I would do anything for it to end.

Gastroparesis kills kids and young adults; it has no prejudice for age. It's a slow killer. People look at you and say, "You're not sick." They have no idea that everything inside your body is slowly shutting down. They have no idea that you wake up every day at war with your stomach. Imagine waking up every day with the worst stomach flu you have ever had. Now imagine having to function like that.

This disease is awful, it has changed my life and my daughter's life. My daughter leaves so early sometimes for the bus stop just because she can't bear to hear me puke anymore. I stay in bed sometimes for three hours after I take a Zofran so I don't puke my guts out. Sometimes it works, sometimes it doesn't. There isn't a magic pill or diet to make this go away. Probiotics aren't the answer to everything. Just because you know one person who has gastroparesis and they were lucky enough that it was manageable by smaller meals, diet or medicine, does not mean that everyone responds so well. Sometimes people's ignorance is okay, except when they don't even want to educate themselves before sharing their opinion about something they couldn't possibly understand. Living it and showing empathy for someone are two entirely different things.

One way for the world to understand gastroparesis is to continue to advocate. Stand up for those who can no longer fight for themselves. I am angry. Angry there aren't enough treatments. Angry there is no cure. Angry that I have no idea what my life will be. I have made a promise to myself that no matter what, I am going to fight this and I will not let this disease take my life. Sometimes we like to ignore reality. I would like to ignore the fact that this disease is destroying my life and appreciate all the wonderful things in life that I can control. My beautiful daughter, my boyfriend, my family and our wacky pug are always there for me. I have friends who have stuck by me. I wake up in the morning, go to work, take a walk. I am thankful for my life and I am not surrendering. This is war and I plan on winning!

*

JENNIFER ZUBIK
Jennifer was diagnosed with idiopathic
gastroparesis in 2010 at age 27

Gastroparesis is evil and understated. Many do not understand the real battles you suffer and try to overcome. It is debilitating, both emotionally and physically. It follows the domino effect, as one problem leads to another in your body, as well as another obstacle in life. My story may be different from others. I was able to overcome my battles and can now continue to live my life to the fullest, at least at this moment, yet hopefully forever.

However, the risks and fears are real. I still have what ifs and unknowns to deal with. I was lucky to be given a second chance, and am not going to take it for granted. I feel for those who are still struggling and I wish nothing but for them to be given the chance I was presented with. I still have regrets and guilt for what my family and I had to experience. I wish I could go back and change the years we struggled into good memories. I conclude this experience has made me stronger, us stronger. We are closer and have learned so much. It has molded us into the people, the family, we are today. We now have a different outlook on life and new meanings to hope and courage.

Life is unfortunately full of lessons and trials and tribulations, but those experiences shape us into who we are. There is nothing easy about being ill, or watching a loved one lose hope. But love, support, understanding, prayers, and hope is all that can be asked for during these trying times. We can also ask for answers and miracles, but those unfortunately aren't always given. I faithfully hope my experience can give others "HOPE." My journey began almost eight years ago and continues to venture on. Live, laugh, love. Have strength and believe. Don't ever give up.

*

CHAPTER TWENTY

Meet the writers

Shared sorrow is half a sorrow.

SWEDISH PROVERB

*

*

MELISSA ADAMS VANHOUTEN

Melissa was diagnosed with
gastroparesis in 2014 at age 47
www.curegp.com | gpfightingforchange@gmail.com

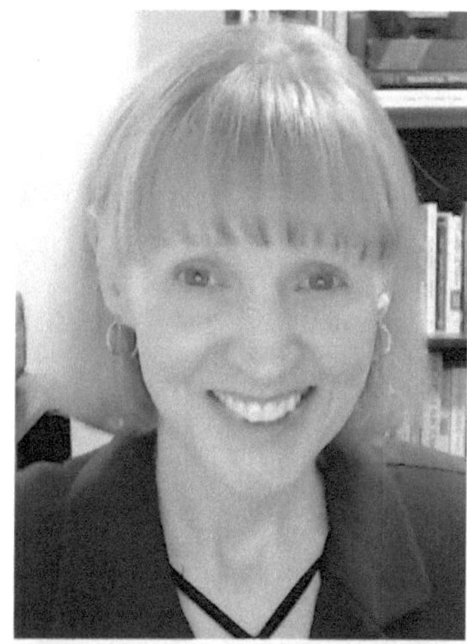

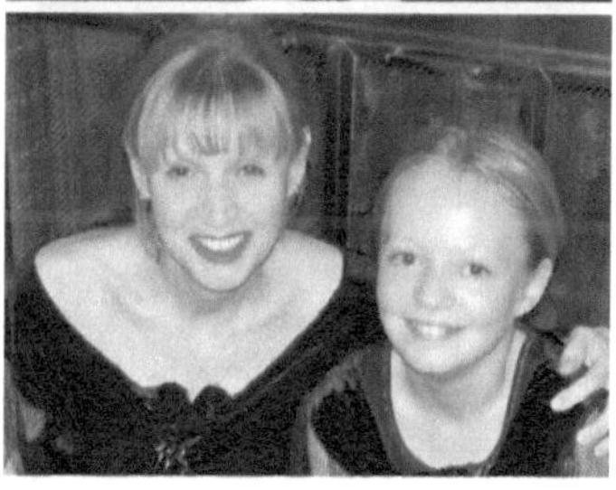

Melissa Adams VanHouten is a dedicated wife and mother who was diagnosed with gastroparesis in February 2014. She holds a bachelor of science degree in political science from St. Joseph's College and a master of arts degree in political science from Indiana State University. She is a former university political science instructor and corporate trainer who currently resides in Indianapolis. Melissa enjoys reading, writing, and intelligent debates. She values her family and relishes the small moments spent in their company. As the creator and administrator of several online support and advocacy groups, she now spends her days advancing the cause of those who struggle to live with the sometimes devastating and life-altering effects of gastroparesis. Over the past two years, her advocacy group, Gastroparesis: Fighting for Change, has made huge strides, passing awareness proclamations in twenty-three states, contributing to the implementation of a national awareness month, and starting a petition drive to advance a congressional bill that would greatly benefit the gastroparesis community. It is her deepest desire to empower others to advocate for awareness, better treatments, and, ultimately, a cure.

*

SAMANTHA ANDERSON

Samantha was diagnosed with idiopathic gastroparesis in 2012 at age 26

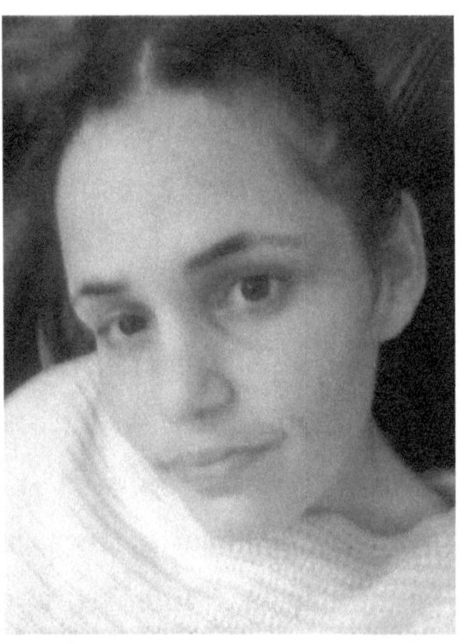

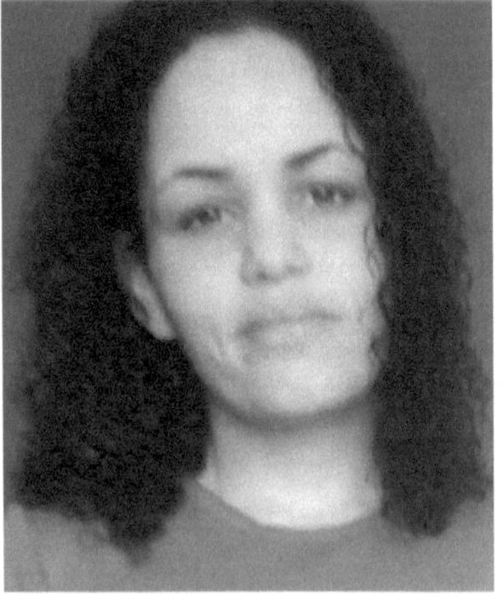

Samantha Jayne Anderson was born in April 1985, and raised in London, England. She gained a 2:1 in bachelor of science (honors) psychology at Sheffield Hallam University in 2006. While at university, she did a variety of jobs (most were enjoyed) to get her through her studies. She went on to become a teaching assistant working with children both with and without special educational needs. It was a job she really enjoyed. She learned a lot about a range of children, and gained more of an understanding of disabilities such as autism and global learning delay; it fueled her passion for teaching. After two years, Sam decided to get a primary school teaching degree at Institute of Education in 2008-2009. She continued to teach until she was ill for ten months in 2012, an illness that changed her life forever. Sam loved going to the gym, exercising regularly five to six times a week, and cycling. She also loved socializing with her amazing family and friends.

*

JOLI ATKINS
Joli was diagnosed with
gastroparesis in 2015 at age 36

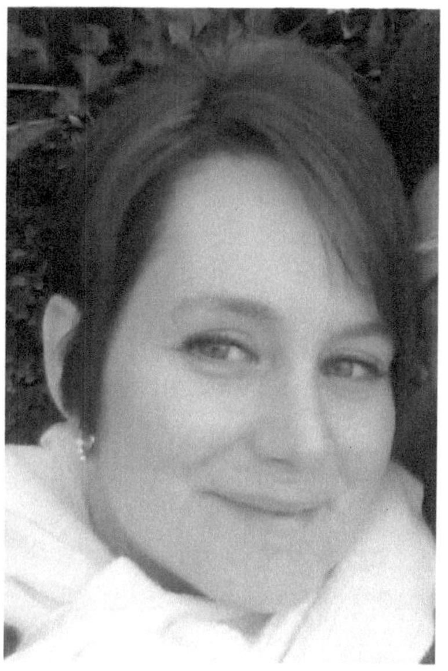

Joli Atkins was born and raised in Southwest Virginia. She graduated from Salem High School in 1995. She earned two associate degrees from Virginia Western Community College, one in administration of justice and the second in general studies. She continued her studies through Southern New Hampshire University and gained her bachelor's degree in psychology in 2017. She had a son in 1998, who in 2016 also graduated from Salem High School, and is a successful dealership mechanic in their hometown. She met an amazing man in 2011 and settled down in a small country town. She enjoys photography, hunting, and reading.

*

MEGAN BOGGS
Megan was diagnosed with
gastroparesis in 2017 at age 38

Megan Boggs was born and raised in Buffalo, New York. She earned her Master's degree in education in 2015. She has an amazing husband and eighteen-year-old son.

*

TRISHA BUNDY

Trisha was diagnosed with gastroparesis in 2013 at age 35

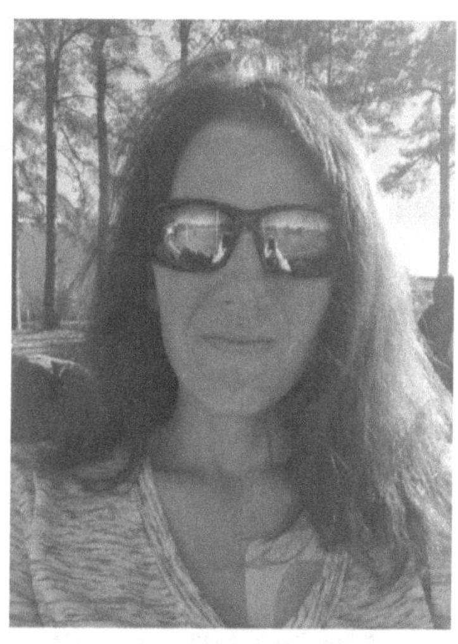

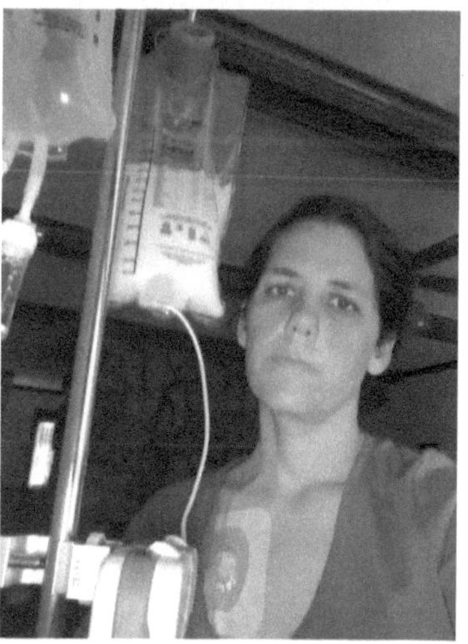

Trisha is a proud parent and sports enthusiast from North Carolina. She earned her bachelor's degree for elementary education, married her high school sweetheart, and embarked on her dream career as an elementary teacher in 2000. In May 2012, Trisha earned her master's degree in reading education. Unfortunately, she became sick in February 2013. After continuous sickness, she reluctantly had to resign in 2016. As a result of her illness, she chose to become a volunteer patient advocate and co-admin for the Gastroparesis: Fighting for Change advocacy group. Trisha is using her personal medical experiences to help bring awareness to functional gastrointestinal motility disorders such as gastroparesis and colonic inertia. Being a tubie since May 2013 and an ileostomate since January 2016, it's important to her that others know they are not alone in their health battles. You can read more about Trisha's health journey by reading her blog at GastroparesisCrusader.weebly.com.

*

LISA COLANDREA
Lisa was diagnosed with gastroparesis in 2016 at age 42

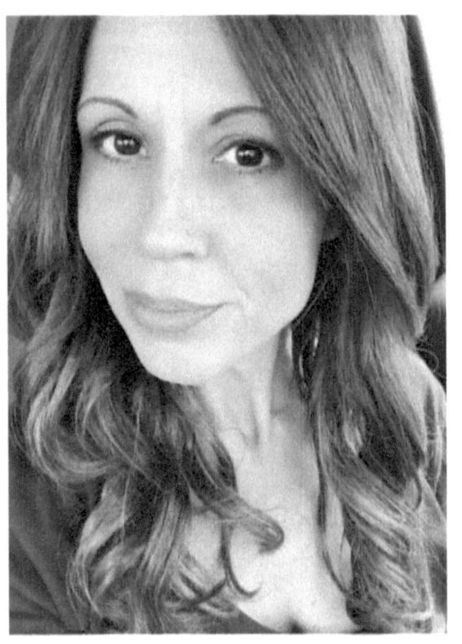

Lisa Colandrea was born and raised in Maynard, Massachusetts. Lisa spent years working as a nursing assistant as well as a case manager in the social services field. Later, after raising her two oldest children, Lisa followed her passion for photography, and attended the New England School of Photography in Boston. Lisa and her wife then followed their dream to move to San Diego, California where they raise their four-year-old and six-year-old and enjoy all of what San Diego has to offer.

*

TAMMY DOWNS

Tammy was diagnosed with Crohn's disease, irritable bowel syndrome, spastic colon, gastroesophageal reflux disease, and gastritis in 2006 at age 46, gastroparesis in 2015 at age 56, and motility dysfunction disorder of the rectum and pelvic floor in 2016 at age 58

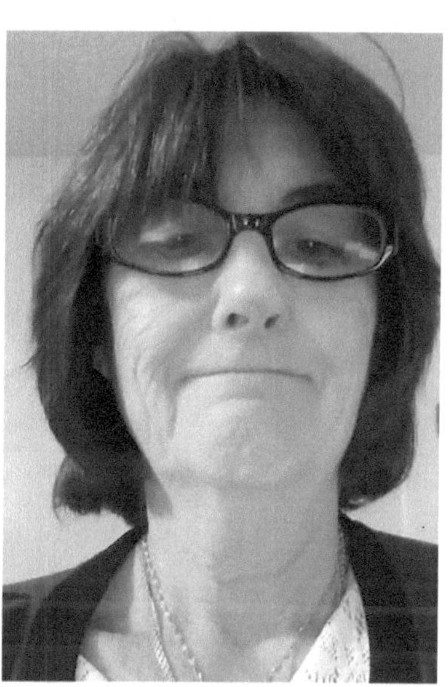

Tammy Downs is a mother of two young men and grandmother of two. She has an amazing man who has been a big supporter, who has done his best to be there and understand what Tammy goes through. Tammy was an emergency room registration clerk and later become a mortgage processor for twelve years before her job became too stressful and her doctors recommended she quit. Her body breaks down easily, and she one day hopes for a cure.

*

SKYE FALCON

Skye was diagnosed with gastroparesis and other autoimmune diseases in 2006 at age 25

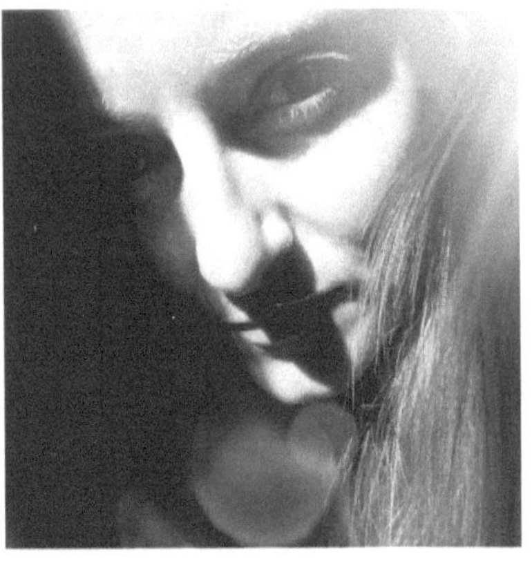

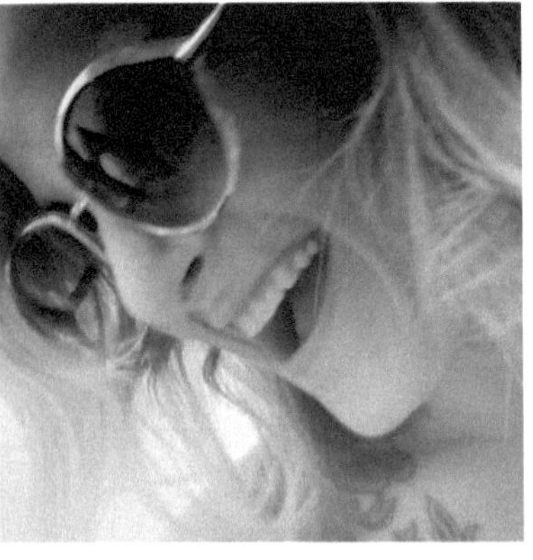

Skye Falcon is a mother, wife, daughter, friend, and multi-business owner. She is bold, driven, and an entrepreneur. She's a right-fighter, standing up for those who have no voice. She is the comforting, wise smile you seek when troubled. Skye Falcon resides in Northern Indiana, and holds degrees in business and education. She works tirelessly on the Justice for Nancy charity which she began after her grandmother was brutally beaten in a home invasion in 2014. She owns a health food company called OH, Forks!™ that frequents farmer's markets in the Midwest. She is also the lead educator and manager of the School of Loving Arts in Fort Wayne, an adult education center for adults, cancer patients and the ill, to help reclaim their intimacy, human needs, and sexual being. She herself knows the struggle of illness in life, works hard on awareness causes and fundraising, and gives compassion and empathy to others. In her spare time, she enjoys being an author, creating new celiac safe recipes, and spending every extra moment with her kids. She believes that being good is the way to turn our world to the light, and giving is the key to happiness.

*

ROBIN MCNAMARA
Robin was diagnosed with
gastroparesis in 2013 at age 55

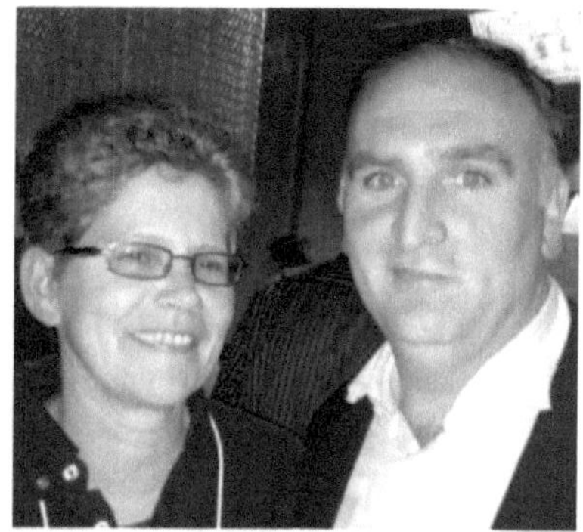

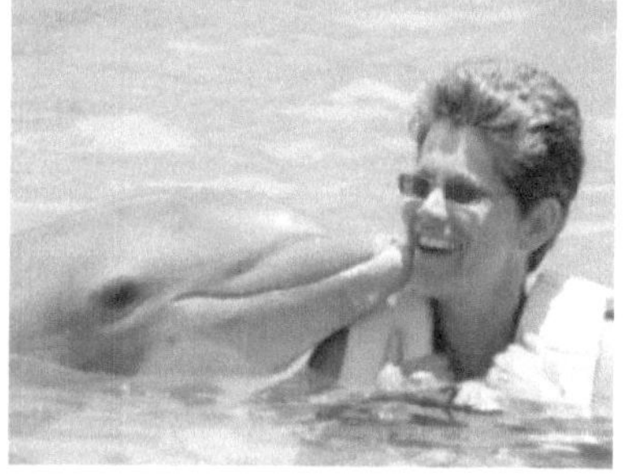

Robin McNamara was born in Westwood, Massachusetts. She earned her master's degree at Cambridge College. She currently works for a family owned supermarket, where she has worked since high school (yes, almost forty-two years with the same company). Robin has two sisters, as well as nieces, nephews, great nieces and nephews, and is the proud mom of two four-legged kitties.

*

TAMMY PITTMAN

Tammy was diagnosed with gastroparesis and irritable bowel syndrome in 2014 at age 34

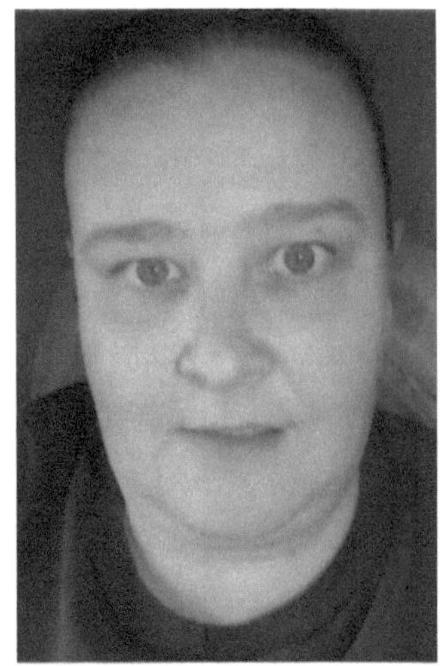

Tammy is a thirty-seven-year-old mother of a twenty-two-year-old. She's a nurse but has been unable to work since 2010. She's been married twice. She enjoys playing pool, singing karaoke and multiple crafts. She enjoys a good book. She's a Christian and very strong in her faith.

*

TAYLOR SCHMITZ

Taylor was diagnosed with idiopathic gastroparesis in 2014 at age 22

Taylor Schmitz was born in Kettering, Ohio, and grew up in the small town of Franklin. After she graduated high school, she decided to join the Ohio Army National Guard, and deployed to Afghanistan in 2012. When she arrived home, she began attending the University of Toledo for criminal justice with a focus on psychology. Unfortunately, during her first two years of college, her mother, who lived three hours away in Franklin, was fighting breast cancer. She ended up passing away in December 2012. Taylor was also pregnant at this time, with her and her husband, Bradley's, first child. She gave birth in 2013 to a beautiful baby girl, Avery. They moved into their first home in October of the same year.

*

DEB SHRADER-TROTTER
Deb was diagnosed with
gastroparesis in 1999 at age 37

Deb Shrader-Trotter was in her first year of teaching in 1990. She was teaching, writing grants, doing youth groups at church, majorette lessons, brownies, and about to pursue her master's in education with an eye toward a doctorate in education. Her life began to slowly unravel at a fast rate, with symptoms jumping and gathering steam like a locomotive train that had lost its air brakes. She had two major sinus surgeries and walking pneumonia, and thought mold in the school was a contributing factor to these health issues. She changed schools but the train kept coming. She began teaching at the new school where she helped create a gifted and talented science fair with judges. An appendectomy and hysterectomy, and a school board with parents fighting to keep her, saved her job—the first time. The second round? The job was over. She then went to the local museum as an educational coordinator. The train was still rolling. While she was in a hospital bed, dehydrated, in her ninety-day probation phase, in a right to work state, she was fired—while in the hospital bed.

*

JESSICA SPENCE
Jessica was diagnosed with
gastroparesis in 2016 at age 25

Jessica Spence was born in Orem, Utah, and grew up in Dane County, Wisconsin. She traveled to New York every summer to visit her paternal grandparents. Jessica learned to love the thirteen-hour ride, and dreamed of traveling the world one day. She had a vivid imagination and sense of adventure. Much of her childhood was spent having these adventures with her many, many cousins at her maternal grandmother's house. At seventeen, she decided to follow in her father's footsteps and enlisted in the National Guard. She served for a year before she was medically discharged due to a mysterious, pre-existing stomach condition. Currently she volunteers at the food pantry her mother runs in Fox Lake, Wisconsin.

*

NICOLE STARZYNSKI

Nicole was diagnosed with gastroparesis in 2016 at age 33

Nicole Lynn Starzynski was raised in South Park, Pennsylvania, a rural town south of Pittsburgh where she owns a home now. A domestic abuse survivor, Nicole is raising her daughter Kirstin (age twelve going on forty) with the help of their loveable pug Zoey. When she's feeling well enough, Nicole loves camping, biking, and hiking in the rolling hills of Pennsylvania with her partner, Josh. Nicole's parents live close by and co-parent Kirstin, who's proud of being a nerd (like her mom) and an All-Star softball player. Nicole is also close with her younger brother and sister, who share her love of John Hughes movies and 90s hits. They are also susceptible to Nicole's infectious sense of humor and fits of laughter. Nicole graduated as president of the student body and top of her class from Pittsburgh Technical Institute with an associate's degree in computer and network systems. Like many women, she has pioneered her career path in technology and is now a director of information technology for a tech company in Pittsburgh.

*

JENNIFER ZUBIK
Jennifer was diagnosed with idiopathic gastroparesis in 2010 at age 27

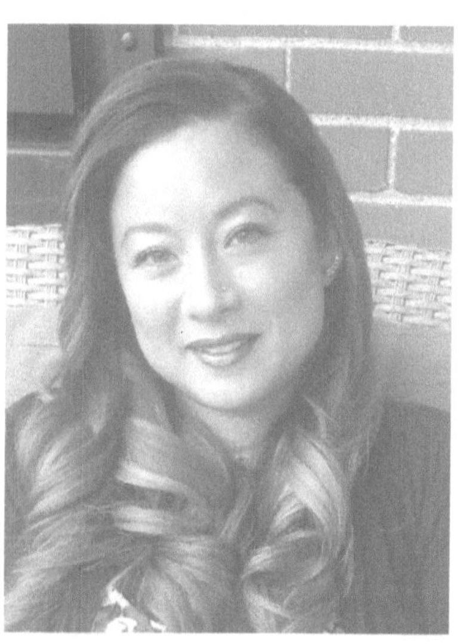

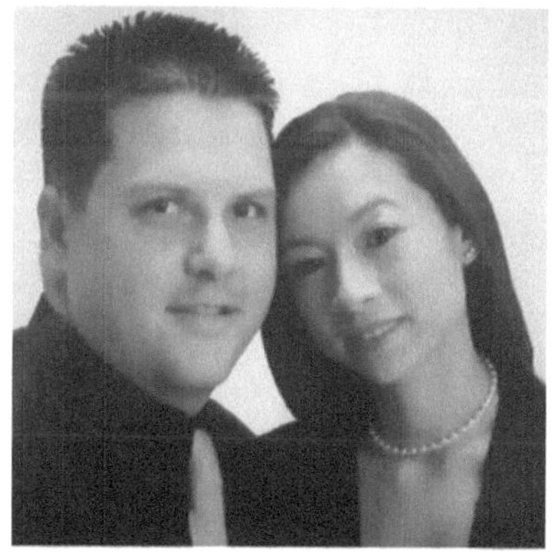

Jennifer Zubik was born in the south hills area outside of Pittsburgh, Pennsylvania. She became a mother at the age of seventeen and has overcome many obstacles with raising a child when so young, yet has loved every moment of it. Jennifer earned her associate's degree in business and accounting, while working a full-time job and raising her daughter. She is married to her amazingly supportive husband, whom she met in high school, and developed a relationship within three years after graduation. Jennifer is currently an accounts receivable manager and billing specialist for an energy service company in the oil and gas industry. She still resides outside of Pittsburgh as a proud mother of her extraordinary seventeen-year-old daughter, happily married, and surrounded by her wonderful family and friends.

FROM LYNDA CHELDELIN FELL

THANK YOU

I am deeply indebted to the writers of Real Life Diaries: Living with Gastroparesis. It takes tremendous courage to bare such vulnerability about a topic so misunderstood. The individual and collective dedication to seeing this book project to the end is a legacy to be proud of. I'm especially grateful to coauthor Melissa Adams VanHouten, a tireless advocate I admire immensely for her hard work to raise awareness and bring this book project to fruition. With very little nonclinical information available about motility disorders, it is my sincere hope that readers who share the same path will find hope and compassion, family and friends will gain better understanding, and professionals will appreciate the candid insight.

Helen Keller once said, "Walking with a friend in the dark is better than walking alone in the light." By sharing our struggles we learn that we aren't truly alone as we travel our journey, for there are others ahead of us, behind us, and right beside us. That is what this book is all about.

Lynda Cheldelin Fell

There's a bright future for you at every turn,
even if you miss one.

*

ABOUT

LYNDA CHELDELIN FELL

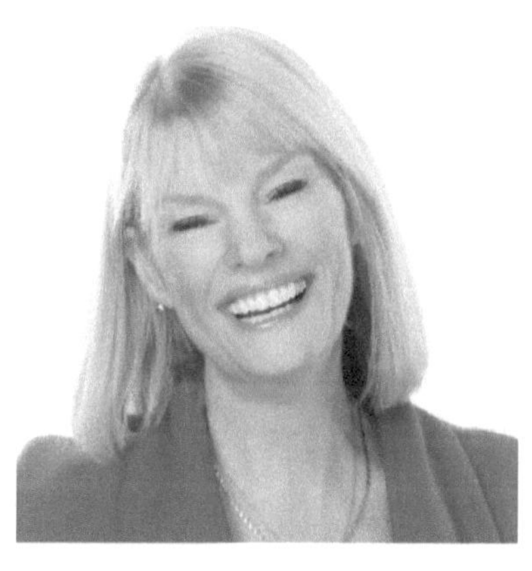

Considered a pioneer in the field of inspirational hope in the aftermath of loss, Lynda Cheldelin Fell has a passion for creating and producing groundbreaking projects that create a legacy of help, healing, and hope.

Her story began when she had an alarming dream about Aly, her young teenage daughter. In the dream, Aly was a backseat passenger in a car that veered off the road and landed in a lake. Aly sank with the car, leaving behind an open book floating face down on the water. Two years later Lynda's dream became reality when her daughter was killed as a backseat passenger in a car accident while coming home from a swim meet. Overcome with grief, Lynda's forty-six-year-old husband suffered a major stroke that left him with severe disabilities.

The following year, Lynda was invited to share her remarkable story, and that inspired her to create groundbreaking projects spanning national events, radio, film and books to help others who share the same journey feel less alone. She has now authored 25 books, earned four literary awards, and sat with Dr. Martin Luther King's daughter, Trayvon Martin's mother, sisters of the late Nicole Brown Simpson, Pastor Todd Burpo of Heaven Is For Real, and other societal newsmakers.

Because of that dream and the book floating where her daughter disappeared, Lynda is dedicated to helping ordinary people share their own extraordinary stories, and bring comfort, healing and hope to people around the world.

lynda@lyndafell.com | www.lyndafell.com

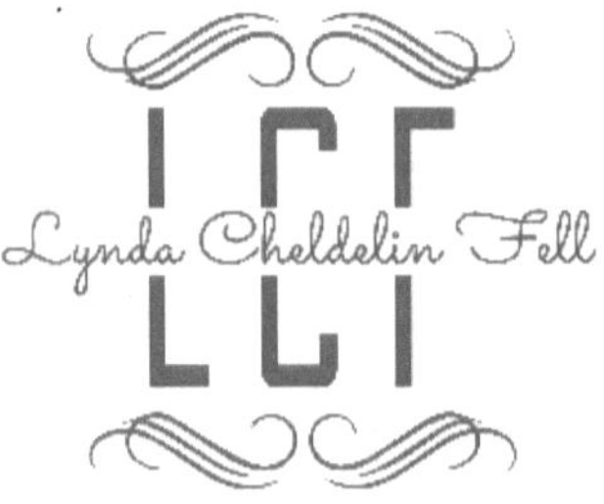

ALYBLUE MEDIA TITLES

Real Life Diaries: Living with Gastroparesis
Real Life Diaries: Living with a Brain Injury
Real Life Diaries: Through the Eyes of DID
Real Life Diaries: Through the Eyes of an Eating Disorder
Real Life Diaries: Living with Endometriosis
Real Life Diaries: Living with Mental Illness
Grief Diaries: Victim Impact Statement
Grief Diaries: Hit by Impaired Driver
Grief Diaries: Surviving Loss of a Spouse
Grief Diaries: Surviving Loss of a Child
Grief Diaries: Surviving Loss of a Sibling
Grief Diaries: Surviving Loss of a Parent
Grief Diaries: Surviving Loss of an Infant
Grief Diaries: Surviving Loss of a Loved One
Grief Diaries: Surviving Loss by Suicide
Grief Diaries: Surviving Loss of Health
Grief Diaries: How to Help the Newly Bereaved
Grief Diaries: Loss by Impaired Driving
Grief Diaries: Loss by Homicide
Grief Diaries: Loss of a Pregnancy
Grief Diaries: Hello from Heaven
Grief Diaries: Grieving for the Living
Grief Diaries: Shattered
Grief Diaries: Project Cold Case
Grief Diaries: Poetry & Prose and More
Grief Diaries: Through the Eyes of Men
Grief Diaries: Will We Survive?
Grammy Visits From Heaven
Grandpa Visits From Heaven
Faith, Grief & Pass the Chocolate Pudding
Heaven Talks to Children
Color My Soul Whole
A Child is Missing: A True Story
A Child is Missing: Searching for Justice
Grief Reiki

Humanity's legacy of stories and storytelling
is the most precious we have.

DORIS LESSING

*

To share your story, visit
www.griefdiaries.com
www.RealLifeDiaries.com

PUBLISHED BY ALYBLUE MEDIA
Explore. Educate. Inspire.
www.AlyBlueMedia.com

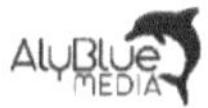

www.ingramcontent.com/pod-product-compliance
Lightning Source LLC
LaVergne TN
LVHW091246150826
845673LV00006B/1331

* 9 7 8 1 9 4 4 3 2 8 8 0 1 *